WITHDRAWN

Neurodevelopmental Outcomes of Preterm Birth

From Childhood to Adult Life

Neurodevelopmental Outcomes of Preterm Birth

From Childhood to Adult Life

Edited by

Chiara Nosarti
Institute of Psychiatry, London

Robin M. Murray
Institute of Psychiatry, London

Maureen Hack
Case Western Reserve University, Ohio

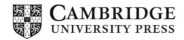

CAMBRIDGE UNIVERSITY PRESS
Cambridge, New York, Melbourne, Madrid, Cape Town, Singapore,
São Paulo, Delhi, Dubai, Tokyo

Cambridge University Press
The Edinburgh Building, Cambridge CB2 8RU, UK

Published in the United States of America by Cambridge University Press, New York

www.cambridge.org
Information on this title: www.cambridge.org/9780521871792

First published 2010

Printed in the United Kingdom at the University Press, Cambridge

A catalog record for this publication is available from the British Library

Library of Congress Cataloging in Publication data
Neurodevelopmental outcomes of preterm birth / [edited by] Chiara Nosarti, Robin M. Murray, Maureen Hack.
    p. ; cm.
  Includes bibliographical references and index.
  ISBN 978-0-521-87179-2 (hardback)
  1. Premature infants–Development.   2. Nervous system–Growth.   3. Brain–Diseases.   I. Nosarti,
  Chiara.   II. Murray, Robin, MD, M Phil, MRCP, MRC Psych.   III. Hack, Maureen.
  [DNLM: 1. Mental Disorders–etiology.   2. Brain Damage, Chronic.   3. Diagnostic Imaging.
  4. Infant, Low Birth Weight.   5. Mental Disorders–diagnosis.   6. Premature Birth. WS 350 N4935 2010]
  RJ250.3.N48 2010
  618.92′011–dc22   2009050377

ISBN 978-0-521-87179-2 Hardback

Contents

Contents

Section 6: Conclusions

Contributors

Matthew P. G. Allin MRCP MRCPsych DM
Clinical Lecturer in Psychiatry and Honorary
Consultant Psychiatrist, Institute of
Psychiatry at the Maudsley, King's College
London, London, UK

Peter J. Anderson BA GradDip (AppPsych) PhD
C. R. Roper Fellow, School of Behavioural Science,
The University of Melbourne; Co-Director,
Victorian Infant Brain Studies Team; Co-Director,
Australian Centre for Child Neuropsychological
Studies, Melbourne, Australia

Glen P. Aylward PhD ABPP
Professor of Developmental and Behavioral
Pediatrics; Director, Division of Developmental and
Behavioral Pediatrics, Southern Illinois University
School of Medicine, Springfield, IL, USA

Sven Cnattigius MD PhD
Professor of Reproductive Epidemiology,
Department of Medical Epidemiology and
Biostatistics, Karolinska Institute, Stockholm,
Sweden

Richard W. I. Cooke MD FRCP FRCPCH
Professor, School of Reproductive and
Developmental Medicine, University of
Liverpool, Liverpool Women's Hospital,
Liverpool, UK

Michelle de Haan PhD
Reader in Developmental Neuropsychology,
University College London Institute of Child
Health, London, UK

Lex W. Doyle MD BS MSc FRACP
Professor, Department of Obstetrics &
Gynaecology, University of Melbourne, Parkville,
Australia

Maureen Hack MB ChB
Professor of Pediatrics, Case Western Reserve
University, Rainbow Babies & Children's Hospital,
Cleveland, OH, USA

Elaine Healy MRCPsych PhD
Consultant Child and Adolescent Psychiatrist,
Lucena Clinic, Dublin, Ireland

Kelly Howard PhD
Postdoctoral Researcher, School of Behavioural
Science, The University of Melbourne,
Melbourne, Australia

Christina M. Hultman PhD PsychD
Professor of Psychiatric Epidemiology,
Department of Medical Epidemiology and
Biostatistics, Karolinska Institute, Stockholm,
Sweden

Terrie E. Inder MD PhD
Professor of Neuroimaging, Washington
University School of Medicine, St Louis, MO,
USA

Stefan Johansson MD PhD
Pediatrician and Neonatologist,
Department of Medical Epidemiology and
Biostatistics, Karolinska Institute, Stockholm,
Sweden

Ingeborg Krägeloh-Mann MD
Professor of Pediatric and Developmental
Neurology, University Children's Hospital,
Tübingen, Germany

Russell K. Lawrence MD
Instructor in Pediatrics, Department of
Pediatrics, Washington University School of
Medicine, St Louis, MO, USA

Marie C. McCormick MD ScD
Sumner and Esther Feldberg Professor of
Maternal and Child Health, Department of
Society, Human Development and Health,
Harvard School of Public Health, Boston, MA,
USA

Beth McManus PT MS MPH ScD
Robert Wood Johnson Health and
Society Postdoctoral Fellow,
University of Wisconsin,
WI, USA

Michael E. Msall MD
Professor of Pediatrics, Section of Developmental
and Behavioral Pediatrics, University of Chicago
Pritzker School of Medicine, Comer and
LaRabadia Children's Hospitals, Chicago, IL, USA

Robin M. Murray MD DSc FRCP FRCPsych FMedSci
Professor of Psychiatric Research, Institute
of Psychiatry at the Maudsley, King's College
London, London, UK

Jeffrey J. Neil MD PhD
Allen P. and Josephine B. Green Professor of
Neurology, Washington University School of
Medicine, St. Louis, MO, USA

Chiara Nosarti PhD
Senior Lecturer in Mental Health Studies and
Neuroimaging, Institute of Psychiatry at the
Maudsley, King's College London, London, UK

Jennifer Park MA
Research Project Professional, University of
Chicago Pritzker School of Medicine, Kennedy
Center on Neurodevelopmental Disability,
Institute of Molecular Pediatric Sciences, Section
of Community Health, Ethics, and Policy, Comer
and La Rabida Children's Hospitals, IL, USA

Larry Rifkin MRCPsych
Honorary Senior Lecturer in Psychiatry and
Consultant Psychiatrist, Institute of Psychiatry at
the Maudsley, King's College London, London,
UK

Teresa M. Rushe PhD
Senior Lecturer in Psychology, University of
Ulster, Londonderry, UK

Mary C. Sullivan PhD RN
Professor of Nursing and Maternal and Child
Health, University of Rhode Island College of
Nursing, Kingston, RI, USA

H. Gerry Taylor PhD
Professor of Pediatrics, Case Western Reserve
University, Rainbow Babies & Children's Hospital,
Cleveland, OH, USA

Betty R. Vohr MD
Professor of Pediatrics, Department of
Pediatrics, Brown University Medical School;
Medical Director, Rhode Island Hearing
Assessment Program; Director, Women & Infants'
Hospital Neonatal Follow-up Clinic, Providence,
RI, USA

Muriel Walshe PhD
Lecturer, Institute of Psychiatry at the Maudsley,
King's College London, London, UK

John Wyatt FRCP FRCPCH
Professor of Neonatal Paediatrics, Department
of Paediatrics, University College London,
London, UK

Preface

At a time of exciting advances in neonatal intensive care and neuroimaging methods, when surviving preterm children represent an increasing percentage of the population, we conceived the current volume to provide the first single-source reference on the latest findings from research into the neurodevelopmental outcome following preterm birth.

New knowledge about the long-term cognitive, neurosensory, neurobiological, social, and behavioral correlates of preterm birth has emerged in the past decade mainly from two sources. Firstly, from "historical" studies of the initial preterm survivors who were examined from birth and have now reached adulthood. Secondly, from more recent studies using sophisticated neurodevelopmental assessments of the preterm infant at term, including neonatal magnetic resonance imaging techniques, which may potentially be used to identify the mechanisms underlying variations in outcome later in life; this may enable subgroups of individuals who are at increased risk of neurodevelopmental problems to benefit from appropriate intervention strategies which may be devised.

In this volume, many of the most admired and prolific investigators in different areas of preterm research present a comprehensive and up-to-date perspective on their work and areas of expertise, including directions for the future. We have been extremely fortunate to secure contributions from these researchers who have been instrumental in increasing the existing knowledge of the neurodevelopmental sequelae of preterm birth.

The volume is divided into six sections. The first introductory section presents an overview of the epidemiology of preterm birth and associated environmental and biological risk factors (Chapter 1). A historical account of the developments in neonatal care for preterm infants over the past 50 years is then provided, together with an exploration of the mechanisms of brain injury in the vulnerable preterm brain, which provides a powerful means for the development of preventative strategies (Chapter 2). A summary of the current state of knowledge of the clinical outcomes following various types and degrees of brain injury from a neurological perspective is then given (Chapter 3). Here we need to remember not only the importance of studying patterns of neurological and developmental disorders associated with very preterm birth, but also the context of the constantly changing and improving nature of neonatal intensive care.

The second section of the volume documents progress in neuroimaging research using various techniques, such as neonatal cranial ultrasound (Chapter 4), structural (Chapter 5) and functional (Chapter 7) magnetic resonance imaging, and diffusion tensor imaging (Chapter 8). Neonatal neuroimaging studies have identified several types of white and gray matter alterations in preterm infants compared to controls, and have also shown that severely abnormal findings can help to predict adverse neurodevelopmental outcomes. Valuable guidelines for the use of the various neonatal imaging techniques are provided (Chapter 4). Existing knowledge concerning longitudinal changes in the preterm brain in the framework of normal brain development is discussed in Chapter 6. Apart from the identification of injury–impairment relationships, an encouraging finding which emerges from neuroimaging data is the suggestion that processes of brain plasticity may enable the preterm brain to compensate, to an extent, for injuries that would cause severe loss of function in an adult, but often only result in mild impairment of functioning in preterm-born individuals.

The third section addresses research into the behavioral outcome following preterm birth, with specific chapters on childhood and adolescent (Chapter 9) and adult outcomes (Chapter 10). Although intrauterine and neonatal factors seem to be important in the pathogenesis of psychiatric disorders, no consensus has yet been reached concerning the interpretation of the association between preterm birth and psychopathology. Some methodological challenges in the field are discussed here.

The fourth section considers research on neuropsychological functioning following preterm birth.

Individual chapters provide summaries of research into the cognitive domains which have been found to be affected in preterm populations, such as language (Chapter 13), memory and learning (Chapter 14), and executive function (Chapter 15). Furthermore, this section includes an overview on the cognitive and functional profile of the preterm child (Chapter 11). Issues concerning neuropsychological outcomes as possible mediators of the effects of biological risks are also discussed. In addition to potential cause–effect inferences, Chapter 12 outlines methodological considerations which readers need to take into account when interpreting the results of outcome studies of individuals born very preterm/very low birth weight .

The fifth section links the current knowledge of the neurodevelopmental processes in preterm individuals with the environment in which they grow up. Chapter 16 summarizes studies investigating the educational attainment of preterm children and describes the substantial social impact of the often reported academic problems, both in terms of economic costs associated with educational resources and in terms of psychosocial adjustment of the preterm-born individual later in life. The impact of environmental variables, which may interact with and affect educational as well as neurodevelopmental outcome, sometimes independent of biological risks, are discussed in Chapter 17. A detailed overview of the results of intervention programs aimed at improving the neurodevelopmental outcome of very preterm individuals by limiting cognitive and behavioral complications, and providing cognitive enhancers, is given in Chapter 18. The results of published studies support the effectiveness of early intervention programs in improving the short- and medium-term cognitive outcomes, but they appear too heterogeneous to provide guidance on what may be the optimal duration and intensity of the intervention. Further research into ways of minimizing the impact of perinatal complications, especially in infants at greater biological (the extremely immature and low birth weight infants) and environmental risk (the socioeconomically disadvantaged), is warranted.

In the final section we summarize what is known to date about the neurodevelopmental sequelae of preterm birth, what the findings explain, and what research challenges are still unmet. We highlight some areas of research which could help further our understanding of the pathways to risk as well as resilience after preterm birth. These include the study of the molecular basis and genetic contribution to susceptibility to brain injury and of ways to modify the sociodemographic environment in which preterm infants grow and develop, including wider availability of and accessibility to intervention programs (Chapter 19).

We hope that this volume will be a valuable source of reference for pediatricians and neurologists, psychiatrists and psychologists, educators and neuroscientists alike, as we have attempted to discuss the implications of research findings for clinical practice. Apart from providing an up-to-date and concise summary of the explosion of research in this field, this volume aims to provide an accessible source of information across several disciplines. This book will have served its purpose if it succeeds in inspiring the next generation of researchers and clinicians to further knowledge of the pathophysiology of preterm birth and its neurodevelopmental sequelae, and lead on to the design and implementation of appropriate intervention services for individuals at risk of short- and long-term complications.

Introduction
Epidemiology of preterm birth

Stefan Johansson and Sven Cnattigius

Introduction

In humans, pregnancy normally lasts nine months, ending with term birth after approximately 40 gestational weeks. Preterm birth is arbitrarily defined as delivery before 37 weeks, and could be further classified as moderately, very or extremely preterm, occurring at 32–36, 28–31, and ≤ 27 weeks, respectively.

Historically, there has been some confusion regarding the diverse concepts of "low birth weight" and "preterm birth." In 1946, the American obstetrician Raymond D McBurney stated on a congress in San Francisco "… it is extremely annoying to have a pediatrician insist that the baby is premature because it may weigh only … five pounds" [1]. McBurney correctly emphasized that birth weight is not only a function of gestational age, but also fetal growth.

In research, the definitions of low, very low and extremely low birth weight (birth weights of < 2500 g, < 1500 g, and < 1000 g, respectively) have been widely used as proxys for preterm birth. However, studies defining preterm infants solely on birth weight criteria are limited by some degree of misclassification, i.e. growth restricted infants with more advanced gestational ages are probably over-represented in such studies.

In outcome research including preterm children and adults, it is important to distinguish preterm birth from intrauterine growth retardation, since gestational age and fetal growth may have differential impacts on outcome. One example is the associations between perinatal risk factors and cardiovascular disease. Studies have shown that preterm birth as well as fetal growth restriction is associated with hypertension in adulthood. In adults born very preterm, decreasing gestational age is associated with an increasing risk of high blood pressure regardless of fetal growth. In contrast, intrauterine growth retardation is the principal perinatal risk factor for hypertension in adults born moderately preterm and term [2].

Few fields in medicine have gone through such a rapid and remarkable development as neonatal medicine. Mortality of preterm infants has decreased dramatically during recent decades, and it is now possible to save the lives of extremely immature infants, born just more than half way through a normal pregnancy. Nevertheless, mortality rates increase substantially with decreasing gestational age, and especially extremely preterm infants face a high mortality risk.

Similar to mortality, neonatal morbidity is inversely related to gestational age. The most immature infants commonly suffer from multiple and interacting medical conditions, such as respiratory problems, infections, and brain hemorrhages, which may lead to permanent impairments. Among the new and growing generation of survivors of preterm birth, cognitive and behavioral problems are not uncommon.

Already during childhood, preterm birth has public health implications, related to pediatric healthcare resources, family support, and school education. In addition, if problems emerging in school age persist into adulthood, the need for societal assistance may also be increased later in life.

Researchers in perinatal epidemiology and neonatal medicine face several challenges. Increased knowledge on risk factors and biological mechanisms is needed to develop efficient strategies to prevent preterm birth. Further refinement of neonatal care is necessary to improve short-term mortality and morbidity among preterm infants. Well-designed follow-up studies are essential to learn more about long-term outcomes, in particular for the growing number of children surviving very and extremely preterm birth in the current era of neonatal medicine.

Definitions of preterm birth

Gestational length to non-elective delivery in humans has been estimated as being 282–283 days [3].

Neurodevelopmental Outcomes of Preterm Birth, ed. Chiara Nosarti, Robin M. Murray, and Maureen Hack. Published by Cambridge University Press. © Cambridge University Press 2010.

Preterm birth ≤ 36 weeks			Term birth 37–41 weeks	Post-term birth ≥ 42 weeks
extremely preterm ≤ 27 weeks				
	very preterm 28–31 weeks			
		moderately preterm 32–36 weeks		

Fig. 1.1 Categorization of gestational age by completed gestational weeks at birth.

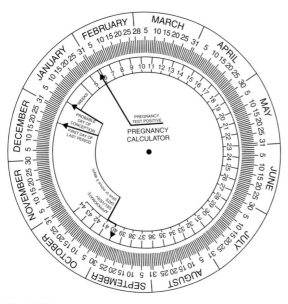

Fig. 1.2 The pregnancy wheel.

Gestational age of a newborn infant is categorized as preterm, term, or post-term (Fig. 1.1), as proposed by the World Health Organization in the 1970s [4]. Preterm birth occurs before 37 completed gestational weeks and could further be subdivided into moderately preterm, very preterm, and extremely preterm. As in this chapter, "very preterm birth" usually refers to all births at ≤ 31 weeks, including also extremely preterm births at ≤ 27 weeks.

To determine gestational age at birth, it is necessary to date the pregnancy and calculate the expected date of delivery (EDD) occurring at 40 completed gestational weeks. One commonly used method is to define EDD as 280 days from the last menstrual period (LMP), using the so-called pregnancy wheel (Fig. 1.2) [5].

The simplicity of this method makes it well suited for low-resource communities. Despite problems of recalling the correct date of LMP [6] the estimations

of gestational age are reasonably good [5,7] and can be used in perinatal epidemiology research when other dating methods are unavailable.

A more accurate way to date the pregnancy is to measure fetal size in early pregnancy, using ultrasound techniques [8]. Fetal growth velocity is constant during early pregnancy [9], and measures such as femoral length and head circumference are proportional to gestational length. Hence, such measures can be used to predict EDD and calculate gestational age in clinical practice [10]. Gestational age derived from LMP typically results in overestimates of about 2–3 days [7]. Importantly, changing the pregnancy dating method from LMP to ultrasound could have an impact on gestational age distribution, leading to an increase in preterm birth rate and a concomitant decrease in post-term birth rate [11]. Hence, rates of preterm birth may not be comparable if these are based on different methods of estimating gestational age.

Rates of preterm birth

Contrary to the general belief, preterm birth is a common pregnancy complication. Internationally, the variation of preterm birth rates is striking. About 6% of all pregnancies end preterm in Sweden (2003) [12], whereas the corresponding figure for the USA is reported to be almost 13% (2005) [13]. In developing countries, rates may be even higher. In a study including ultrasound-dated pregnancies in Malawi, 20% of women delivered preterm [14].

Very preterm births, occurring before 32 completed gestational weeks, account for about 15% of preterm births, which means that 1–2% of all pregnancies end very preterm [12,13].

Rates of preterm birth seem to be constant or even decreasing in the UK and Sweden [15,16], but several countries report increasing rates over recent decades [13,17,18]. This observation has been attributed to a number of factors, such as the introduction of ultrasound pregnancy dating, more frequent medically

Table 1.1 Risk factors for preterm birth

- Ethnicity
- Family history
- Infections
- Maternal characteristics
- Socioeconomic status
- Multiple pregnancies
- Smoking and substance abuse
- Air pollution

induced preterm deliveries, assisted reproduction, and more frequent twin births [17,18]. Increasing preterm birth rates seem to be explained by a greater number of moderately preterm births, since rates of very preterm birth have been stable over time [13,16].

Risk factors for preterm birth

Preterm birth has been associated with a number of risk factors (Table 1.1).

Ethnicity

Epidemiological studies have shown differences in rates of preterm birth among different ethnic groups [19]. In the USA during 2005, 19% of pregnancies ended preterm among black non-Hispanic women, whereas only 12% of white non-Hispanic women delivered preterm [13]. Corresponding rates for very preterm birth were 2.3% and 1.1%, respectively. In addition, black women do not only face an increased risk of preterm birth. Compared to white women, they are also at an increased risk of repeated preterm birth [19]. Although such findings may be explained by environmental or/ and/ socioeconomic factors, they could also indicate that some ethnic groups have a genetic predisposition for preterm birth [20].

Family history

One preterm delivery increases the risk of preterm deliveries in subsequent pregnancies [21,22] and the risk of repeating a preterm delivery is especially high for very preterm birth [21]. The heritability of preeclampsia, a common cause of preterm delivery, has been estimated to approximate 31%, and genetic factors may account for one third of all preterm deliveries [23,24]. The mechanisms underlying such genetic influences remain to be determined, but case-control studies

support the idea that inflammatory responses may be influenced by genetic factors [25–27].

Infections

Bacterial vaginosis and intrauterine bacterial infections are well-established risk factors of preterm delivery [28]. Bacterial vaginosis may increase the risk of very preterm delivery more than two fold [29], and intrauterine infection is reported to be associated with even higher risks, especially for extremely preterm birth [30]. Infections localized to organ systems other than the reproductive tract may also be important. Periodontal infections have been reported to more than double the risk of very preterm birth [31].

The uterus and amniotic membranes can become infected in several ways. Bacteria can migrate to the uterus from the vagina or the abdominal cavity, be introduced during invasive procedures such as chorionic villi sampling [32], or through hematogenous spread [33]. If chorioamnionitis develops, the risk of very preterm delivery is increased, especially if an inflammatory response is also elicited in the fetus, when the risk of extremely preterm birth may increase ten fold [30].

A number of bacteria have been cultured from amniotic fluid and chorioamniotic membranes in preterm deliveries; vaginal organisms with low virulence, such as *Ureaplasma urealyticum, Mycoplasma hominis, Gardnerella vaginalis,* and *Bacteroides* species, and several other bacteria such as *Escherichia coli, Enterococcus faecalis, Streptococcus* species, and *Chlamydia trachomatis* [28].

While much focus has been on bacteria, less is known about the role of viral infections. The only larger epidemiological study suggested that *Parvovirus B19* may be associated with an increased risk of late spontaneous abortion and stillbirth [34]. The prevalence of immunoglobulin M (IgM) seropositivity for *Parvovirus B19* among women with such pregnancy complications was 13% as compared with 1.5% in the remaining pregnant population [34]. Smaller clinical studies and case-series also report that viral infections may increase the risk of preterm delivery. Levels of antibodies against *Cytomegalovirus* were found to be higher in women with early onset preeclampsia and preterm delivery, compared to women with normal pregnancies ending at term [35]. *Cytomegalovirus* was also more commonly detected in dried neonatal blood spots, sampled after birth, in infants born preterm than in term infants (prevalence 33% versus 24%)[36].

Maternal characteristics

Several maternal characteristics have been associated with preterm birth. Firstly, as already described, preterm birth rates differ by ethnicity. Secondly, maternal age is reported to influence pregnancy outcome. Low and high maternal age increase the risk of preterm birth [37,38]. Moreover, maternal age has been shown to interact with parity, i.e., the risk of preterm birth being highest in younger multiparae and older primiparae [39]. Compared with 25- to 29-year-old primiparae, the risk of preterm birth is approximately doubled for multiparae aged less than 18 years and for primiparae aged more than 40 years. One may speculate that teenage mothers with several children are exposed to less favorable socioeconomic conditions [40]. Delayed childbearing at an older age is related to more prevalent assisted reproduction, higher risk of preeclampsia, and more frequent twin pregnancies [41].

Finally, reproductive history may be important. Previous induced abortions may increase the risk of very preterm births with spontaneous onset [42]. Women with a previous second trimester spontaneous abortion or a previous very preterm delivery are at increased risk of very preterm delivery in a subsequent pregnancy [19,21]. A short interval between subsequent pregnancies (< 6 months) has also been reported to be a risk factor, doubling the risk of extremely preterm delivery in subsequent pregnancies [43]. However, the association between a short interpregnancy interval and other adverse pregnancy outcomes including preterm birth may be confounded by socioeconomic factors [44] or adverse outcomes in previous pregnancies [45].

Socioeconomic status

There are marked socioeconomic inequalities in preterm birth rates. The differences in preterm birth rates between countries like Sweden, USA, and Malawi are probably partly explained by different socioeconomic contexts [12–14]. Within developed countries, socioeconomic status is also related to risk of preterm birth. A recent British study demonstrated that very preterm birth was twice as common among women living in the most deprived areas compared to women in the least deprived areas [46]. Similar conclusions were drawn in Norway, where maternal characteristics such as single motherhood and low education were associated

with a 25% and 50% increase in risk of preterm birth, respectively [47].

Multiple pregnancies

An American study reported that 54% of twins were born preterm [48]. In Europe, preterm birth rates in twin pregnancies vary from 42% in Ireland to 68% in Austria, amounting to 20% of all preterm births [49]. Twins resulting from subfertility treatment are more commonly born preterm compared to naturally concieved twins [50]. The majority of preterm births in singletons are due to spontaneous onset of labor, but induced deliveries account for about half of preterm births among twins [49].

In absolute terms, neonatal outcome of multiple pregnancies is generally worse than in singleton pregnancies [51]. However, besides intrauterine growth retardation, prematurity is the principal factor responsible for increased mortality and morbidity rates in twins and triplets. When gestational age is taken into account, risks of neonatal mortality and morbidity are not increased in multiple pregnancies compared to single pregnancies [52].

Smoking and substance abuse

Maternal smoking has a dose-dependent impact on risk of preterm birth [53]. Heavy smoking ($\geq$ 10 cigarettes per day) may increase the risk of very preterm delivery more than two fold. Exposure to environmental tobacco smoke (passive smoking) has also been associated with an increased risk, yet lower than for active smoking [54]. The association between snuff (smokeless tobacco) and preterm birth is less well studied, but an investigation from Sweden found that snuff increased the risk of preterm birth by 79% [55]. A South African study concluded that snuff did not affect the rate of preterm birth, although women using snuff had slightly shorter gestational length in term births compared to women not using snuff [56].

Abuse of other drugs during pregnancy, including narcotics and alcohol, is associated with a number of poor perinatal outcomes, including preterm birth [57]. Prenatal drug exposure to tobacco and cocaine has been estimated to account for 5.7% of preterm births in American settings [58]. Excessive alcohol use is also reported to be more common among women who deliver preterm [59]. However, narcotics and alcohol may be part of a low socioeconomic lifestyle, and it is difficult to disentangle the independent roles of substance abuse versus deprived socioeconomic circumstances.

Air pollution

Exposure to ambient air pollution, such as particulate matter, ozone, carbon monoxide, and nitric dioxide, has been reported in several studies to increase the risk of preterm birth in a dose-dependent manner [60,61]. However, there are also published studies which reported negative results [62]. Despite attempts to adjust for socioeconomic status in studies reporting positive findings [60,61], one cannot exclude that residual socioeconomic confounders may contribute to explain the association between air pollutants and preterm birth.

Etiologies and biological mechanisms

The variety of identified risk factors could be translated into different etiologies of preterm birth (Table 1.2).

Firstly, one needs to consider two principally different etiological concepts; spontaneous preterm birth and medically induced preterm birth [63]. The majority of preterm births have spontaneous onset, initiated by premature labor, rupture of membranes, or vaginal bleeding [49]. The remaining preterm births are medically induced on maternal or fetal indications, typically due to preeclampsia. This heterogeneity of preterm births needs to be considered in research on etiological concepts and biological mechanisms [63]. Neonatal outcome may be more dependent on gestational age at birth than on the etiology of preterm birth [64], but risk factors may have differential impact on spontaneous and induced preterm birth, respectively [65].

Secondly, the various etiologies of preterm birth are related to several biological pathways (Table 1.3).

Genetic mechanisms

Ethnic differences [19], risk of repeated preterm delivery [21,22], and familial aggregation of preeclampsia and preterm birth [23,24] indicate that genetic mechanisms are important for preterm birth.

One may speculate about genetic influences on several physiological processes leading to preterm delivery. Polymorphisms of genes involved in the immune system could be related to preterm delivery. One genotype of a promotor gene for interleukin (IL)-6, regulating responses to stressful stimuli, was found in 38% of mothers with very preterm deliveries, and in 29% of mothers

Table 1.2 Main etiologies of preterm birth

- Premature labor
- Preterm premature rupture of membranes
- Placental abruption and vaginal bleeding
- Preeclampsia and other maternal illnesses

Table 1.3 Biological pathways for preterm birth

- Genetic mechanisms
- Inflammation
- Vascular mechanisms
- Neuroendocrine stress responses
- Mechanical stress

with term deliveries [25]. Tandem repeat polymorphism of the gene for the IL-1 receptor antagonist, involved in duration and severity of inflammation, was found in 27% of women with preterm deliveries, compared to 12% of women with term deliveries [26]. Polymorphisms of immunoregulatory genes for IL-10 and mannose-binding protein 2 (MBL2) have also been more commonly found in women with preterm births and may increase the risk of chorioamnionitis [27], a pregnancy complication often preceding spontaneous preterm birth.

A low intake of dietary vitamin C may increase the risk of preterm birth [66], and genetic variants of a membrane-bound vitamin C transporter may double the risk of spontaneous preterm delivery [67]. Polymorphisms in folate-metabolizing genes, affecting homocysteine levels, may also play a role for spontaneous preterm delivery, especially in black women with low folate intake [68].

Inflammation

The association between intrauterine infections and preterm birth involves biological pathways related to inflammation [28]. Bacterial colonization and release of toxins activates the production of cytokines, such as tumor necrosis factor α (TNFα) and IL-6. Cytokines stimulate prostaglandin production in the chorioamniotic membranes and placenta and lead to infiltration of neutrophilic white blood cells. Activation of metalloproteases leads to weakening of chorioamniotic membranes and cervical ripening. Prostaglandins also stimulate myometrial contractions. The inflammatory response culminates in preterm labor and rupture of the membranes.

An inflammatory response in the fetus also contributes to preterm labor and rupture of membranes.

5

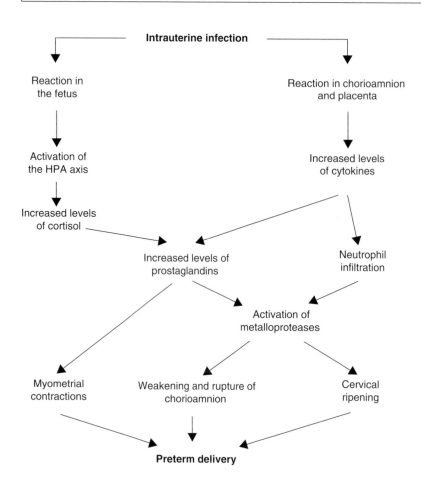

Fig. 1.3 Potential pathways from intrauterine infection to preterm delivery. Adapted from Goldenberg *et al.* [28].

Chorioamnionitis could result in fetal stress involving the hypothalamic–pituitary–adrenal axis (HPA axis). Fetal release of cortisol contributes to increased levels of prostaglandins.

A schematic view of inflammatory pathways leading to preterm delivery is shown in Fig. 1.3.

Vascular mechanisms

Preeclampsia and placental abruption are pregnancy complications often resulting in medically induced preterm delivery. Although principally different, both complications can be attributed to impaired placental vascular function.

Preeclampsia, affecting 3–5% of pregnant women, is a complex disorder initiating already during the critical process of implantation and placentation shortly after conception [69,70]. Inadequate invasion of endovascular cells, placental production of anti-angiogenic factors, and development of endothelial dysfunction leads to small-bore, high-resistant placental vessels that cannot respond to the

increasing demand of blood supply and nutrition to the fetus. Clinical manifestations of preeclampsia, such as hypertension, renal dysfunction, and neurological symptoms, may necessitate preterm delivery on maternal indication. More commonly, delivery is induced on fetal indication, due to signs of fetal stress including abnormal umbilical blood flow and growth restriction.

Placental abruption, complicating 0.5–1% of pregnancies, is a too early separation of the placenta from the uterine wall, diagnosed by a combination of ultrasound findings and clinical signs, such as vaginal bleeding, abdominal pain, and fetal distress [71]. Clinical outcome depends on the degree of placental detachment, the degree of fetal distress, and gestational age at abruption, but the risk of perinatal mortality in very preterm deliveries following abruption is substantially increased [72].

Neuroendocrine stress responses

The association between low socioeconomic status and preterm delivery could be mediated by psychological distress during pregnancy [73]. Maternal stress activates the HPA axis, illustrated by elevated cortisol levels in gestational week 15 in women who later delivered preterm [74]. Increased secretion of cortisol stimulates placental secretion of corticotropin-releasing hormone (CRH), interacting with prostaglandins and oxytocin, which mediate uterine contractions. Secretion of CRH is reported to be elevated in pregnant women who later deliver preterm [75] and it has been suggested that serum levels of CRH may be a useful marker in the clinical assessment of the risk of parturition in women presenting with preterm contractions [76].

Mechanical stress

Finally, mechanical stress of the uterus and cervix could be associated with preterm delivery. Cesarian section in a first pregnancy increases the risk of preterm birth in a second pregnancy [77]. Uterine overdistension is assumed to increase the risk of preterm delivery, exemplified by shorter gestations in twin pregnancies, especially in those with excessive amniotic fluid (polyhydramnios) [78]. Leiomyomata, benign neoplasms in the uterine wall, are associated with an increased risk of preterm delivery, supposedly due to increased mechanical strain on the uterus [79]. One proposed mechanism is that stretching of fetal membranes increases IL-8 concentrations and collagenase activity, implicated in cervical ripening [80]. Finally, incompetence of the cervix has been regarded to be casually related to preterm delivery, and cervical cerclage (tracheloplasty) has been widely used in attempts to prevent preterm birth. However, cervical cerclage is largely an unsuccessful strategy [81], which suggests that the cervix plays more than just a mechanical role [82].

Relations between risk and biology

There are probably complex relationships between risk factors of preterm birth and biological mechanisms. One risk factor may be important for several pathways and vice versa. In Fig. 1.4 we have made an attempt to summarize these relationships.

Prevention efforts

The ultimate goal of research on risk factors, etiologies, and biological mechanisms of preterm birth is to develop preventive strategies. Especially very preterm infants face substantial risks of mortality or long-term neurological sequels [83,84]. There are also economic implications. Neonatal intensive care is associated with significant costs, which increase exponentially with decreasing gestational age [85]. Preventing preterm deliveries would not only save lives, but also yield large cost savings.

The majority of preterm births have a spontaneous onset [49]. Given the association between preterm delivery and infections [28], antibiotic treatment could provide a potential strategy for prevention. However, large randomized controlled trials have drawn rather disappointing conclusions. Antibiotic treatment of women in preterm labor with intact membranes does not delay or prevent preterm delivery [86]. Similarly, treatment does not prevent preterm birth in pregnant women with bacterial vaginosis [87]. Antibiotic treatment of women with premature rupture of the membranes does not reduce the rate of preterm births, but can to some extent delay preterm delivery [88]. Still, it is possible that antibiotic treatment could be beneficial if offered to high-risk groups, as indicated by a large American study: in black urban women screened for reproductive tract infections, antibiotics reduced

Risk factor \ Biological pathway	Genes	Inflammation	Vascular	Neuroendocrine	Mechanical
Ethnicity	+++	+		+	
Family history	++	+		+	
Infections	+	+++		+	
Low maternal age		+		+	
High maternal age		+	+	+	
Reproductive history	+	+	+		+
Socioeconomic status	+	+		++	
Multiple pregnancy			+	+	++
Smoking		+	++	+	
Air pollution		+		+	

Fig. 1.4 Relationships between risk factors and biological mechanisms of preterm birth.

the risk of preterm delivery (relative risk = 0.16, 95% confidence interval [CI] = 0.04–0.66) [89].

Maternal periodontal disease is associated with an increased risk of preterm birth [31]. If bacterial load in the oral cavity contributes to chorioamnionitis, through hematogeneous spread or due to increased systemic inflammatory activity, treatment of periodontal disease could be beneficial for pregnancy outcome. One small pilot study showed that treatment of periodontal disease during pregnancy reduced systemic inflammation, measured by levels of IL-6, and reduced the risk of preterm birth (odds ratio = 0.26, 95% CI = 0.08–0.85)[90]. However, in a larger study treatment of periodontitis had no effect on risk of preterm birth, despite improved periodontal health in treated women [91].

Prevention of preeclampsia, as a means to prevent preterm birth, has been extensively studied [92]. Many strategies have been tested, including lifestyle choices (rest or exercise), various nutritional measures, and drugs. However, almost all strategies have been unsuccessful, with the exception of moderate benefits of low-dose aspirin and calcium supplementation [93, 94]. Antioxidants seem to decrease the risk of preeclampsia, but results should be interpreted cautiously, especially since antioxidants may increase the risk of preterm birth [95]. Treatment of preeclamptic women with antihypertensive drugs is widely used, but there are limited data supporting that such treatment may reduce the risk of preterm delivery [96].

Smoking and substance abuse are potentially preventable factors associated with preterm birth. Women who stop smoking from their first their to second pregnancy reduce their risk of preterm birth to that of non-smoking women [21]. A recent meta-analysis including randomized controlled trials concluded that smoking cessation during pregnancy was associated with a 16% reduction of risk of preterm delivery [97]. Studies on treatment of substance abuse with regard to infant outcomes are scarce, but two small studies have found that gestational length increases somewhat in women undergoing such treatment [98, 99].

Similarly, social disadvantage may be a target for intervention programs. However, a large randomized trial of psychosocial support and health education during high-risk pregnancies could not find that such interventions reduced the risk of preterm birth [100]. A recent meta-analysis of studies on social support during pregnancy came to the same conclusion [101].

Mortality during the neonatal period and during infancy

Infant mortality (death during the first year of life) has decreased during the last four decades for all infants, as demonstrated by national birth statistics from Sweden (Fig. 1.5, unpublished data from the Medical Birth Register). The reduction in infant mortality over time is mainly explained by decreased neonatal mortality (death during the first four weeks of life), although postneonatal mortality (death after the first four weeks of life but before one year of life) has declined somewhat.

The same pattern of improved survival during the neonatal period is seen among term, moderately preterm and very preterm infants, but in absolute numbers, the improvement is most dramatic for very preterm infants (≤ 31 weeks) (Fig. 1.6). From 1973 to 2002, neonatal mortality rates decreased from 401 to 90 per 1000 live-born very preterm infants, whereas the corresponding rates per 1000 live-born moderately preterm infants (32–36 weeks) and term infants (≥37 weeks) decreased from 34 to 8 and from 3 to 1, respectively. This improvement in survival among very preterm infants during the neonatal period has primarily been attributed to improvements of neonatal intensive care, including the introduction of antenatal corticosteroids and surfactant for prevention and treatment of respiratory distress syndrome [102].

Mortality in very preterm infants is inversely related to gestational age. Despite the overall reduction, the most immature infants still face a substantial risk of death, as illustrated by recently reported mortality rates from Sweden, and the Australia and New Zealand Neonatal Network (Fig. 1.7) [103,104].

Another way to express the relation over time between mortality and gestational age is that the so-called "border-of-viability" has shifted to the left. Today, extremely small and immature infants could be considered as candidates for resuscitation and admission to neonatal intensive care units. However, as demonstrated by data from the Vermont Oxford Network,[1] mortality rates are exceptionally high among the tiniest infants [105]. Of infants born with a birth weight of 401–500 g (mean gestational age of 23 weeks), overall survival was only 17%.

---

1 The Vermont Oxford Network is a worldwide network of neonatal intensive care units, which report their outcome data to a central database. Any neonatal intensive care unit can join the Vermont Oxford Network.

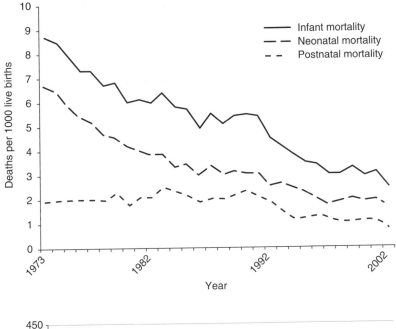

Fig. 1.5 Infant, neonatal, and postnatal mortality in infants born in Sweden 1973 to 2002.

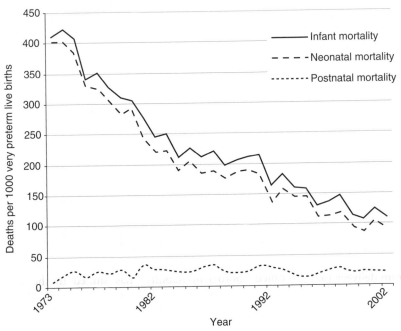

Fig. 1.6 Infant, neonatal and postnatal mortality in very preterm infants born in Sweden 1973 to 2002.

A large proportion of infants born at the "border-of-viability" die because of decisions taken shortly after delivery to limit intensive care and provide only palliative treatment [106]. Therefore, management policies could be important for survival in the most immature infants. Studies from Sweden and Germany support that proactive management promotes survival in infants born at 22–25 gestational weeks [107,108].

To improve survival, the regional and/or national organization of neonatal intensive care also needs to be considered. The complex nature of neonatal intensive care demands highly qualified staffing as well as access to advanced technologies. In several studies from different countries, level-III neonatal intensive care units, i.e. university hospitals, have had lower mortality rates when compared with smaller level-II units. However,

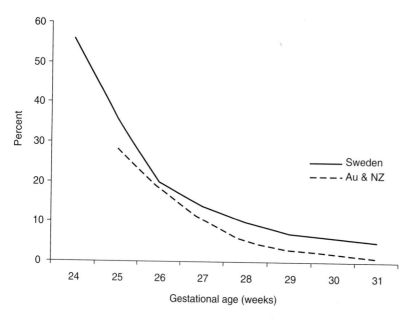

Fig. 1.7 Infant mortality rates in Sweden 1992–8, and mortality rates before discharge from neonatal intensive care in Australia and New Zealand 1998–2001, by gestational week.

the older studies have limitations. They categorized infants according to birth weight instead of gestational age [109,110], were performed before recent improvements of neonatal practice [111,112], or did not adjust for potential confounders such as obstetric complications [109,112]. Still, more recent studies also support that centralization of neonatal intensive care is associated with reduced mortality. A large American study, including 48 237 very low birth weight infants (< 1500 g, 75% born at ≤ 31 weeks), found that both volume of care (number of admissions) and level of care were associated with risk of neonatal mortality [113]. According to a report from Finland, 69 of 170 annual deaths could be prevented if all very preterm infants (≤ 31 weeks) were born in university hospitals [114]. A British study investigating variations in standards of neonatal care showed that poor quality of ventilatory support, cardiovascular support, and thermal care increased the risk of mortality two- to threefold for infants born at 27 and 28 weeks [115]. In addition, poor quality of care was especially associated with deaths among infants in good condition at birth (see also Chapter 2).

Neonatal morbidity

Preterm infants face high morbidity risks during the neonatal period, although advances in neonatal care during recent decades have led to reduced rates of some conditions. For instance, the introduction of antenatal corticosteroids has almost halved risks of respiratory distress syndrome and brain hemorrhage [116]. However,

improvements in neonatal care and nursing are not only related to new treatments, but also due to implementation of refined strategies, such as improved nutrition, better infection control, and more gentle ventilatory support. Thus, neonatology has learnt to better deal with the medical problems related to preterm birth.

Similar to mortality, morbidity risks are inversely related to gestational age [107,117]. Compared to term infants, infants born close to term (34–36 weeks) are at risk of developing problems related to immaturity, such as feeding difficulties, temperature instability, infections and respiratory distress, occasionally even necessitating mechanical ventilation [118,119]. Nevertheless, moderately preterm infants are generally spared from complicated morbidity. In contrast, very and extremely preterm infants commonly suffer from multiple and interacting morbidities. Medical problems are especially prevalent among 23–25 week infants [105,107,108], since their extremely immature organs at birth ill-equip them to make the transition from intrauterine to extrauterine life.

A number of different medical conditions may affect preterm infants (Table 1.4) [120]. Although those conditions are separate clinical entities, they are also strongly correlated. For example, acute lung problems shortly after birth (RDS) are correlated with circulatory problems (PDA), brain hemorrhage (IVH) and later lung disease (BPD).

While some studies report relatively low or decreasing morbidity rates among survivors after extremely preterm birth (≤ 27 weeks) [121–123],

Table 1.4 Common medical problems in preterm infants

Clinical entity	Synopsis
Respiratory distress syndrome (RDS)	Lung problem developing shortly after birth due to lack of endogenous surfactant in the lungs. Surface tension increases in the smallest airways and lungs get non-compliant (stiff). Treated with instillation of exogenous surfactant in the airway. Common reason for mechanical ventilation
Patent ductus arteriosus (PDA)	The duct is a blood vessel between the pulmonary artery and the aorta, essential for fetal blood circulation. The duct should close after birth but can stay open in preterm infants, shunting too much blood to the lungs and leaving too little blood for other organs. Can be closed with drugs or surgery
Necrotizing enterocolitis (NEC)	Inflammation and necrosis of the bowel, leading to various abdominal symptoms. Treated with bowel rest and antibiotics, but surgical bowel resection is commonly performed in cases of bowel necrosis and/or perforation
Bronchopulmonary dysplasia (BPD)	A more chronic lung problem, related to short gestational age, RDS, PDA, and mechanical ventilation. Months of ventilatory support and supplementary oxygen may be needed in severe cases. Some, but not all, children can be prone to asthma-like problems and have reduced lung function
Retinopathy of prematurity (ROP)	Overgrowth of blood vessels in the immature retina of the eye, related to factors such as short gestational age and oxygen administration. Low-grade retinopathy usually resolve without specific therapy but laser treatment may be needed in severe forms. Worst-case scenario includes retinal detachment and blindness
Intraventricular hemorrhage (IVH)	Bleedings originating in the germinal matrix, a highly vascularized and cellularly active tissue beside the brain ventricles. Localized bleedings may not be associated with poor outcomes, but those extending into the brain tissue may have a poor prognosis, and could contribute to decisions to withdraw care (end-of-life decisions).
Periventricular leukomalacia (PVL)	Damage of brain white matter, related to hypoxia and inflammation. The initial insults may usually occur shortly after birth or during a sudden clinical deterioration and PVL then develops over the following weeks. Some forms of PVL are strongly associated with cerebral paresis. Can be diagnosed with ultrasound of the brain
Infections	Very common, due to an immature immune system and much exposure to bacteria from the environment (including staff). Bacteria of low virulence and fungi are common pathogens. Can usually be treated successfully with antibiotics, but infection-related mortality is significant

Table 1.5 Neonatal morbidity in extremely preterm infants surviving till discharge. Data presented as numbers (%)

	Serenius et al.[121]	Markestad et al. [122]	Vanhaesebrouck et al. [124]	Wilson-Costello et al. [123]
Study characteristics				
Setting	Sweden	Norway	Belgium	Cleveland, USA
Time period	1992–8	1999–2000	1999–2000	2000–2
Gestational age	23–25 weeks	22–27 weeks	22–26 weeks	500–999 grams
Total no. of births	224	502	525	not reported
Admissions	213	366	303	233
Survivors till discharge	140 (66%)	290 (79%)	175 (58%)	165 (71%)
Morbidity in survivors				
BPD (oxygen at 36 w)	50 (36%)	106 (36%)	78 (44%)	84 (51%)
ROP (treated)	21 (15%)	14 (5%)	35 (20%)	not reported
Any IVH or PVL	33 (24%)	124 (43%)	84 (48%)	43 (26%)

other studies conclude that the improved survival over recent decades have led to increased morbidity rates [117,124]. Table 1.5 provides neonatal morbidity rates among extremely preterm infants, reported in studies from Europe and the USA.

As already mentioned, neonatal morbidity rates are inversely related to gestational age. Compared to the most immature infants (≤ 27 weeks), very preterm infants born at 28–31 weeks have less medical problems during the neonatal period. For example, a

Dutch study reported 87% survival until discharge in very preterm infants and a rate of BPD in only 10% of survivors [125].

With regard to preterm birth and outcomes in adulthood, one needs to consider that modern neonatal intensive care has a short history. Antenatal corticosteroids and surfactant for prevention and treatment of RDS were broadly implemented less than 20 years ago. Consequently, very little is known about health in adult life for the growing number of children who have survived very and extremely preterm birth since the 1990s. Chapter 2 will provide a wide overview of developments in neonatal care for preterm infants over the last 50 years, and discuss the mechanisms of brain injury in this vulnerable population.

References

1. McBurney RD. The undernourished full term infant. *West J Surg Obstet Gynecol* 1947; **55**: 363–70.

2. Johansson S, Iliadou A, Bergvall N, *et al*. Risk of high blood pressure among young men increases with the degree of immaturity at birth. *Circulation* 2005; **112**(22): 3430–6.

3. Bergsjo P, Denman DW, 3rd, Hoffman HJ, Meirik O. Duration of human singleton pregnancy. A population-based study. *Acta Obstet Gynecol Scand* 1990; **69**(3): 197–207.

4. WHO: recommended definitions, terminology and format for statistical tables related to the perinatal period, and use of a new certificate for cause of perinatal deaths. Modifications recommended by FIGO as amended October 14, 1976. *Acta Obstet Gynecol Scand* 1977; **56**(3): 247–53.

5. Ross MG. Circle of time: errors in the use of the pregnancy wheel. *J Matern Fetal Neonatal Med* 2003; **14**(6): 370–2.

6. Waller DK, Spears WD, Gu Y, Cunningham GC. Assessing number-specific error in the recall of onset of last menstrual period. *Paediatr Perinat Epidemiol* 2000; **14**(3): 263–7.

7. Savitz DA, Terry JW, Jr., Dole N, *et al*. Comparison of pregnancy dating by last menstrual period, ultrasound scanning, and their combination. *Am J Obstet Gynecol* 2002; **187**(6): 1660–6.

8. Kramer MS, McLean FH, Boyd ME, Usher RH. The validity of gestational age estimation by menstrual dating in term, preterm, and postterm gestations. *JAMA* 1988; **260**(22): 3306–8.

9. Milani S, Bossi A, Bertino E, *et al*. Differences in size at birth are determined by differences in growth velocity during early prenatal life. *Pediatr Res* 2005; **57**(2): 205–10.

10. Persson PH, Weldner BM. Normal range growth curves for fetal biparietal diameter, occipito frontal diameter, mean abdominal diameters and femur length. *Acta Obstet Gynecol Scand* 1986; **65**(7): 759–61.

11. Goldenberg RL, Davis RO, Cutter GR, *et al*. Prematurity, postdates, and growth retardation: the influence of use of ultrasonography on reported gestational age. *Am J Obstet Gynecol* 1989; **160**(2): 462–70.

12. Medical birth registration in 2003. Stockholm: The National Board of Health and Welfare; 2005.

13. Hamilton BE, Minino AM, Martin JA, *et al*. Annual summary of vital statistics: 2005. *Pediatrics* 2007; **119**(2): 345–60.

14. van den Broek N, Ntonya C, Kayira E, White S, Neilson JP. Preterm birth in rural Malawi: high incidence in ultrasound-dated population. *Hum Reprod* 2005; **20**(11): 3235–7.

15. Balchin I, Whittaker JC, Steer PJ, Lamont RF. Are reported preterm birth rates reliable? An analysis of interhospital differences in the calculation of the weeks of gestation at delivery and preterm birth rate. *BJOG* 2004; **111**(2): 160–3.

16. Morken NH, Kallen K, Hagberg H, Jacobsson B. Preterm birth in Sweden 1973–2001: rate, subgroups, and effect of changing patterns in multiple births, maternal age, and smoking. *Acta Obstet Gynecol Scand* 2005; **84**(6): 558–65.

17. Joseph KS, Kramer MS, Marcoux S, *et al*. Determinants of preterm birth rates in Canada from 1981 through 1983 and from 1992 through 1994. *N Engl J Med* 1998; **339**(20): 1434–9.

18. Langhoff-Roos J, Kesmodel U, Jacobsson B, Rasmussen S, Vogel I. Spontaneous preterm delivery in primiparous women at low risk in Denmark: population based study. *BMJ* 2006; **332**(7547): 937–9.

19. Kistka ZA, Palomar L, Lee KA, *et al*. Racial disparity in the frequency of recurrence of preterm birth. *Am J Obstet Gynecol* 2007; **196**(2): 131.e1–6.

20. Nesin M. Genetic basis of preterm birth. *Front Biosci* 2007; **12**: 115–24.

21. Cnattingius S, Granath F, Petersson G, Harlow BL. The influence of gestational age and smoking habits on the risk of subsequent preterm deliveries. *N Engl J Med* 1999; **341**(13): 943–8.

22. Ananth CV, Getahun D, Peltier MR, Salihu HM, Vintzileos AM. Recurrence of spontaneous versus medically indicated preterm birth. *Am J Obstet Gynecol* 2006; **195**(3): 643–50.

23. Clausson B, Lichtenstein P, Cnattingius S. Genetic influence on birthweight and gestational length determined by studies in offspring of twins. *BJOG* 2000; **107**(3): 375–81.

24. Nilsson E, Salonen Ros H, Cnattingius S, Lichtenstein P. The importance of genetic and environmental effects for pre-eclampsia and gestational hypertension: a family study. *BJOG* 2004; **111**(3): 200–6.

25. Hartel C, Finas D, Ahrens P, et al. Polymorphisms of genes involved in innate immunity: association with preterm delivery. *Mol Hum Reprod* 2004; **10**(12): 911–5.

26. Murtha AP, Nieves A, Hauser ER, et al. Association of maternal IL-1 receptor antagonist intron 2 gene polymorphism and preterm birth. *Am J Obstet Gynecol* 2006; **195**(5): 1249–53.

27. Bodamer OA, Mitterer G, Maurer W, et al. Evidence for an association between mannose-binding lectin 2 (MBL2) gene polymorphisms and pre-term birth. *Genet Med* 2006; **8**(8): 518–24.

28. Goldenberg RL, Hauth JC, Andrews WW. Intrauterine infection and preterm delivery. *N Engl J Med* 2000; **342**(20): 1500–7.

29. Svare JA, Schmidt H, Hansen BB, Lose G. Bacterial vaginosis in a cohort of Danish pregnant women: prevalence and relationship with preterm delivery, low birthweight and perinatal infections. *BJOG* 2006; **113**(12): 1419–25.

30. Gupta M, Mestan KK, Martin CR, et al. Impact of clinical and histologic correlates of maternal and fetal inflammatory response on gestational age in preterm births. *J Matern Fetal Neonatal Med* 2007; **20**(1): 39–46.

31. Offenbacher S, Boggess KA, Murtha AP, et al. Progressive periodontal disease and risk of very preterm delivery. *Obstet Gynecol* 2006; **107**(1): 29–36.

32. Hogge WA, Schonberg SA, Golbus MS. Chorionic villus sampling: experience of the first 1000 cases. *Am J Obstet Gynecol* 1986; **154**(6): 1249–52.

33. Shimizu S, Kojima H, Yoshida C, et al. Chorioamnionitis caused by Serratia marcescens in a non-immunocompromised host. *J Clin Pathol* 2003; **56**(11): 871–2.

34. Jensen IP, Thorsen P, Jeune B, Moller BR, Vestergaard BF. An epidemic of parvovirus B19 in a population of 3,596 pregnant women: a study of sociodemographic and medical risk factors. *BJOG* 2000; **107**(5): 637–43.

35. von Dadelszen P, Magee LA, Krajden M, et al. Levels of antibodies against cytomegalovirus and Chlamydophila pneumoniae are increased in early onset pre-eclampsia. *BJOG* 2003; **110**(8): 725–30.

36. Gibson CS, MacLennan AH, Goldwater PN, et al. Neurotropic viruses and cerebral palsy: population based case-control study. *BMJ* 2006; **332**(7533): 76–80.

37. Olausson PO, Cnattingius S, Haglund B. Teenage pregnancies and risk of late fetal death and infant mortality. *BJOG* 1999; **106**(2): 116–21.

38. Hoffman MC, Jeffers S, Carter J, et al. Pregnancy at or beyond age 40 years is associated with an increased risk of fetal death and other adverse outcomes. *Am J Obstet Gynecol* 2007; **196**(5): e11–3.

39. Schempf AH, Branum AM, Lukacs SL, Schoendorf KC. Maternal age and parity-associated risks of preterm birth: differences by race/ethnicity. *Paediatr Perinat Epidemiol* 2007; **21**(1): 34–43.

40. Olausson PO, Lichtenstein P, Cnattingius S. Aetiology of teenage childbearing: reasons for familial effects. *Twin Res* 2000; **3**(1): 23–7.

41. Gilbert WM, Nesbitt TS, Danielsen B. Childbearing beyond age 40: pregnancy outcome in 24,032 cases. *Obstet Gynecol* 1999; **93**(1): 9–14.

42. Moreau C, Kaminski M, Ancel PY, et al. Previous induced abortions and the risk of very preterm delivery: results of the EPIPAGE study. *BJOG* 2005; **112**(4): 430–7.

43. Smith GC, Pell JP, Dobbie R. Interpregnancy interval and risk of preterm birth and neonatal death: retrospective cohort study. *BMJ* 2003; **327**(7410): 313.

44. Klebanoff MA. The interval between pregnancies and the outcome of subsequent births. *N Engl J Med* 1999; **340**(8): 643–4.

45. Stephansson O, Dickman PW, Cnattingius S. The influence of interpregnancy interval on the subsequent risk of stillbirth and early neonatal death. *Obstet Gynecol* 2003; **102**(1): 101–8.

46. Smith LK, Draper ES, Manktelow BN, Dorling JS, Field DJ. Socioeconomic inequalities in very preterm birth rates. *Arch Dis Child Fetal Neonatal Ed* 2007; **92**(1): F11–14.

47. Thompson JM, Irgens LM, Rasmussen S, Daltveit AK. Secular trends in socioeconomic status and the implications for preterm birth. *Paediatr Perinat Epidemiol* 2006; **20**(3): 182–7.

48. Gardner MO, Goldenberg RL, Cliver SP, et al. The origin and outcome of preterm twin pregnancies. *Obstet Gynecol* 1995; **85**(4): 553–7.

49. Blondel B, Macfarlane A, Gissler M, Breart G, Zeitlin J. Preterm birth and multiple pregnancy in European countries participating in the PERISTAT project. *BJOG* 2006; **113**(5): 528–35.

50. Verstraelen H, Goetgeluk S, Derom C, et al. Preterm birth in twins after subfertility treatment: population based cohort study. *BMJ* 2005; **331**(7526): 1173.

51. Blondel B, Kaminski M. Trends in the occurrence, determinants, and consequences of multiple births. *Semin Perinatol* 2002; **26**(4): 239–49.

52. Garite TJ, Clark RH, Elliott JP, Thorp JA. Twins and triplets: the effect of plurality and growth on neonatal outcome compared with singleton infants. *Am J Obstet Gynecol* 2004; **191**(3): 700–7.

13

53. Kyrklund-Blomberg NB, Cnattingius S. Preterm birth and maternal smoking: risks related to gestational age and onset of delivery. *Am J Obstet Gynecol* 1998; **179**(4): 1051–5.

54. Fantuzzi G, Aggazzotti G, Righi E, *et al.* Preterm delivery and exposure to active and passive smoking during pregnancy: a case-control study from Italy. *Paediatr Perinat Epidemiol* 2007; **21**(3): 194–200.

55. England LJ, Levine RJ, Mills JL, *et al.* Adverse pregnancy outcomes in snuff users. *Am J Obstet Gynecol* 2003; **189**(4): 939–43.

56. Steyn K, de Wet T, Saloojee Y, Nel H, Yach D. The influence of maternal cigarette smoking, snuff use and passive smoking on pregnancy outcomes: the Birth To Ten Study. *Paediatr Perinat Epidemiol* 2006; **20**(2): 90–9.

57. Kennare R, Heard A, Chan A. Substance use during pregnancy: risk factors and obstetric and perinatal outcomes in South Australia. *Aust N Z J Obstet Gynaecol* 2005; **45**(3): 220–5.

58. Bada HS, Das A, Bauer CR, *et al.* Low birth weight and preterm births: etiologic fraction attributable to prenatal drug exposure. *J Perinatol* 2005; **25**(10): 631–7.

59. Schoeman J, Grove DV, Odendaal HJ. Are domestic violence and the excessive use of alcohol risk factors for preterm birth? *J Trop Pediatr* 2005; **51**(1): 49–50.

60. Maroziene L, Grazuleviciene R. Maternal exposure to low-level air pollution and pregnancy outcomes: a population-based study. *Environ Health* 2002; **1**(1): 6.

61. Hansen C, Neller A, Williams G, Simpson R. Maternal exposure to low levels of ambient air pollution and preterm birth in Brisbane, Australia. *BJOG* 2006; **113**(8): 935–41.

62. Landgren O. Environmental pollution and delivery outcome in southern Sweden: a study with central registries. *Acta Paediatr* 1996; **85**(11): 1361–4.

63. Moutquin JM. Classification and heterogeneity of preterm birth. *BJOG* 2003; **110** Suppl 20: 30–3.

64. Kimberlin DF, Hauth JC, Owen J, *et al.* Indicated versus spontaneous preterm delivery: An evaluation of neonatal morbidity among infants weighing </=1000 grams at birth. *Am J Obstet Gynecol* 1999; **180**(3 Pt 1): 683–9.

65. Savitz DA, Dole N, Herring AH, *et al.* Should spontaneous and medically indicated preterm births be separated for studying aetiology? *Paediatr Perinat Epidemiol* 2005; **19**(2): 97–105.

66. Siega-Riz AM, Promislow JH, Savitz DA, Thorp JM, Jr., McDonald T. Vitamin C intake and the risk of preterm delivery. *Am J Obstet Gynecol* 2003; **189**(2): 519–25.

67. Erichsen HC, Engel SA, Eck PK, *et al.* Genetic variation in the sodium-dependent vitamin C transporters, SLC23A1, and SLC23A2 and risk for preterm delivery. *Am J Epidemiol* 2006; **163**(3): 245–54.

68. Engel SM, Olshan AF, Siega-Riz AM, Savitz DA, Chanock SJ. Polymorphisms in folate metabolizing genes and risk for spontaneous preterm and small-for-gestational age birth. *Am J Obstet Gynecol* 2006; **195**(5): 1231.e1–11.

69. Norwitz ER. Defective implantation and placentation: laying the blueprint for pregnancy complications. *Reprod Biomed Online* 2006; **13**(4): 591–9.

70. Baumwell S, Karumanchi SA. Pre-eclampsia: clinical manifestations and molecular mechanisms. *Nephron Clin Pract* 2007; **106**(2): c72–81.

71. Kyrklund-Blomberg NB, Gennser G, Cnattingius S. Placental abruption and perinatal death. *Paediatr Perinat Epidemiol* 2001; **15**(3): 290–7.

72. Ananth CV, Wilcox AJ. Placental abruption and perinatal mortality in the United States. *Am J Epidemiol* 2001; **153**(4): 332–7.

73. Copper RL, Goldenberg RL, Das A, *et al.* The preterm prediction study: maternal stress is associated with spontaneous preterm birth at less than thirty-five weeks' gestation. National Institute of Child Health and Human Development Maternal-Fetal Medicine Units Network. *Am J Obstet Gynecol* 1996; **175**(5): 1286–92.

74. Sandman CA, Glynn L, Schetter CD, *et al.* Elevated maternal cortisol early in pregnancy predicts third trimester levels of placental corticotropin releasing hormone (CRH): priming the placental clock. *Peptides* 2006; **27**(6): 1457–63.

75. Mancuso RA, Schetter CD, Rini CM, Roesch SC, Hobel CJ. Maternal prenatal anxiety and corticotropin-releasing hormone associated with timing of delivery. *Psychosom Med* 2004; **66**(5): 762–9.

76. Makrigiannakis A, Semmler M, Briese V, *et al.* Maternal serum corticotropin-releasing hormone and ACTH levels as predictive markers of premature labor. *Int J Gynaecol Obstet* 2007; **97**(2): 115–19.

77. Taylor LK, Simpson JM, Roberts CL, Olive EC, Henderson-Smart DJ. Risk of complications in a second pregnancy following caesarean section in the first pregnancy: a population-based study. *Med J Aust* 2005; **183**(10): 515–19.

78. Orhan A, Kurzel RB, Istwan NB, *et al.* The impact of hydramnios on pregnancy outcome in twin gestations. *J Perinatol* 2005; **25**(1): 8–10.

79. Qidwai GI, Caughey AB, Jacoby AF. Obstetric outcomes in women with sonographically identified uterine leiomyomata. *Obstet Gynecol* 2006; **107**(2 Pt 1): 376–82.

80. Maradny EE, Kanayama N, Halim A, Maehara K, Terao T. Stretching of fetal membranes increases the concentration of interleukin-8 and collagenase activity. *Am J Obstet Gynecol* 1996; **174**(3): 843–9.

81. Berghella V, Odibo AO, To MS, Rust OA, Althuisius SM. Cerclage for short cervix on ultrasonography: meta-analysis of trials using individual patient-level data. *Obstet Gynecol* 2005; **106**(1): 181–9.

82. Noori M, Helmig RB, Hein M, Steer PJ. Could a cervical occlusion suture be effective at improving perinatal outcome? *BJOG* 2007; **114**(5): 532–6.

83. Callaghan WM, MacDorman MF, Rasmussen SA, Qin C, Lackritz EM. The contribution of preterm birth to infant mortality rates in the United States. *Pediatrics* 2006; **118**(4): 1566–73.

84. Platt MJ, Cans C, Johnson A, *et al.* Trends in cerebral palsy among infants of very low birthweight (<1500 g) or born prematurely (< 32 weeks) in 16 European centres: a database study. *Lancet* 2007; **369**(9555): 43–50.

85. Schmitt SK, Sneed L, Phibbs CS. Costs of newborn care in California: a population-based study. *Pediatrics* 2006; **117**(1): 154–60.

86. King. J, Flenady V. Prophylactic antibiotics for inhibiting preterm labour with intact membranes. *Cochrane Database Syst Rev* 2002 4: CD000246. DOI: 10.1002/14651858.CD000246.

87. McDonald H, Brocklehurst P, Gordon A. Antibiotics for treating bacterial vaginosis in pregnancy. *Cochrane Database Syst Rev* 2007 1: CD DOI: 10.1002/14651858. CD000262.pub3.

88. Kenyon S, Boulvain M, Neilson J. Antibiotics for preterm rupture of membranes. *The Cochrane Database Syst Rev* 2003; (2): CD001058. DOI: 10.1002/14651858. CD001058.

89. French JI, McGregor JA, Parker R. Readily treatable reproductive tract infections and preterm birth among black women. *Am J Obstet Gynecol* 2006; **194**(6): 1717–26; discussion 1726–7.

90. Offenbacher S, Lin D, Strauss R, *et al.* Effects of periodontal therapy during pregnancy on periodontal status, biologic parameters, and pregnancy outcomes: a pilot study. *J Periodontol* 2006; **77**(12): 2011–24.

91. Michalowicz BS, Hodges JS, DiAngelis AJ, *et al.* Treatment of periodontal disease and the risk of preterm birth. *N Engl J Med* 2006; **355**(18): 1885–94.

92. Duley L, Meher S, Abalos E. Management of pre-eclampsia. *BMJ* 2006; **332**(7539): 463–8.

93. Hofmeyr GJ, Atallah AN, Duley L. Calcium supplementation during pregnancy for preventing hypertensive disorders and related problems. *Cochrane Database Syst Rev* 2006; (3): CD001059.

94. Duley L, Henderson-Smart DJ, Meher S, King JF. Antiplatelet agents for preventing pre-eclampsia and its complications. *Cochrane Database Syst Rev* 2007; (2): CD004659.

95. Rumbold A, Duley L, Crowther C, Haslam R. Antioxidants for preventing pre-eclampsia. *Cochrane Database Syst Rev* 2005; (4): CD004227.

96. Easterling TR, Carr DB, Brateng D, Diederichs C, Schmucker B. Treatment of hypertension in pregnancy: effect of atenolol on maternal disease, preterm delivery, and fetal growth. *Obstet Gynecol* 2001; **98**(3): 427–33.

97. Lumley J, Oliver SS, Chamberlain C, Oakley L. Interventions for promoting smoking cessation during pregnancy. *Cochrane Database Syst Rev* 2004; (4): CD001055.

98. Sweeney PJ, Schwartz RM, Mattis NG, Vohr B. The effect of integrating substance abuse treatment with prenatal care on birth outcome. *J Perinatol* 2000; **20**(4): 219–24.

99. Little BB, Snell LM, Van Beveren TT, *et al.* Treatment of substance abuse during pregnancy and infant outcome. *Am J Perinatol* 2003; **20**(5): 255–62.

100. Villar J, Farnot U, Barros F, *et al.* A randomized trial of psychosocial support during high-risk pregnancies. The Latin American Network for Perinatal and Reproductive Research. *N Engl J Med* 1992; **327**(18): 1266–71.

101. Hodnett ED, Fredericks S. Support during pregnancy for women at increased risk of low birthweight babies. *Cochrane Database Syst Rev* 2003; (3): CD000198.

102. Fanaroff AA, Hack M, Walsh MC. The NICHD neonatal research network: changes in practice and outcomes during the first 15 years. *Semin Perinatol* 2003; **27**(4): 281–7.

103. Johansson S, Montgomery SM, Ekbom A, *et al.* Preterm delivery, level of care, and infant death in Sweden: a population-based study. *Pediatrics* 2004; **113**(5): 1230–5.

104. Evans N, Hutchinson J, Simpson JM, *et al.* Prenatal predictors of mortality in very preterm infants cared for in the Australian and New Zealand Neonatal Network. *Arch Dis Child Fetal Neonatal Ed* 2007; **92**(1): F34–40.

105. Lucey JF, Rowan CA, Shiono P, *et al.* Fetal infants: the fate of 4172 infants with birth weights of 401 to 500 grams – the Vermont Oxford Network experience (1996–2000). *Pediatrics* 2004; **113**(6): 1559–66.

106. Larroque B, Breart G, Kaminski M, *et al.* Survival of very preterm infants: Epipage, a population based cohort study. *Arch Dis Child Fetal Neonatal Ed* 2004; **89**(2): F139–44.

107. Hakansson S, Farooqi A, Holmgren PA, Serenius F, Hogberg U. Proactive management promotes outcome in extremely preterm infants: a population-based comparison of two perinatal management strategies. *Pediatrics* 2004; **114**(1): 58–64.

108. Herber-Jonat S, Schulze A, Kribs *et al.* Survival and major neonatal complications in infants born between 22 0/7 and 24 6/7 weeks of gestation (1999–2003). *Am J Obstet Gynecol* 2006; **195**(1): 16–22.

109. Phibbs CS, Bronstein JM, Buxton E, Phibbs RH. The effects of patient volume and level of care at the hospital of birth on neonatal mortality. *JAMA* 1996; **276**(13): 1054–9.

110. Cifuentes J, Bronstein J, Phibbs CS, *et al.* Mortality in low birth weight infants according to level of neonatal care at hospital of birth. *Pediatrics* 2002; **109**(5): 745–51.

111. Verloove-Vanhorick SP, Verwey RA, Ebeling MC, Brand R, Ruys JH. Mortality in very preterm and very low birth weight infants according to place of birth and level of care: results of a national collaborative survey of preterm and very low birth weight infants in The Netherlands. *Pediatrics* 1988; **81**(3): 404–11.

112. Field D, Hodges S, Mason E, Burton P. Survival and place of treatment after premature delivery. *Arch Dis Child* 1991; **66**(4 Spec No): 408–10; discussion 410–11.

113. Phibbs CS, Baker LC, Caughey AB, *et al.* Level and volume of neonatal intensive care and mortality in very-low-birth-weight infants. *N Engl J Med* 2007; **356**(21): 2165–75.

114. Rautava L, Lehtonen L, Peltola M, *et al.* The effect of birth in secondary- or tertiary-level hospitals in Finland on mortality in very preterm infants: a birth-register study. *Pediatrics* 2007; **119**(1): e257–63.

115. Acolet D, Elbourne D, McIntosh N, *et al.* Project 27/28: inquiry into quality of neonatal care and its effect on the survival of infants who were born at 27 and 28 weeks in England, Wales, and Northern Ireland. *Pediatrics* 2005; **116**(6): 1457–65.

116. Roberts D, Dalziel S. Antenatal corticosteroids for accelerating fetal lung maturation for women at risk of preterm birth. *Cochrane Database Syst Rev* 2006; (3): CD004454.

117. Stoelhorst GM, Rijken M, Martens SE, *et al.* Changes in neonatology: comparison of two cohorts of very preterm infants (gestational age < 32 weeks): the Project On Preterm and Small for Gestational Age Infants 1983 and the Leiden Follow-Up Project on Prematurity 1996–1997. *Pediatrics* 2005; **115**(2): 396–405.

118. Raju TN, Higgins RD, Stark AR, Leveno KJ. Optimizing care and outcome for late-preterm (near-term) infants: a summary of the workshop sponsored by the National Institute of Child Health and Human Development. *Pediatrics* 2006; **118**(3): 1207–14.

119. Engle WA, Tomashek KM, Wallman C. "Late-preterm" infants: a population at risk. *Pediatrics* 2007; **120**(6): 1390–401.

120. Rennie JM, Roberton NRC. *Textbook of Neonatology*, 4edn. Edinburgh: Churchill Livingstone; 2005.

121. Serenius F, Ewald U, Farooqi A, *et al.* Short-term outcome after active perinatal management at 23–25 weeks of gestation. A study from two Swedish perinatal centres. Part 3: neonatal morbidity. *Acta Paediatr* 2004; **93**(8): 1090–7.

122. Markestad T, Kaaresen PI, Ronnestad A, *et al.* Early death, morbidity, and need of treatment among extremely premature infants. *Pediatrics* 2005; **115**(5): 1289–98.

123. Wilson-Costello D, Friedman H, Minich N, *et al.* Improved neurodevelopmental outcomes for extremely low birth weight infants in 2000–2002. *Pediatrics* 2007; **119**(1): 37–45.

124. Vanhaesebrouck P, Allegaert K, Bottu J, *et al.* The EPIBEL study: outcomes to discharge from hospital for extremely preterm infants in Belgium. *Pediatrics* 2004; **114**(3): 663–75.

125. de Kleine MJ, den Ouden AL, Kollee LA, *et al.* Lower mortality but higher neonatal morbidity over a decade in very preterm infants. *Paediatr Perinat Epidemiol* 2007; **21**(1): 15–25.

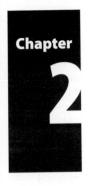

Chapter 2

The changing face of intensive care for preterm newborns

John Wyatt

Introduction

Neonatal intensive care has seen dramatic evolution over the last 50 years. It is natural for psychologists, therapists and developmental pediatricians to assume that "very preterm birth" represents an insult to the developing brain which is relatively constant and unchanging over time. In practice, continually varying trends, developments and fashions in neonatal care over the last 50 years have led to a constantly changing spectrum of insults and pathogenetic processes in the neonatal period. As a consequence, ex-premature survivors who are now entering adolescence and adulthood were exposed to forms of neonatal care which have become outdated and obsolete. A disturbing but recurrent theme over the last 50 years has been the considerable range of standard neonatal practices and therapies which have subsequently been found to lead to iatrogenic brain injury. An important task is to attempt to relate the pattern of neurological and developmental disorders associated with very preterm birth to the nature of care which was received in the neonatal period.

This chapter provides a brief and inevitably selective overview of developments in neonatal care for extremely preterm infants over the last 50 years, and discusses the mechanisms of brain injury in this vulnerable population. A number of more detailed sources on the history of neonatal care are available [1–4].

Neonatal care before 1965

The principles of care for premature babies were first laid down by Pierre Budin, Professor of Obstetrics in the University of Paris. The English edition of his book "The Nursling" was published in 1907 [5]. Budin emphasized the importance of warmth, nutrition, and prevention of contagious infections. Sadly Budin's cardinal principles have frequently been ignored in the history of neonatal care, often with tragic consequences.

Specialized incubators for premature babies were developed initially by Budin and his followers. Dr. Cooney demonstrated infants nursed in incubators in Europe and then at a number of public exhibitions in the USA. However, it was not until the 1950s and 1960s that premature baby units became established in a number of large hospitals.

In the UK a premature baby unit had been set up in Bristol in 1946 [1]. It emphasized the importance of 24-hour nursing care, together with meticulous observation and recording of appearance and behavior. An autopsy service was established and it became apparent that the principal causes of death were immaturity, respiratory distress, kernicterus, and intracranial hemorrhage.

In 1952 Virginia Apgar, an American anesthetist, introduced a system for evaluation of the newborn immediately after birth and in the same year the first evidence of a link between oxygen therapy and retinal damage was demonstrated. Retinopathy had been virtually unknown before 1940, but in the early 1950s it had become the leading cause of blindness in children in the USA. At this time it had become common practice to give high inspired oxygen concentrations to infants with respiratory distress. In 1954 a remarkable scientific innovation, a multicenter randomized clinical trial, showed that infants nursed in high oxygen had a much higher incidence of retinal injury. Tragically it was estimated that by then approximately 10 000 children had been permanently blinded as a consequence of excessive oxygen [6]. Following this, the inspired oxygen concentration was rigorously restricted and the incidence of retinopathy fell markedly. However, it was subsequently noted that deaths from hyaline membrane disease were increasing, suggesting that a blanket and simplistic policy of oxygen restriction was having negative consequences, leading to unrecognized hypoxic-ischemic injury.

Neurodevelopmental Outcomes of Preterm Birth, ed. Chiara Nosarti, Robin M. Murray, and Maureen Hack. Published by Cambridge University Press. © Cambridge University Press 2010.

In 1958 Silverman *et al.* demonstrated that preterm infants nursed in cool incubators had a higher mortality compared with those in warm incubators [7], and subsequent experimental work clarified the importance of thermal homeostasis in preterm care. In the 1950s it was common practice to delay the first feed in premature babies for periods of between 24 and 96 hours. Unfortunately, this bizarre clinical practice led to a high incidence of unrecognized hypoglycemia and dehydration. The work of Drillien published in 1964 indicated that neonatal care for very preterm infants was associated with a very high incidence of neurodisability in the small number of survivors [8]. This led to increased controversy about the wisdom of providing intensive care for ever more premature infants. Some questioned whether the introduction of more active life support techniques was wise. To the pessimists it seemed likely that intensive care for very premature babies would lead to a greatly increased number of disabled survivors. The enthusiasts argued that physiologically based care would lead *both* to improved survival and to a diminution in permanent brain injury due to hypoxia, hypoglycemia and other disturbances. The concerns about the impact of new forms of intensive care were an impetus to the establishment of long-term prospective follow-up studies of very preterm survivors at a number of major centers.

1965 to 1985

In the history of neonatal intensive care there has always been a close connection between new developments in medical technology and improvements in clinical care. In the 1950s the introduction of plastic sterilized intravascular catheters and nasogastric tubes was of critical importance, allowing intravenous fluid management and continuous gastric feeding to be established safely. In the 1960s the development of techniques to measure arterial blood gas levels and the increasing use of mechanical ventilators led to the development of the first neonatal intensive care units (NICUs), in which clinical practice and medical technology were oriented towards the establishment and maintenance of physiological homeostasis. Oxygen therapy could now be controlled in order to achieve satisfactory blood oxygen levels, and ventilator settings could be manipulated on a rational basis. With critical input from bioengineers and medical physicists, non-invasive physiological monitoring was gradually introduced at the bedside. This included continuous recording of electroencephalography (EEG), respiratory function, and blood oxygenation. The development of invasive oxygen-sensing catheters, transcutaneous monitoring electrodes, and pulse oximetry in the 1980s was of critical importance in enabling physiological homeostasis to be achieved and maintained.

With improvements in thermal control, nutrition, and physiological monitoring, there was growing recognition of the importance of respiratory distress due to hyaline membrane disease. Progressive respiratory distress over the first 48 hours was common in preterm babies of less than 37 weeks, and frequently led to death. A number of different methods of artificial ventilation were being attempted but with varying success.

In the early 1970s, the University College Hospital London (UCHL) group, together with a number of other groups, had developed successful methods of using intermittent positive pressure ventilation in infants with severe respiratory distress [1,9]. This led to a significant improvement in survival in preterm infants with hyaline membrane disease. However, chronic lung disease, or bronchopulmonary dysplasia, was now increasingly recognized in survivors who had received mechanical ventilation, leading to many weeks or months of oxygen dependency and hospital care. The use of continuous positive airways pressure (CPAP) to prevent alveolar collapse was also introduced in the USA in the 1970s [10] and nasal CPAP has grown in importance as a means of providing minimally invasive respiratory support. Methods for transporting sick infants by ambulance were being established and this allowed intensive care resources to be centralised in major centers and the beginning of regionalization of care [1].

Jaundice had been recognized as a common problem of premature infants, but the only successful treatment was exchange transfusion which was both hazardous and costly in resources. The widespread introduction of phototherapy, following a controlled clinical trial by Lucey and colleagues in 1968 [11], led to a substantial improvement in care and a reduction in the incidence of kernicterus, which was particularly associated with dyskinetic cerebral palsy and sensorineural hearing loss.

Very preterm infants undergoing intensive care in this period were exposed to huge and damaging fluctuations in physiological variables. Infants were often born in very poor conditions with severe hypoxia, acidosis, and bruising following a traumatic delivery. Severe hyaline membrane disease in the first days of life was very common and it led to major cardiorespiratory collapses due to pneumothorax and ventilation problems. Many infants went through repeated episodes of cardiorespiratory collapse followed by resuscitation and stabilization. Infants were exposed to frequent disturbance, including repeated arterial blood sampling, chest drain insertion and other painful procedures, and pain control methods were rudimentary.

Intraventricular hemorrhage (IVH) was known to be a common autopsy finding in very preterm babies who died in the first days of life, but it was thought to be a catastrophic and agonal event. However, in the late 1970s it became possible to image the infant brain during life, with the introduction of computed tomography (CT) X-ray scanning in a few major centers. In 1979 imaging of the infant brain using real-time ultrasound through the anterior fontanel was described simultaneously by the UCHL group and by Richard Cooke [1]. It became apparent that there was a disturbingly high incidence of IVH in very preterm survivors, with 30–40% of the smallest babies affected. In 1979 Ann Stewart and Osmund Reynolds commenced a prospective follow-up study of very preterm infants at UCHL designed to relate cranial ultrasound appearances in the neonatal period with long-term neurological and developmental outcome [12,13]. Similar follow-up studies were started in a number of perinatal centers worldwide [14,15] and they have confirmed the role of cranial ultrasound as an essential tool of the neonatologist, providing valuable diagnostic and prognostic information at the cotside.

The introduction of cranial ultrasound led to a new interest in the mechanisms of brain injury and to an awareness of the central importance of minimizing neurological damage during the critical first days and weeks of life. Magnetic resonance imaging (MRI) of the newborn brain was first described at the Hammersmith Hospital in 1982 [16] and in the same year the first magnetic resonance spectroscopy data from the newborn were obtained at UCHL [17]. These new modalities had the potential to provide unparalleled information on the structure of the developing nervous structure and on its underlying metabolism, and the role of magnetic resonance brain imaging is discussed in detail in Chapters 4 to 8.

1985 to 1995

The causal relationship between surfactant deficiency and hyaline membrane disease had been first demonstrated by Avery and Mead in 1959 [18]. Antenatal steroids in preterm labor were first shown to be effective in reducing the severity of respiratory distress by Liggins and Howie in 1972 in a landmark placebo-controlled clinical trial [19]. A large number of other trials confirmed these findings but there was continuing concern about possible side effects from the use of steroids. However, there was a remarkable delay before the use of antenatal steroids became universally accepted. It was not until 1990 that this treatment was generally adopted by obstetricians following the publication of a detailed meta-analysis of existing trials [20].

The first successful use of exogenous surfactant for the treatment of neonatal respiratory distress syndrome was described by Fujiwara and colleagues in Japan in 1980 [21], but again there was a long delay before the findings of an initial research trial were translated into a widely accepted clinical therapy. By the early 1990s there was overwhelming evidence that the use of exogenous surfactant in the first hours of life led to a significant reduction both in mortality and in the incidence of severe IVH [22]. The combination of antenatal steroids and surfactant therapy after birth led to a dramatic reduction in the severity of respiratory distress and its consequences.

However, this period was also characterized by increasing use of the artificial corticosteroid dexamethasone for treatment of chronic lung disease. A randomized trial in 1989 in preterm infants who were ventilator dependent and at high risk of lung disease had demonstrated that a prolonged course of high-dose dexamethasone led to faster weaning from the ventilator compared with control infants [23]. Following this study, dexamethasone in high dose was increasingly adopted by neonatologists across the world as the treatment of choice for infants with chronic lung disease. In retrospect, the body of experimental data showing that prolonged courses of high-dose steroids could have detrimental effects on the developing nervous system should have instilled caution, but little concern was expressed at the time.

In this period the importance of asymptomatic hypoglycemia as a potential source of brain injury was increasingly recognized. As measurement techniques improved, it became apparent that blood glucose levels were frequently low in the first few days of life. A study by Lucas and colleagues in the Cambridge (UK) region published in 1988 found that moderate asymptomatic hypoglycemia was present in over 60% of preterm infants and that low glucose levels often persisted for many hours or days [24]. It was appreciated that deprivation of this primary metabolic fuel might be contributing to significant brain injury, despite the lack of any clinical symptoms or signs, and there was continuing controversy about the safe blood levels which should be achieved. By this time the role of early enteral feeding was again emphasized, together with frequent bedside testing of blood glucose levels and active management to avoid hypoglycemia.

1995 to present

The combination of antenatal steroids to improve lung maturation prior to delivery and improved and more proactive obstetric management has had the result that many very preterm infants are now delivered in remarkably good condition. The widespread use of exogenous surfactant after birth and improvements in ventilator management have meant that a significant proportion of infants can be rapidly stabilized in the first minutes and hours of life. In the modern era prolonged intubation and mechanical ventilation is often not required, and many extremely preterm infants may be supported with CPAP from the first days of life. This has meant that the severe and damaging fluctuations in oxygen, carbon dioxide, blood pressure, and other physiological variables are avoided. The frequent episodes of cardiorespiratory collapse and recovery, which were a feature of care in the 1970s and 1980s, are now mercifully unusual. Unfortunately, chronic lung disease is still a substantial problem, and many infants still require weeks of CPAP support and additional inspired oxygen until lung function has recovered sufficiently to allow air breathing.

There is anecdotal evidence to suggest that infection may have become an increasing problem over the last decade. Antenatal infection is increasingly recognized both as an important cause of preterm labor and as a causal mechanism underlying a significant proportion of perinatal brain injury (see Chapter 1). In addition, postnatal infection with hospital-acquired organisms is an important factor in extremely preterm infants who undergo many weeks of care in a neonatal intensive care unit. Invasive infection with *Staphylococcus*, *Candida*, and other skin commensals is common as a result of indwelling venous and arterial catheters and other instrumentation. The use of broad-spectrum intravenous antibiotics has led to a marked increase in multi-resistant organisms, leading to a further spiral of increasing antibiotic exposure. Necrotizing enterocolitis has remained a significant clinical problem and an association between sepsis in the neonatal period and white matter injury has been demonstrated. Ensuring adequate nutrition for very low birth weight infants during weeks of intensive care has remained a major problem. Impaired growth of both body and head is common over the first weeks of life and the problem is exacerbated by frequent episodes of sepsis, leading to interruptions in enteral and parenteral nutrition. This is particularly important because impaired brain growth in the neonatal period has been found to have a strong association with impaired neurological development (see below).

By 2000, increasing evidence was accumulating that dexamethasone, particularly when given early in the neonatal course, was associated with an increased risk of cerebral palsy and abnormal neurological functioning in survivors. A meta-analysis published in the Cochrane Library in 2003 gave an increased relative risk of 1.69 for cerebral palsy with early dexamethasone treatment [25]. More recently, a range of MRI studies have indicated that treatment is associated with reduced cortical gray matter and white matter volumes. In 2002 the American Academy of Pediatrics published guidelines stating that postnatal dexamethasone should not be given routinely to very low birth weight infants and that its use should be largely restricted to randomized control trials with long-term neurodevelopmental follow-up.

Mechanisms of brain injury

The mechanisms of brain injury in extremely preterm infants are uniquely related to the stage of brain development during the time when the brain is exposed to a range of pathological processes.

The formation of the cortex depends initially on the processes of neuronal proliferation and migration. From approximately 10 weeks of gestation, radial glial cells provide a structural guide between the subventricular zone and the pial surface. Neurons generated from stem cells within the subventricular zone of the lateral ventricles physically migrate in radial direction through the substance of the cerebral hemisphere until they achieve their final position within the cerebral cortex. This process of neuronal migration has largely concluded by 22–24 weeks of gestation. Once migration is complete, the process of *cortical organization* commences. This includes the development of subplate neurons, which appear to have a crucial role in establishing synaptic contact with axons ascending from the thalamus, the development of dendritic and axonal ramifications, synaptogenesis, and glial cell proliferation and differentiation [26].

The process of synaptogenesis is particularly remarkable with each cortical neuron establishing an average of approximately 1000 synaptic connections, creating the great bulk of corticocortical connections within the cerebral hemispheres. This is sometimes described as the "flowering" of the dendritic tree. It is estimated that there are approximately 10 [11] neurons and 10 [14] synapses within the human central nervous system. It appears that a very substantial proportion of these synapses are created between 24 and 40 weeks of gestation, although maximal synaptic density is not achieved until late in the first year of life. A back of the envelope calculation gives the astonishing figure of around a hundred million synapses which are being created *every minute* during the third trimester of pregnancy. It is not surprising therefore that extremely premature delivery followed by prolonged intensive care may lead to pervasive and wide-ranging disturbances of cortical development and organization.

Germinal matrix: intraventricular hemorrhage (IVH)

The germinal or subependymal matrix, just ventrolateral to the lateral ventricles, is the site at which cerebral neuroblasts are formed during the phase of neuronal proliferation. During the third trimester it is also a source of primitive glial cells. The germinal matrix has a rich but immature microvascular network which is continuous with the deep venous drainage of the cerebrum. In extremely preterm infants, the germinal matrix is extensive and highly vascular. It gradually involutes over the third trimester and vascular remodeling occurs. The site of origin of germinal matrix hemorrhage is thought to be within the microvascular network or at the capillary venule junction. Hence, the initiation of IVH may be particularly associated with fluctuations in cerebral perfusion and cerebral venous pressure [26].

Following initiation of bleeding within the germinal matrix, free blood may enter the lateral ventricles and spread throughout the ventricular system then occurs. Any significant hemorrhage within the germinal matrix leads to its disruption and it seems likely that subsequent glial cell proliferation from this site will be affected. The most serious complication of IVH is hemorrhagic infarction within the parenchyma of the periventricular white matter. This occurs in approximately 15% of infants with IVH and its incidence rises with increasing immaturity [27]. The region affected is highly variable and the lesion is nearly always strikingly asymmetrical. The size of infarction may range from a few millimeters to a large proportion of the periventricular white matter within one hemisphere. The process of infarction is thought to be mainly the result of mechanical obstruction of the venous drainage of a region of cerebral white matter, due to the presence of a germinal matrix hemorrhage on the same side [26,28]. The presence of old hemorrhage within the brain parenchyma leads to the presence of free iron which may enhance the production of activated oxygen radicals leading to white matter injury.

Hemorrhagic infarction is almost invariably followed by the development of a porencephalic cyst which becomes continuous with the lateral ventricle, leading to permanent asymmetry of the ventricular system. Another important complication of IVH is the development of posthemorrhagic ventricular dilatation, which may lead to rapidly progressive hydrocephalus requiring neurosurgical intervention.

The pathogenesis of IVH has been a matter of extensive investigation for more than 20 years. Using repeated cranial ultrasound examinations from the time of birth, it is possible to time the initiation and development of the hemorrhage. It is unusual for bleeding to be detected in the first four hours following delivery, but hemorrhage within the germinal matrix is normally visualized within the first 48 hours and IVH reaches its maximum extent within the first week of life. Fluctuations in blood pressure in both the cerebral arterial and venous systems are thought to be of central importance in the initiation of bleeding [26]. Studies of cerebral oxygenation using near infrared spectroscopy in extremely premature babies undergoing intensive care have provided new insights into impaired vascular control mechanisms which may underlie IVH [29,30]. Sick infants who are receiving mechanical ventilation may show a strong correlation between second-to-second changes in arterial blood pressure and indices of cerebral oxygenation. This is thought to indicate the loss of normal cerebral vascular control mechanisms, and the presence of a pressure-passive cerebral circulation. In this clinical context it is likely that rapid fluctuations in arterial blood pressure will be transmitted directly to the cerebral vasculature, and this may result in the rupture of vulnerable vessels within the germinal matrix.

Studies of cerebral blood flow have tended to show low levels of cerebral perfusion over the first 24 hours of life followed by a progressive rise over the first few

21

days of life [31]. It may be that in many infants the onset of detectable hemorrhage is related to the increase in cerebral blood flow seen on the second and third days of life. It is of interest that a study of preterm infants on the first day of life found that those who subsequently developed IVH had lower cerebral blood flow compared with those who did not develop intracranial bleeding [31]. It is thus plausible that in some infants IVH may represent the consequence of a period of relative cerebral ischemia followed by reperfusion leading to rupture of the vulnerable vasculature of the germinal matrix.

Other clinical factors which have been shown to be associated with IVH include rapid volume expansion, hypercarbia, severe respiratory disease, pneumothorax, disturbances of platelet function, and abnormal blood coagulation. Hence it is not surprising that severe IVH was common in infants who underwent intensive care in the 1970s and 1980s [26].

Prevention of IVH

The most effective pharmacological intervention which has been shown to reduce the incidence of IVH is the administration of antenatal corticosteroids. The primary rationale behind this treatment is the beneficial effect of steroids on lung maturation leading to a reduction in severe respiratory illness after birth. A recent meta-analysis of the effects of antenatal corticosteroids found that the relative risk of cerebral hemorrhage in treated infants was approximately halved compared with controls [32]. Interestingly, multivariate analysis suggested that part of the effect of antenatal steroids may be independent of improved lung maturation and it has been suggested that the treatment may have a direct protective effect on the cerebral microvasculature.

Early postnatal administration of indomethacin has been shown to be associated with a significant reduction in IVH, especially in the most severe grades of hemorrhage [33]. Indomethacin has been shown to decrease baseline cerebral blood flow presumably by a direct vasoconstrictor action and also to reduce the sensitivity of the cerebral circulation to changing carbon dioxide tension. It may therefore exert a protective effect on the cerebral vasculature. Secondly, studies in the beagle puppy have indicated that indomethacin may have a direct action on the germinal matrix leading to maturation of microvessels and reducing the likelihood of rupture [34].

Indomethacin may have pervasive effects on cerebral development. A recent functional MRI study of preterm survivors at 8 years of age has demonstrated a differential effect between males and females of indomethacin administration [35]. Male children who had been randomly exposed to indomethacin demonstrated activation patterns to phonological stimuli which were more similar to term control subjects than those randomized to saline. Female children did not demonstrate a differential effect. For more details on this and other functional MRI studies please refer to Chapter 7.

Ethamsylate, an agent with complex effects on prostaglandin synthesis and platelet function, led to a reduction in the incidence of IVH in a number of clinical trials but its efficacy was not confirmed in a large multicenter randomized trial and its value remains uncertain. Other pharmacological agents including phenobarbitone and vitamin E have also been suggested to have a protective role but their clinical role is unproven.

Several authors have reported a decline in the incidence in IVH over the last 20 years [36]. Volpe reported an incidence of 35–50% in studies from the late 1970s and early 1980s, a lower incidence of 20% in the late 1980s and only 15% in the 1990s [26]. It seems plausible that this significant reduction is a consequence of a range of factors including improvements in obstetric care, greater use of antenatal corticosteroids and postnatal surfactant therapy, and other improvements in respiratory and fluid management in the critical first hours and days of life. However it is notable that white matter injury has not shown a similar decline in incidence, suggesting that the pathophysiological mechanisms are distinct.

White matter injury

Injury to the cerebral white matter of preterm infants was first described more than a century ago and the classical description of periventricular leukomalacia (PVL) was given by Banker and Larroche in 1962 [37]. This lesion is characterized by focal areas of cystic necrosis in the periventricular white matter, especially in the parieto-occipito or frontal regions. This classical appearance can be easily identified by cranial ultrasound imaging, but it is a relatively unusual finding in prospective studies of extremely preterm infants, occurring in 5% or less. However, both autopsy studies and MRI studies have shown a much higher incidence of diffuse white matter injury in extremely preterm infants who survive the first days of life [38,39]. In magnetic resonance imaging studies of preterm infants scanned at term, signal abnormalities in the white matter have been identified in up to three quarters of infants [40–42]. Signal abnormalities have also been associated with an increase in the apparent diffusion coefficient (ADC) values [43,44], suggesting that there is an underlying microstructural abnormality in the white matter regions. It is plausible that injury to oligodendrocyte precursors and subsequent abnormalities in myelination of axons may underlie these MRI findings. Of particular importance is the consistent observation that abnormalities of cerebral white matter are frequently accompanied by volumetric and microstructural changes in the overlying cortex [45,46], suggesting that white matter injury may have secondary consequences on cortical development.

Neuropathological autopsy studies from preterm infants with white matter injury have demonstrated the presence of activated microglia and evidence of lipid peroxidation and protein nitration in affected brain regions. These findings support the role of reactive oxygen species (such as hydroxyl ion) and reactive nitrogen species (such as peroxynitrite) in the pathogenesis of oligodendrocyte injury [47,48]. It seems likely that microglial activation is of central importance in the underlying pathological process.

Both clinical and experimental data support the importance of cerebral hypoxia-ischemia and infection in the causation of white matter injury. Both hypoxia-ischemia and infection can cause activation of microglia and the generation of cytotoxic free radicals. It is of particular significance that hypoxia-ischemia and infection may exercise a synergistic action in causing brain injury. In the immature rat, pre-exposure to lipopolysaccharide causes increased sensitivity of the brain to subsequent hypoxia-ischemia [49]. A number of clinical studies have shown an association between maternal intrauterine infection and white matter injury after birth [50] and asymptomatic maternal infection may be an important cause of unexplained preterm delivery. It is therefore plausible that antenatal infection may combine synergistically with mild cerebral ischemia caused by fluctuations in cerebral blood flow after birth, leading to microglial activation and diffuse white matter injury.

There is strong epidemiological evidence that markedly low arterial carbon dioxide tensions are associated with an increased risk of adverse neurodevelopmental outcome. This is assumed to reflect cerebral arterial vasoconstriction leading to ischemia in the vulnerable periventricular regions. However, other factors including changes in intracellular pH may be relevant in the pathogenetic sequence. Little is known about the magnitude or duration of hypocarbia which is associated with white matter injury. A recent study from the Neonatal Network of the National Institutes of Health calculated the time integral of exposure to low carbon dioxide levels over the first 7 days of life in a cohort of very low birth weight infants undergoing intensive care [51]. Infants with the highest quartile of exposure to hypocarbia had a fivefold incidence of PVL compared with the lowest quartile. Paradoxically, infants with relatively minor lung disease may be more at risk of inadvertent hypocarbia due to accidental hyperventilation than those with severe respiratory distress. These data emphasize the importance of obsessional attention to detail in ventilator management and the ever-present risk of iatrogenic brain injury from unskilled care. There is clear evidence of a temporal shift in the nature of white matter injury over the last 20 years. As the classic form of cystic PVL has become less common, diffuse white matter injury, affecting a large area of the cerebral hemispheres has become increasingly recognized, especially in the extremely preterm infant [41,42]. It is not clear whether this change is primarily a reflection of the increased numbers of infants who are now surviving at extremely low gestational ages or whether other pathogenetic factors are responsible.

Neuronal injury

Volumetric magnetic resonance studies of ex-preterm infants have demonstrated significant reductions in cerebral gray matter volumes compared with term infants and quantitative deficits in the complexity of cortical folding [52–54]. It is therefore increasingly evident that significant abnormalities of cortical development may occur in preterm infants in the absence of significant white matter injury. In addition, reduced volume of deep nuclear structures has also been detected in preterm infants and the volumetric deficit was greatest in the most immature infants. The underlying processes leading to loss of gray matter volume have not been delineated. It is known that subplate neurons play a critical role in cerebral development in the third trimester. They are involved in the development of thalamocortical and corticocortical connections and contribute to the functional maturation of cortical and thalamic structures [52]. Recent experimental evidence suggests that subplate neurons are selectively vulnerable to hypoxia-ischemia, and hence subplate injury may mediate some of the abnormalities in cortical development

23

which are observed by MRI. Human autopsy studies have also shown evidence of injury in cortical neurons and abnormal cortical organization overlying areas of deep white matter injury. It is therefore possible that a primary injury to the deep white matter may lead to secondary abnormalities in cortical development due to interruption of afferent or efferent axonal connections. Alternatively, a primary injury to cortical neurons may lead to impaired axonal development. Hence, development of the gray and white matter regions of the brain during the third trimester are intimately interconnected and causal pathological mechanisms may operate in a range of directions.

Epidemiological studies have found a consistent relationship between duration of exposure to additional oxygen because of bronchopulmonary dysplasia and impaired cognitive function at school age [55]. Since the duration of exposure to additional oxygen is directly related to the severity of the underlying lung disease, it is not possible to isolate the causal mechanisms underlying this association. Some of the neuropathological findings associated with bronchopulmonary disease, including gliosis and neuronal loss in the central gray matter, may be a consequence of chronic hypoxia rather than elevated oxygen levels. Infants with chronic lung disease are also likely to have increased episodes of infection, impaired nutrition, and abnormal environmental stimulation. It seems likely therefore that multiple causal mechanisms underlie this epidemiological association.

Metabolic and nutritional causes of brain injury

Since glucose is the primary metabolic fuel of the developing brain, the importance of hypoglycemia as a potential cause of neonatal brain injury has been recognized since the 1960s. In 1988 Lucas and coworkers found a statistical association between moderate levels of hypoglycemia and adverse neurodevelopmental outcome (a composite measure including cerebral palsy or developmental delay) in a large prospective study of preterm infants [24]. The risk of neurodevelopmental impairment increased with the duration of exposure to moderate hypoglycemia in the neonatal period. A recent study of preterm infants who were small for gestational age showed a correlation between repeated episodes of hypoglycemia, reduced head growth, and impaired neurodevelopmental outcome [56].

The furious pace of brain growth and development which occurs in the third trimester of pregnancy implies the central importance of delivering adequate nutritional substrate to the brain. Brain growth is maximal during the third trimester and first six postnatal months. Yet there are immense practical problems in delivering satisfactory nutrition to sick preterm infants undergoing neonatal intensive care and many infants suffer profound and prolonged nutritional deprivation. It is only relatively recently that the obvious and important connection between nutrition in the neonatal period and impaired brain development has been highlighted.

In a cohort of very low birth weight infants born between 1977 and 1979, Maureen Hack and colleagues demonstrated a strong correlation between head circumference at 8 months of age and impaired cognitive function at 8–9 years of age. This association persisted with multiple regression analysis to account for socioeconomic status, intrauterine growth deprivation, neonatal risk factors, and neuromotor impairment. Other workers have confirmed the importance of impaired brain growth both before and after delivery in the causation of cognitive and behavioral difficulties at school age. In a group of small-for-gestational-age infants, those with impaired growth during both the intrauterine and postnatal phases had the worst outcome, whereas intrauterine growth restriction followed by restoration of normal brain growth after birth was associated with less risk of impairment. Richard Cooke, in a cohort of very low birth weight infants born between 1981 and 1982, has reported that cognitive outcome correlated strongly with head circumference at 4 and 15 years of age, after correction for intrauterine growth retardation and socioeconomic status [57]. In contrast, mild motor impairment correlated most strongly with brain growth between birth and discharge from hospital. These data suggest that early postnatal brain growth failure is more likely to be causally associated with impaired motor function, whereas minor cognitive deficits are related to prolonged restriction of brain growth over childhood. It is clear that nutritional deprivation may have profound differences on eventual neurological and cognitive functioning, depending upon the precise phase of brain development at which it occurs.

Environmental influences on brain development

The last decade has been characterized by increasing awareness of the adverse effects of the environment of the NICU on the developing central nervous system.

A recent study from the Netherlands indicated that infants in a NICU were subjected to an average of 14 painful procedures per day. There is a substantial body of experimental evidence showing that exposure to multiple painful experiences in the newborn period leads to abnormal development of nociceptive circuits and permanent alteration in behavioral responses to pain [58]. Exposure to noxious stimuli in early life is also associated with later abnormalities in the stress response system. Recent clinical studies have demonstrated that even extremely preterm infants have complex patterns of cortical activation and behavioral responses to painful procedures.

In addition to painful stimuli, infants undergoing intensive care are exposed to a grossly abnormal range of other sensory stimuli. In place of the relative sensory deprivation of the uterus, the infant is exposed to high levels of light intensity with abolition of normal circadian rhythms. Mechanical sound exposure is considerable, especially within incubators, where peak noise levels may exceed internationally accepted safety limits. Continuous high frequency sound exposure from CPAP and ventilator equipment may continue for weeks and months. Interruption of normal sleep–wake cycling is inevitable and all phases of sleep are disturbed. This may be particularly important in the development of normal cortical visual connections. Studies in newborn rodents have suggested that rapid eye movement (REM) sleep may provide neuronal stimuli for shaping synaptic connections in visual pathways. In the newborn rodent 7 days of REM sleep deprivation led to alterations in synaptic plasticity in the visual cortex [59]. Enhanced endocrine stress responses are also seen in infants undergoing intensive care and endogenous corticosteroid and catecholamine plasma levels are often substantially elevated over prolonged periods. In addition, infants are frequently exposed to prolonged courses of analgesics including opiates and sedatives including benzodiazepines. The long-term consequences of this abnormal sensory, endocrine and pharmacological exposure in humans are still unknown, but it seems inevitable that permanent structural and functional changes in the central and peripheral nervous system will result.

Growing awareness of the vulnerability of premature babies to the NICU environment has led to a movement, especially amongst neonatal nurses and therapists, to minimize harmful interventions and stimuli and explore alternative methods of providing care (see also Chapter 18). One approach, the Neonatal Individualized Developmental Care Program (NIDCAP) is designed to minimize interference with the baby's own individual behavioral cycles and responses whilst intensive care is given. Preliminary studies have indicated that this approach, although requiring intensive staffing and high levels of resources, may be associated with improved neurodevelopmental outcome and with an improvement in white matter imaging appearances and connectivity [60].

Future developments in neonatal care

It seems unlikely that the current limits of viability at 22–23 weeks' gestation will change significantly within the next decade. The goal of neonatal staff is to ensure that infants who can benefit from conventional methods of intensive care have the best possible chance of intact survival with normal brain development. The concept of "brain-oriented intensive care," where all interventions are optimized to protect and enhance brain development, is not new. However, in current neonatal practice, the brain is still seen largely as a "black box" and apart from intermittent cranial ultrasound scanning, direct monitoring of the brain is not possible. Optical techniques using near infrared light have the potential to provide continuous information on brain oxygenation and perfusion at the cotside. In addition, cortical activation to a range of stimuli can be detected and monitored [61]. At present these techniques are limited to research use in a small number of centers, but with further development they could become widely available, providing continuous information on important aspects of cerebral function at the bedside, and allowing nursing and other therapeutic interventions to be optimized. Continuous EEG recording from the neonatal brain is also feasible and this technique has the potential to provide valuable information to neonatal staff, including monitoring of sleep–wake cycling and behavioral states.

The growing trend to modify the environment of the NICU to minimize adverse stimuli is likely to continue, and it may be that detailed non-invasive monitoring of brain function combined with behavioral observation would allow methods of care to be optimized to individual babies.

There is obvious potential in neuroprotective interventions in very preterm infants. Although moderate hypothermia has been shown to be protective in term infants with acute encephalopathy following perinatal asphyxia, there is understandable caution about the deliberate manipulation of body and brain temperature in extremely preterm infants. A particular problem is the lack of suitable animal models which replicate the complex nature of brain injury in premature infants undergoing intensive care. The recent development of a preterm baboon model of neonatal intensive care is especially promising [62], but other experimental paradigms are required. The long history of well-meaning therapies that turn out to have disastrous long-term consequences, and the delay in obtaining outcome measures, make clinical trials of new therapies complex, expensive, and hazardous. It has been suggested that neuroimaging methods, especially using MRI, may provide early surrogate outcome markers for trials of neuroprotective agents in preterm infants. However, the multiple factors which influence cognitive outcome following discharge from hospital imply that early neuroimaging will always have limitations as an outcome predictor.

Finally, there is the growing potential of therapeutic interventions following discharge from hospital which can improve long-term neurological, neurosensory, and cognitive outcome. Developmental biologists have emphasized the central importance of environmentally dependent remodeling of the central nervous system throughout childhood. On the negative side, impaired parental input can have pervasive effects on neurodevelopment. Maternal depression is associated with an increased risk of cognitive impairment in children, especially when the infant is already at increased risk of adverse outcome. Since maternal depression is more likely when infants are born very preterm, it is possible that this provides another causal pathway by which preterm delivery is associated with cognitive and behavioral problems.

On the positive side, studies in rodents have demonstrated the remarkable effects of rearing immature animals in an "enriched environment," providing enhanced sensory stimuli and opportunities for exploratory play. Animals reared in this environment demonstrate improved memory and motor skills following a range of insults including perinatal brain injury. The enriched environment leads to marked structural and functional changes within the developing central nervous system, including increased brain weight and dendritic branching, enhanced neurogenesis and improved cortical synaptic plasticity [63]. The challenge of the next decade will be to translate these promising experimental findings into practical therapies for the growing number of surviving extremely preterm children.

Conclusion

Neonatal intensive care has seen dramatic evolution over the last 50 years. This means that all long-term outcome studies of very preterm infants are documenting the consequences of neonatal care which has since become outdated and obsolete. It is important to relate the pattern of neurological and developmental disorders associated with very preterm birth to the constantly changing nature of care which was received in the neonatal period. Preterm infants born in the period before 1965 were exposed to a high risk of injury due to unregulated oxygen therapy, hypoxia-ischemia, unrecognized hypoglycemia, jaundice, and poor nutrition. Between 1965 and 1985, survival improved dramatically, but there was a high incidence of IVH and hypoxic-ischemic brain injury, both associated with severe lung disease and its complications. Between 1985 and 2000, IVH declined in incidence and respiratory morbidity became much less severe. However, widespread and prolonged dexamethasone usage towards the end of this era was associated with impaired brain growth and cortical development. In the most recent period, IVH has continued to decline but diffuse white matter injury, together with associated cortical and cerebellar abnormalities, is now recognized as an extremely common and poorly understood accompaniment of extremely preterm birth and current methods of neonatal care.

Future developments in care are likely to lead to greater concentration on minimizing the adverse effects of the environment of the intensive care unit on the developing brain and on the use of non-invasive cerebral monitoring techniques to provide a brain-oriented focus of care. At the same time, novel neuroprotective interventions both before and after discharge from hospital will be developed and tested. The challenge of the next decade will be to find practical ways to minimize injury and optimize brain development for the growing number of surviving extremely preterm children.

Acknowledgments

The author acknowledges the major contribution of his colleagues at University College London in improving care for premature infants and the understanding of perinatal brain injury, especially Osmund Reynolds, David Delpy, David Edwards, Nikki Robertson,

Donald Peebles, Judith Meek, Topun Austin and Ann Stewart (deceased).

References

1. Origins of neonatal intensive care in the UK. A Witness Seminar held at the Welcome Institute for the History of Medicine, London on 27 April 1999. Welcome Witnesses to Twentieth Century Medicine Vol. 9; 2001. Available from: http://eprints.ucl.ac.uk/2071/. Accessed September 2009.

2. The history of neonatology. Available from: www.neonatology.org/tour/history.html. Accessed July 2009.

3. Philip AG. The evolution of neonatology. *Pediatr Res* 2005; **58**(4): 799–815.

4. Robertson AF. Reflections on errors in neonatology: I. The "Hands-Off" years, 1920 to 1950. *J Perinatol* 2003; **23**(1): 48–55.

5. Budin PC. *The Nursling. The Feeding and Hygiene of Premature and Full-term Infants*. London, England: Caxton Publishing Co.; 1907.

6. Silverman WA. A cautionary tale about supplemental oxygen: the albatross of neonatal medicine. *Pediatrics* 2004; **113**(2): 394–6.

7. Silverman WA, Fertig JW, Berger AP. The influence of the thermal environment upon the survival of newly born premature infants. *Pediatrics* 1958; **22**(5): 876–86.

8. Drillien CM. *The Growth and Development of the Prematurely Born Infant*. Baltimore, MD: Williams & Wilkins; 1964.

9. Reynolds EO. Effect of alterations in mechanical ventilator settings on pulmonary gas exchange in hyaline membrane disease. *Arch Dis Child* 1971; **46**(246): 152–9.

10. Gregory GA, Kitterman JA, Phibbs RH, Tooley WH, Hamilton WK. Treatment of the idiopathic respiratory-distress syndrome with continuous positive airway pressure. *N Engl J Med* 1971; **284**(24): 1333–40.

11. Lucey J, Ferriero M, Hewitt J. Prevention of hyperbilirubinemia of prematurity by phototherapy. *Pediatrics* 1968; **41**(6): 1047–54.

12. Stewart AL, Reynolds EO, Lipscomb AP. Outcome for infants of very low birthweight: survey of world literature. *Lancet* 1981; **1**(8228): 1038–40.

13. Stewart AL, Reynolds EO, Hope PL, *et al*. Probability of neurodevelopmental disorders estimated from ultrasound appearance of brains of very preterm infants. *Dev Med Child Neurol* 1987; **29**(1): 3–11.

14. Hack M, Horbar JD, Malloy MH, *et al*. Very low birth weight outcomes of the National Institute of Child Health and Human Development Neonatal Network. *Pediatrics* 1991; **87**(5): 587–97.

15. Wilson-Costello D, Borawski E, Friedman H, *et al*. Perinatal correlates of cerebral palsy and other neurologic impairment among very low birth weight children. *Pediatrics* 1998; **102**(2 Pt 1): 315–22.

16. Levene MI, Whitelaw A, Dubowitz V, *et al*. Nuclear magnetic resonance imaging of the brain in children. *Br Med J (Clin Res Ed)* 1982; **285**(6344): 774–6.

17. Cady EB, Costello AM, Dawson MJ, *et al*. Non-invasive investigation of cerebral metabolism in newborn infants by phosphorus nuclear magnetic resonance spectroscopy. *Lancet* 1983; **1**(8333): 1059–62.

18. Avery ME, Mead J. Surface properties in relation to atelectasis and hyaline membrane disease. *Am J Dis Child* 1959; **97**(5 pt 1): 517–23.

19. Liggins GC, Howie RN. A controlled trial of antepartum glucocorticoid treatment for prevention of the respiratory distress syndrome in premature infants. *Pediatrics* 1972; **50**(4): 515–25.

20. Crowley P, Chalmers I, Keirse MJ. The effects of corticosteroid administration before preterm delivery: an overview of the evidence from controlled trials. *Br J Obstet Gynaecol* 1990; **97**(1): 11–25.

21. Fujiwara T, Maeta H, Chida S, *et al*. Artificial surfactant therapy in hyaline membrane disease. *Lancet* 1980; **1**(8159): 55–9.

22. Hennes HM, Lee MB, Rimm AA, Shapiro DL. Surfactant replacement therapy in respiratory distress syndrome. Meta-analysis of clinical trials of single-dose surfactant extracts. *Am J Dis Child* 1991; **145**(1): 102–4.

23. Cummings JJ, D'Eugenio DB, Gross SJ. A controlled trial of dexamethasone in preterm infants at high risk for bronchopulmonary dysplasia. *N Engl J Med* 1989; **320**(23): 1505–10.

24. Lucas A, Morley R, Cole TJ. Adverse neurodevelopmental outcome of moderate neonatal hypoglycemia. *BMJ* 1988; **297**(6659): 1304–8.

25. Halliday HL, Ehrenkranz RA, Doyle LW. Early postnatal (< 96 hours) corticosteroids for preventing chronic lung disease in preterm infants. *Cochrane Database Syst Rev* 2003; (1): CD001146.

26. Volpe JJ. Intracranial hemorrhage: germinal matrix-intraventricular hemorrhage of the premature infant. In: *Neurology of the Newborn*, 4th edn. Philadelphia, PA: W.B. Saunders Company; 2001: 428–93.

27. Vollmer B, Roth S, Baudin J, *et al*. Predictors of long-term outcome in very preterm infants: gestational age versus neonatal cranial ultrasound. *Pediatrics* 2003; **112**(5): 1108–14.

28. Gould SJ, Howard S, Hope PL, Reynolds EO. Periventricular intraparenchymal cerebral hemorrhage in preterm infants: the role of venous infarction. *J Pathol* 1987; **151**(3): 197–202.

29. Meek JH, Tyszczuk L, Elwell CE, Wyatt JS. Low cerebral blood flow is a risk factor for severe intraventricular haemorrhage. *Arch Dis Child Fetal Neonatal Ed* 1999; **81**(1): F15–18.

30. Tsuji M, Saul JP, du Plessis A, *et al.* Cerebral intravascular oxygenation correlates with mean arterial pressure in critically ill premature infants. *Pediatrics* 2000; **106**(4): 625–32.

31. Meek JH, Tyszczuk L, Elwell CE, Wyatt JS. Cerebral blood flow increases over the first three days of life in extremely preterm neonates. *Arch Dis Child Fetal Neonatal Ed* 1998; **78**(1): F33–7.

32. Roberts D, Dalziel S. Antenatal corticosteroids for accelerating fetal lung maturation for women at risk of preterm birth. *Cochrane Database Syst Rev.* 2006; (3): CD004454.

33. Fowlie PW, Davis PG. Prophylactic indomethacin for preterm infants: a systematic review and meta-analysis. *Arch Dis Child Fetal Neonatal Ed* 2003; **88**(6): F464–6.

34. Ment LR, Stewart WB, Ardito TA, Huang E, Madri JA. Indomethacin promotes germinal matrix microvessel maturation in the newborn beagle pup. *Stroke* 1992; **23**(8): 1132–7.

35. Ment LR, Peterson BS, Vohr B, *et al.* Cortical recruitment patterns in children born prematurely compared with control subjects during a passive listening functional magnetic resonance imaging task. *J Pediatr* 2006; **149**(4): 490–8.

36. Philip AG, Allan WC, Tito AM, Wheeler LR. Intraventricular hemorrhage in preterm infants: declining incidence in the 1980s. *Pediatrics* 1989; **84**(5): 797–801.

37. Banker BQ, Larroche JC. Periventricular leucomalacia in infancy: a form of neonatal anoxic encephalopathy. *Arch Neurol* 1962; **7**: 386–410.

38. Hope PL, Gould SJ, Howard S, *et al.* Precision of ultrasound diagnosis of pathologically verified lesions in the brains of very preterm infants. *Dev Med Child Neurol* 1988; **30**(4): 457–71.

39. Paneth N, Rudelli R, Monte W, *et al.* White matter necrosis in very low birth weight infants: neuropathologic and ultrasonographic findings in infants surviving six days or longer. *J Pediatr* 1990; **116**(6): 975–84.

40. Maalouf EF, Duggan PJ, Rutherford MA, *et al.* Magnetic resonance imaging of the brain in a cohort of extremely preterm infants. *J Pediatr* 1999; **135**(3): 351–7.

41. Counsell SJ, Rutherford MA, Cowan FM, Edwards AD. Magnetic resonance imaging of preterm brain injury. *Arch Dis Child Fetal Neonatal Ed* 2003; **88**(4): F269–74.

42. Inder TE, Wells SJ, Mogridge NB, Spencer C, Volpe JJ. Defining the nature of the cerebral abnormalities in the premature infant: a qualitative magnetic resonance imaging study. *J Pediatr* 2003; **143**(2): 171–9.

43. Inder T, Huppi PS, Zientara GP, *et al.* Early detection of periventricular leukomalacia by diffusion-weighted magnetic resonance imaging techniques. *J Pediatr* 1999; **134**(5): 631–4.

44. Counsell SJ, Allsop JM, Harrison MC, *et al.* Diffusion-weighted imaging of the brain in preterm infants with focal and diffuse white matter abnormality. *Pediatrics* 2003; **112**(1 Pt 1): 1–7.

45. Hüppi PS, Warfield S, Kikinis R, *et al.* Quantitative magnetic resonance imaging of brain development in premature and mature newborns. *Ann Neurol* 1998; **43**(2): 224–35.

46. Hüppi PS, Murphy B, Maier SE, *et al.* Microstructural brain development after perinatal cerebral white matter injury assessed by diffusion tensor magnetic resonance imaging. *Pediatrics* 2001; **107**(3): 455–60.

47. Volpe JJ. Neurobiology of periventricular leukomalacia in the premature infant. *Pediatr Res* 2001; **50**(5): 553–62.

48. Haynes RL, Baud O, Li J, *et al.* Oxidative and nitrative injury in periventricular leukomalacia: a review. *Brain Pathol* 2005; **15**(3): 225–33.

49. Kendall G, Peebles D. Acute fetal hypoxia: the modulating effect of infection. *Early Hum Dev* 2005; **81**(1): 27–34.

50. Dammann O, Leviton A. Inflammatory brain damage in preterm newborns – dry numbers, wet lab, and causal inferences. *Early Hum Dev* 2004; **79**(1): 1–15.

51. Shankaran S, Langer JC, Kazzi SN, Laptook AR, Walsh M. Cumulative index of exposure to hypocarbia and hyperoxia as risk factors for periventricular leukomalacia in low birth weight infants. *Pediatrics* 2006; **118**(4): 1654–9.

52. Volpe JJ. Encephalopathy of prematurity includes neuronal abnormalities. *Pediatrics* 2005; **116**(1): 221–5.

53. Kapellou O, Counsell SJ, Kennea N, *et al.* Abnormal cortical development after premature birth shown by altered allometric scaling of brain growth. *PLoS Med* 2006; **3**(8): e265.

54. Inder TE, Warfield SK, Wang H, Huppi PS, Volpe JJ. Abnormal cerebral structure is present at term in premature infants. *Pediatrics* 2005; **115**(2): 286–94.

55. Anderson PJ, Doyle LW. Neurodevelopmental outcome of bronchopulmonary dysplasia. *Semin Perinatol* 2006; **30**(4): 227–32.

56. Duvanel CB, Fawer CL, Cotting J, Hohlfeld P, Matthieu JM. Long-term effects of neonatal hypoglycemia on brain growth and psychomotor development in

small-for-gestational-age preterm infants. *J Pediatr* 1999; **134**(4): 492–8.

57. Cooke RW. Are there critical periods for brain growth in children born preterm? *Arch Dis Child Fetal Neonatal Ed* 2006; **91**(1): F17–20.

58. Fitzgerald M. The development of nociceptive circuits. *Nat Rev Neurosci* 2005; **6**(7): 507–20.

59. Shaffery JP, Sinton CM, Bissette G, Roffwarg HP, Marks GA. Rapid eye movement sleep deprivation modifies expression of long-term potentiation in visual cortex of immature rats. *Neuroscience* 2002; **110**(3): 431–43.

60. Als H, Duffy FH, McAnulty GB, *et al.* Early experience alters brain function and structure. *Pediatrics* 2004; **113**(4): 846–57.

61. Austin T. Optical imaging of the neonatal brain. *Arch Dis Child Fetal Neonatal Ed* 2007; **92**(4): F238–41.

62. Dieni S, Inder T, Yoder B, *et al.* The pattern of cerebral injury in a primate model of preterm birth and neonatal intensive care. *J Neuropathol Exp Neurol* 2004; **63**(12): 1297–309.

63. van Praag H, Kempermann G, Gage FH. Neural consequences of environmental enrichment. *Nat Rev Neurosci* 2000; **1**(3): 191–8.

Chapter 3

Clinical outcome: neurological sequelae following preterm birth

Ingeborg Krägeloh-Mann

Introduction

Neurological outcome after preterm birth refers to neurologically defined conditions due to disorders of the motor system – e.g. spasticity, dyskinesia or ataxia – which are commonly summarized under the term "cerebral palsy" (CP). Studies of CP in relation to birth weight (BW) and gestational age (GA) estimate that infants of very low birth weight (VLBW); i.e., of BW less than 1500 g, or very immature infants; i.e., with GA less than 32 weeks, are between 40 and 100 times more likely to have CP than normal BW infants or infants born at term [1,2]. No other disability associated with preterm birth, such as learning impairments, mental retardation, behavioral problems or sensorineural deficits, shows such a high difference in prevalence in relation to birth at term or normal BW. This means that CP following preterm birth, or brain compromise affecting the motor system, is probably related to a pathomechanism specifically affecting the immature brain, which stresses the importance of gaining insight into the following questions:

- What is the prevalence of CP following preterm birth with respect to mortality and during the course of development? A hypothesis suggests that increasing survival rates are associated with increasing CP rates as more preexistingly damaged children are brought to survival. The competing hypothesis assumes that increasing survival rates first lead to increasing, but then to decreasing or at least stable CP rates, as progress in pre-, peri-, and neonatal care first reduces mortality, and subsequently also morbidity.
- Does CP prevalence per live births (LB) and also per neonatal survivors (NNS) show a linear increase with lower BW and GA? The hypothesis being that the pathomechanism underlying CP becomes more relevant with higher immaturity.
- What is the potential of neuroimaging to depict the lesions/abnormalities of the motor systems causing CP and thus to elucidate the origin or at least the pathogenesis of CP following preterm birth? The assumption here is that non-progressive disorders of the motor systems affecting the immature brain leave indelible traces which can be detected by neuroimaging techniques, especially magnetic resonance imaging (MRI).

Before discussing these questions, CP and its clinical features will be defined and described.

Definition and classification of CP

Key elements of the current CP definitions involve the following features:

- CP is a group of disorders;
- it involves a disorder of movement and posture and of motor function;
- it is permanent but not unchanging;
- it is due to a non-progressive interference/lesion/abnormality;
- this interference/lesion/abnormality is in the developing/immature brain.

A European network of health professionals working in the domain of CP has agreed on this definition – the SCPE: Surveillance of CP in Europe [3] – which is also in line with a recently proposed international definition [4]. Both underline that accompanying disabilities of cognitive, behavioral, and sensory functions are frequent, and agree that the disorders of posture and motor function must be neurologically defined. The predominant feature of CP determines classification, and pure hypotonicity is not a feature of CP. Subtypes of CP are thus defined as spastic, dyskinetic, and ataxic. The SCPE divides spastic CP into unilateral spastic CP (US-CP), covering the terms spastic hemiplegia or

Neurodevelopmental Outcomes of Preterm Birth, ed. Chiara Nosarti, Robin M. Murray, and Maureen Hack. Published by Cambridge University Press. © Cambridge University Press 2010.

hemiparesis, and bilateral spastic CP (BS-CP), covering the terms di- or tetraplegia or -paresis, which is usually employed to distinguish a more leg-dominated form from a complete form. The distinction between di- and tetraplegia has proven to be very difficult to define, and it may vary from 20% vs. 80% to 80% vs. 20%, respectively, between centers [5]. The SCPE therefore recommended to describe functional severity in legs and arms according to standardized scores [3], such as the Gross Motor Function Classification System (GMFCS) [6] and the Bimanual Fine Motor Function System (BFMFS) [7] or the Manual Ability Classification System (MACS) [8].

The typical neurological signs take time to develop and it is generally agreed that the child should at least be 3 years of age before the CP diagnosis is established; CP registers unquestionably accept children only at age 5[3,9]. Early diagnosis is difficult to establish, as early neurological signs may be transitory or may change. Furthermore, a disease starting early and progressing slowly may take time to become apparent, in terms of manifesting in clearly progressive loss of acquired skills. This does not preclude that a diagnosis of CP can be established earlier in an individual situation, but it is important to take these facts into account for the discussion of prevalence data [10].

Clinical features of CP

As indicated above, the clinical picture of CP is often not only characterized by motor function problems but also by additional disturbances of cognition, communication, perception, and/or behavior, and/or by a seizure disorder. These features determine prognosis and treatment, and have to be taken into account in both the patient's assessment and the multidisciplinary therapeutical approach.

Spastic cerebral palsy is by far the predominant characteristic of CP, accounting for around 85% of cases, in preterm-born children for even more than 90% [1]. The neurological symptoms in spastic CP are as follows:

- *increased tone,* characterized by increased resistance to passive movement which is velocity dependent;
- *pathological reflexes,* e.g., increased reflexes or hyperreflexia and pyramidal signs, e.g., Babinski response;
- *abnormal pattern of movement and posture,* characterized in lower limbs by equinus foot, crouch gait, internal rotation, and hip adduction,

in upper limbs by arms in flexion, fisted hands with adducted thumb, or stiff and poorly directed finger movements.

The bilateral form, BS-CP, is especially predominant in preterm-born children (see below). Leg-dominated forms or diplegia are most common in most studies and account for around 75% of cases [11,12]. The symptoms of BS-CP are as follows:

- *Motor deficit* is found in around 50% of the preterm children and it is severe in that affected individuals cannot walk without aid at the age of 5 years. This illustrates that diplegia can take a severe form. Secondary motor problems with contractures – in equinus position, hip adduction, and knee flexion – are frequent, especially in children who have not learnt to walk.
- *Cognitive problems,* in terms of learning difficulties or mental retardation, are less often seen in preterm-born or low birth weight (LBW – less than 2500 g) than in term-born children – around 30–40% have mental retardation and around 25% have learning difficulties, whereas the figures are 70% and 15%, respectively, for children with normal BW and BS-CP. Mental retardation is encountered especially in the children with severe forms of BS-CP.
- *Severe cerebral visual problems* are encountered in around 15% of VLBW children and in 10% of LBW children with BS-CP. Around half of the children with severe forms of the condition are blind or nearly blind.
- *Hearing problems* (deaf or near deaf) are, however, not frequent, occurring only in around 3% of affected individuals [11].
- *Epilepsy* is encountered in around 20% of VLBW and LBW children with BS-CP; whereas West syndrome, characterized by infantile spasms, in less than 10% – again, only half as often as in BS-CP children with normal BW. Epilepsy is mainly symptomatic and is related to the severity of functional disability.

The unilateral form, US-CP is characterized by:
- *Motor deficit,* which is rarely severe. Less than 2% of the population-based series of Uvebrant [13] did not walk at the age of 5 years; more than half could walk without much restrictions. Secondary motor problems with contractures are mainly seen in the paretic foot with equinus position, and hip subluxation, a symptom where the ball of

the ball-and-socket hip joint is pushed part of the way out of joint, is not a frequent problem [14]. Hypotrophy of the affected limbs is often seen, correction of leg length is seldomly necessary.

- *Cognitive problems,* in terms of learning difficulties or mental retardation, are less often found in children with US-CP than in other forms of CP. Uvebrant [13] found mild mental retardation in 12% of his preterm children with US-CP.
- *Severe cerebral visual problems* are also especially rare in preterm-born children (e.g., around 5%). There is no gross difference in language according to hemisphere affected [15–17], although children with left hemispheric lesions are reported to be slower in language development [18], which indicates that reorganization of language to the right "takes some time" but can well be reached.
- *Epilepsy* is not a rare problem in US-CP, but found mainly in term-born children.

Prevalence trends over time and in different BW and GA groups

Incidence looks at the occurrence of new cases of a condition, while *prevalence* looks at those cases who currently have the condition. In CP, it is typically prevalence that is measured and compared, the reference basis being mainly birth periods and place of residence at birth. This relates to the fact that the CP diagnosis is only possible with some delay between brain compromise and its obvious clinical signs, and some children may have died within this period before CP diagnosis could be established.

As indicated above, the risk to develop CP is higher in infants with lower BW or lower GA. For infants with a BW between 1500 and 2500 g (LBW) or a GA between 32 and 36 weeks, CP prevalence is around 10 per 1000 LB in contrast to 1 per 1000 in normal BW or mature infants. Very low birth weight infants (BW less than 1500 g) or very immature infants have prevalence between 40 and 100 per 1000 live birth [9, 19–21]. The decreased neonatal mortality of VLBW infants in the past decades are associated with an improved understanding of the care of the premature infant that has altered clinicians' perceptions of viability. During this time, there has also been an increase in multiple births. Both these changes have resulted in a rise in the absolute number of VLBW infants at risk of CP.

Trends over time in LBW children

These children are often somewhat neglected when discussing CP prevalence, as their risk is lower than that for the very small infants. It is, however, definitely higher than in the term-born or normal BW child. Low birth weight groups could even be used as a model of what may happen in the even more immature child, assuming similar pathogenetic mechanisms for CP in both groups. Changes in outcome in the less immature child may precede those in the very immature individual. Indeed, CP prevalence data in this group indicate a trend in this direction. Data from population-based studies in the late 1970s and 1980s were somewhat discrepant in reporting an increase in prevalence in these children [22], a leveling off [23], or even a decrease in prevalence [24,25]. In the 1980s and early 1990s, the decreasing trend was however predominant [20,21,26]. This is supported by the findings from the SCPE database showing a significant decrease between 1982 and 1996 from 12 to 8 per 1000 LB (C. Cans, personal communication, 2008).

Trends over time in VLBW children

Evidence from CP registers suggests that the prevalence of CP among VLBW infants has risen in the 1980s [1,22,24]. This is reported in some studies also for the 1990s [19,27]. Others, however, indicate that the rates of CP in VLBW infants are now beginning to fall ([25] for BS-CP; [20], [21,28] for total CP). Thus, these data suggest a similar pattern of prevalence rates to that observed in the LBW group, although in more recent years and definitely to a greater extent.

These studies, although covering large geographical areas, are still limited by their small number of cases, affecting the precision of any estimate. Even less information is available on the subset of infants weighing less than 1000g at birth (whose survival has also improved substantially during the 1980s). The SCPE database with data from 16 European population-based centers described CP prevalence in the period 1980–96 [3]. A decline in CP rate was seen initially in infants of 1000–1499 g from 60 per 1000 LB in 1980 to 40 per 1000 LB in 1996 (or from 90 per 1000 NNS to 44 per 1000 NNS), but a decreasing trend was also seen in infants of BW < 1000 g in more recent times. Cerebral palsy rates in the 1990s in this European cohort were similar for infants with a BW < 1000 g and children with BW 1000–1500 g, e.g., around 40 per 1000 LB; they differed, however, in terms of neonatal survival, e.g., 80 per 1000 NNS in the former group versus 50 per 1000 NNS in the latter. Towards the end of

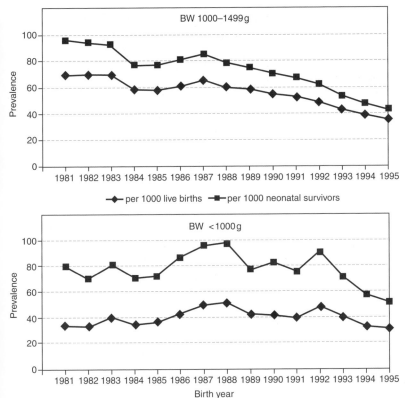

Fig 3.1 Cerebral palsy rates (3-years moving average) from nine European countries in infants born with a BW < 1000 g (lower) and 1000–1499 g (upper). Adapted from Platt MJ *et al. Lancet* 2007; **369**: 43–50.

the observation period, however, the prevalence became more similar also per NNS, e.g. around 50 in the former and around 40 in the latter group, reflecting a more pronounced fall in mortality in the extremely and very low weight groups (Fig. 3.1). Trends in the rate of CP by GA mirrored those of BW, with a significant fall over the time period for those of GA 28–31 weeks, but with no significant trend in those of < 28 weeks' gestation, suggesting that a shift in proportion of small-for-gestational-age infants may not provide a comprehensive explanation for the fall in prevalence.

The significant reduction in the birth prevalence of CP per 1000 LB was mostly due to a reduction in BS-CP among 1000–1499 g infants. Unilateral spastic CP did not change significantly over the study period .

CP rates in the extremely immature infants born in recent years

Survival of extremely immature infants, i.e., infants of less than 27 weeks of gestation, is increasing and the above-discussed data do not specifically respond to concerns about their outcome, as they are included in the larger group of infants with a BW < 1000 g or a GA < 28 weeks. A number of studies have reported CP rates in births during the late 1990s. Two large European cohort studies report a CP prevalence per NNS of 19.6% and 15.9%, respectively, in infants born at 25 weeks of gestation and below; the first figures are provided by the Epicure study involving infants born in 1995 in the UK and Ireland, and the second figures by the EPIPAGE study, referring to infants born in 1997 in nine regions of France [29]. Similar rates are reported from the USA [30]: 19% CP per NNS was found in infants born in 1997–8 with a GA between 22 and 26 weeks and cared for in 14 tertiary care centers; rates were unchanged in comparison to 1993–4 and were higher than those in infants born between 27 and 32 weeks. More specifically, CP rates in even more immature infants, born before 25 weeks, were 23% in those born in 1993–6 and 21% in those born in 1996–9 [31], thus higher than in the entire group born before 27 weeks and not changing over time. Promising results are reported from Alberta in West Canada [32] for infants born at a GA of 20–25 weeks. Cerebral palsy rates increased from 0 to 110 per 1000 LB between 1974 and 1994, but decreased thereafter to 22 per 1000 LB in the years 2001–3. In the GA groups 26 and 27 weeks the increase was from 15 to 155, followed by a decrease to 16 thereafter. Rates per 2-years survivors mirrored these trends on a higher level, reaching rates of nearly 25% in 1993 and falling to below 5% in 2003. Survival increased in the two GA groups from 4% to 31% and from 23% to 75–80%, respectively. Thus, stable or reduced mortality of extremely immature babies was associated first with an increase in CP prevalence, although in the last observation period the trend was reversed.

These prevalence data indicate that not only the survival of LBW or mildly preterm infants, but also of those with a BW < 1500 g or a GA < 32 weeks, continues to improve, and that this continuous improvement in survival is not at the expense of increased morbidity. It has to be kept in mind, however, that the CP rates increase with lower BW and more severe immaturity, especially with respect to NNS (Fig. 3.2). Population-based studies can provide a more global view of the impact of the neonatal intensive care on survival and quality of survival in the last two decades. It is not yet possible, however, to associate the trends reported here with the introduction or withdrawal of specific perinatal management strategies, for example antenatal steroids and surfactant therapy.

Pathogenesis of CP in children born preterm and the role of neuroimaging

The CP definition describes its origin very broadly as "non-progressive lesions or abnormality of the developing/immature brain." In earlier times these changes used to be described by the medical branch of postmortem neuropathology. When investigating living individuals, risk factors indicative of brain compromise need to be used as substitutes. Since the advent of neuroimaging techniques, such as ultrasound (US) or MRI, gross morphological brain abnormalities can readily be described in vivo. Specifically, MRI techniques have the potential to comprehensively visualize brain lesions or maldevelopments.

The major neuropathological complications arising in the early to mid third trimester are periventricular lesions, e.g., periventricular leukomalacia (PVL) or complications of intraventricular hemorrhage (IVH), that is periventricular hemorrhagic infarction (PHI). They constitute the main lesional patterns in preterm children [33–38]. Please refer to Chapters 4 to 8 for

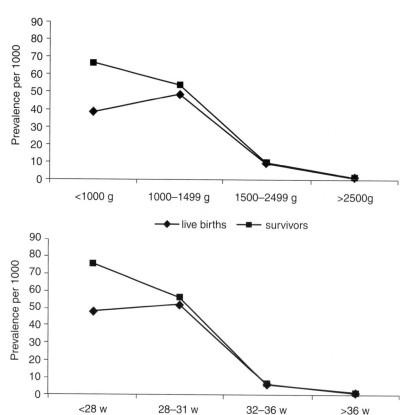

Fig 3.2 Cerebral palsy rates per live births and neonatal survivors in different birth weight (upper) and gestational age groups (lower) in 1990–8 from nine European countries showing increasing rates especially when referring to neonatal survivors; the rates per live births, however, show a levelling off, reflecting the higher mortality in the lightest and most immature groups (SCPE database, C. Cans, personal communication, 2008).

further discussion of neuroimaging studies in preterm and LBW samples.

Neonatal imaging is mainly done by routine US in neonatal units caring for the very preterm newborn. Bleedings are relatively easy to identify and timing of IVH is usually not difficult to determine with sequential US, which can immediately detect at least the hemorrhagic component of a lesion (see also Chapter 4). It is more difficult to clearly identify PVL or the parenchymal component of an IVH, e.g., periventricular hemorrhage (PVH). Changes – focal in PVH and mainly bilateral in PVL – develop over time. Increased periventricular echogenicity is a common finding during the first days of life, and it becomes indicative of leukomalacia only when lasting more than 7–10 days. Neonatal imaging is probably less sensitive for depicting the lesions behind CP than later imaging (see below). Ultrasound was judged as normal in 35% of children with CP in the entire cohort of the EPIPAGE study, all preterm children having a GA below 33 weeks [39]. In earlier birth years this insensitivity was probably even higher, e.g., only a third of the preterm children born in the late 1980s who were identified as having periventricular lesions by MRI between 5 and 7 years had a neonatal US diagnosis of PVL [37].

Late MRI of PVL is characterized by periventricular gliosis, usually involving the peritrigonal region and extending towards the region around the bodies of the lateral ventricles and then towards the periventricular white matter. This is best seen when myelination has progressed to near mature patterns, e.g. after the age of 2 years. In the more extensive forms, gliosis is accompanied by periventricular tissue loss, the end stage of cystic necrosis; some small cysts may still be seen. This results in periventricular white matter loss and ventricular dilatation with irregular borders [37,40,41]. In most severe forms, this can result in the pattern of multicystic encephalomalacia. The late MRI of PVL is characterized by porencephalic focal ventricular enlargement, often accompanied by some gliosis. In a systematic review of MRI studies in children with CP, 90% of preterm-born children had periventricular lesions, maldevelopments indicating an earlier origin (mostly before 24 weeks) were found in 2.5% and "more mature" lesional patterns (cortical and deep gray matter lesions) were found in 3.5% of the sample, mainly in the more mature children [42]. Please refer to Chapter 4 for further discussion on neonatal neuroimaging and to Chapters 5 to 8 for further discussion on neuroimaging studies in preterm and LBW samples in adolescence and early adulthood.

Morphology–function correlates after periventricular lesions

The clinical consequences of periventricular white matter lesions are dependent on the topography and extent of the lesions (Figs. 3.3 and 3.4). In unilateral lesions, or

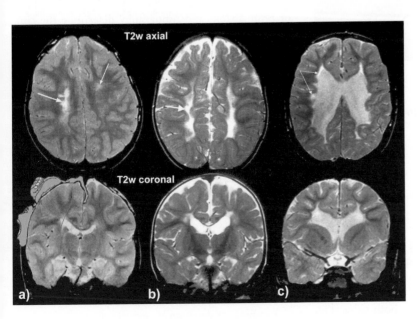

Fig. 3.3 Morphology–function in periventricular leukomalacia with respect to motor tracts/CP. Magnetic resonance imaging of three 6-year-old children with different degrees of periventricular leukomalacia (the bottom images are in coronal orientation in the domain of the motor tracks). Images are displayed in radiological view (Right = Left, Left = right). (a) A very mild and asymmetrical form with periventricular gliosis only, which affects only the right side (thick arrow) of the motor tracts, on the left only frontal involvement is seen (thin arrow), thus gives rise to **unilateral spastic CP** on the left. (b) Mild PVL, again characterized by gliosis (arrow), but more symmetrical and affecting both motor tracts, thus causes **mild, leg-dominated BS-CP**. (c) Severe PVL with gliosis (arrows) and tissue loss, affecting, thus, motor tracts on both sides **severely and causes spastic CP** not only affecting legs but also trunk, arms, and face (usually also associated with cognitive problems and visual deficits, see Fig. 3.4). See plate section for color version.

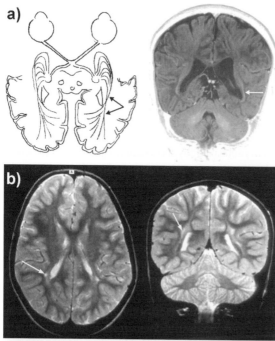

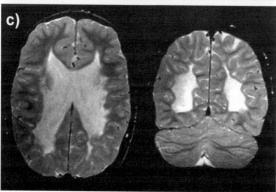

Fig 3.4 Morphology–function in periventricular leukomalacia with respect to visual system/visual function. (a) Schematic view of the visual system in axial (left) and coronal (right) orientation in the brain of a 3-month-old child, where white matter is not yet myelinated with the exception of the optic radiation, which can be visualized circumventing the lower part of the posterior horns only (arrow). (b) Example for mild PVL (arrow) situated in the peritrigonal area superior to the optic radiation, thus not affecting visual acuity (but with a risk to influence visuoperceptive functions). This child has no spasticity as motor tracts are not involved. (c) Severe PVL affecting the optic radiation and causing severe cerebral visual deficits (same child as Fig. 3.3c).

very asymmetrical lesions involving motor tracts only on one side (Fig. 3.3a), the typical sequela is US-CP. An early sign on MRI is signal abnormalities in the posterior limb of the internal capsule (PLIC) [43]. In lesions with involvement of motor tracts on both sides (Fig. 3.3b, 3.3c), the typical neurological manifestation is again spastic CP, but bilateral. The extent of the lesions within the motor tracts mainly determines the neurological and functional sequelae, e.g., leg-dominated or complete, mild or severe motor deficits [41,44]. Severe PVL with extensive tissue loss within the peritrigonal area (usually accompanied by severe spastic CP) often involves the optic radiation and leads to severe cerebral visual impairment [37,45] (Fig. 3.4c). Bilateral extensive white matter loss is also related to severe cognitive impairment [37]. However, the high prevalence of mild cognitive deficits in preterm individuals can probably not be accounted for by mild PVL [34,36–38,46]. There is only evidence that PVL within the parieto-occipital area, even when it does not affect the optic radiation and thus visual acuity, is related to specific visuoperceptive deficits [47,48] (Fig. 3.4b).

Conclusion

Neurological outcome after preterm birth is characterized by CP. Its prevalence increases with lower BW and higher immaturity. Increase of survival after preterm birth has also increased CP rates. However, already in the 1980s this trend was reversed for LBW infants and in the 1990s also for VLBW or very immature infants. The outcome with respect to CP in the group of extremely LBW or immature infants is, however, a matter of specific concern, as prevalence seems to be rather stable on a high level.

Cerebral palsy is caused in more than 90% of cases by periventricular lesions – PVL or sequelae of IVH, or both. Extent and topography determine the clinical subtype of CP and also the presence and severity of associated disabilities, such as mental retardation or cerebral visual problems. An exception is learning disability, which seems not to be clearly related to these lesions, thus, other pathogenetic mechanisms than those responsible for periventricular lesions may play a role in contributing to this outcome and need further investigation.

References

1. Hagberg B, Hagberg G. The origins of cerebral palsy. In: David TJ, ed. *Recent Advances in Paediatrics,* Vol. 11. Edinburgh: Churchill Livingstone. 1993; 67–83.

2. Platt MJ, Cans C, Johnson A, *et al.* Trends in cerebral palsy among infants of very low birthweight (<1500g) or born prematurely (<32 weeks) in 16 European centres: a data base study. *Lancet* 2007; **369**: 43–50.

3. SCPE Working group. Surveillance of cerebral palsy in Europe: a collaboration of cerebral palsy surveys and registers. *Dev Med Child Neurol* 2000; **42**: 816–24.

4. Rosenbaum P, Paneth N, Leviton A, *et al.* A report: the definition and classification of cerebral palsy. *Dev Med Child Neurol* 2007; **109**: 8–14.

5. Colver AF, Gibson M, Hey EN, *et al.* Increasing rates of cerebral palsy across the severity spectrum in north-east England 1964–1993. The North of England Collaborative Cerebral Palsy Survey. *Arch Dis Child Fetal Neonatal Ed* 2000; **83**: F7–12.

6. Palisano R, Rosenbaum P, Walter S, *et al.* Gross motor function classification system for cerebral palsy. *Dev Med Child Neurol* 1997; **37**: 214–23

7. Beckung E, Hagberg G. Bimanual fine motor function in children with cerebral palsy. *Dev Med Child Neurol* 2002; **44**: 309–16.

8. Eliasson AC, Krumlinde-Sundholm L, Rösblad B, *et al.* The Manual Ability Classification System (MACS) for children with cerebral palsy: scale development and evidence of validity and reliability. *Dev Med Child Neurol* 2006; **48**: 549–54.

9. Stanley F, Blair E, Alberman E. *Cerebral Palsies: Epidemiology & Causal Pathways.* London: MacKeith Press; 2000.

10. Krägeloh-Mann I Bax M. Cerebral palsy. In: Aicardi J, ed. *Diseases of the Nervous System in Childhood* London: Mac Keith Press. 2009; 210–42.

11. Krägeloh-Mann I, Hagberg G, Meisner Ch, *et al.* Bilateral spastic cerebral palsy – A comparative study between south-west Germany and western Sweden. I. Clinical patterns and disabilities. *Dev Med Child Neurol* 1993; **35**: 1037–47.

12. Gorter JW, Rosenbaum PL, Hanna SE, *et al.* Limb distribution, motor impairment, and functional classification of cerebral palsy. *Dev Med Child Neurol* 2004; **46**: 461–7.

13. Uvebrant P. Hemiplegic cerebral palsy, aetiology and outcome. *Acta Paediatr Scand* 1988; Suppl 1988; **345**: 1–100.

14. Hägglund G, Lauge-Pedersen H, Wagner P. Characteristics of children with hip displacement in cerebral palsy. *BMC Musculoskelet Disord*, **8**: 101.

15. Carlsson G, Uvebrant, P, Hugdahl K, *et al.* Verbal and nonverbal function of children with right- versus left-hemiplegic cerebral palsy of pre- and perinatal origin. *Dev Med Child Neurol* 1994; **36**: 503–12.

16. Staudt M, Grodd W, Niemann G, *et al.* Early left periventricular brain lesions induce right hemispheric organization of speech. *Neurology* 2001; **57**: 122–5.

17. Lidzba K, Krägeloh-Mann I. Development and lateralization of language in the presence of early brain lesions. *Dev Med Child Neurol* 2005; **47**: 724.

18. Chilosi AM, Cipriani PP, Bertuccelli B, Pfanner PL, Cioni PG. Early cognitive and communication development in children with focal brain lesions. *J Child Neurol* 2001; **16**(5): 309–16.

19. Blair E, Watson L, Badawi N, Stanley FJ, Life expectancy among people with cerebral palsy in Western Australia. *Dev Med Child Neurol* 2001; **43**(8): 508–15.

20. Topp M, Uldall P, Greisen G. Cerebral palsy births in eastern Denmark, 1987–90: implications for neonatal care. *Paediatr Perinat Epidemiol* 2001; **15**: 271–7.

21. Himmelmann K, Hagberg G, Beckung E, Hagberg B, Uvebrant P. The changing panorama of cerebral palsy in Sweden. IX. Prevalence and origin in the birth-year period 1995–1998. *Acta Paediatr* 2005; **94**: 287–94.

22. Pharoah POD, Cooke T, Cooke RWI, Rosenbloom L. Birthweight specific trends in cerebral palsy. *Arch Dis Child* 1990; **65**: 602–6.

23. Hagberg B, Hagberg G, Olow I, von Wendt L. The changing panorama of cerebral palsy in Sweden. V. The birth year period 1979–82. *Acta Paediatr Scand* 1989; **78**: 283–90.

24. Stanley FJ, Watson L. Trends in perinatal mortality and cerebral palsy in Western Australia, 1967 to 1985. *BMJ* 1992; **304**: 1658–63.

25. Krägeloh-Mann I, Hagberg G, Meisner Ch, *et al.* Bilateral spastic cerebral palsy – A comparative study between south-west Germany and western Sweden. II. Epidemiology. *Dev Med Child Neurol* 1994; **36**: 473–83.

26. Hagberg B, Hagberg G, Beckung E, Uvebrant P. Changing panorama of cerebral palsy in Sweden. VIII. Prevalence and origin in the birth year period 1991–94. *Acta Paediatr* 2001; **90**: 271–7.

27. Doyle LW, Betheras FR, Ford GW, Davis NM, Callanan C. Survival, cranial ultrasound and cerebral palsy in very low birthweight infants: 1980s versus 1990s. *J Paediatr Child Health* 2000; **36**: 7–12.

28. Surman G, Newdick H, Johnson A; Oxford Register of Early Childhood Impairments Management Group. Cerebral palsy rates among low-birthweight infants fell in the 1990s. *Dev Med Child Neurol* **45**: 456–62.

29. Bodeau-Livinec F, Marlow N, Ancel P-Y, *et al.* The impact of intensive care practices on short and long-term outcomes for extremely preterm babies: a comparison between the British Isles and France. *Pediatrics* 2008; **122**: e1014–21.

30. Vohr BR, Wright LL, Poole WK, McDonald, SA. Neurodevelopmental outcomes of extremely low birth weight infants <32 weeks' gestation between 1993 and 1998. *Pediatrics* 2005; **116**: 635–43.

31. Hintz SR, Kendrick DE, Vohr BR, Poole WK., Higgins RD; National Institute of Child Health and Human Development Neonatal Research Network. Changes in neurodevelopmental outcomes at 18 to 22 months' corrected age among infants of less than 25 weeks' gestational age born in 1993–1999. *Pediatrics* 2005; **115**: 1645–51.

32. Robertson CM, Watt MJ, Yasui Y. Changes in the prevalence of cerebral palsy for children born very prematurely within a population-based program over 30 years. *JAMA* 2007; **297**: 2733–40.

33. de Vries LS. Neurological assessment of the preterm infant. *Acta Paediatr* 1996; **85**: 765–71.

34. Skranes JS, Vik T, Nilsen G, *et al.* Cerebral magnetic resonance imaging and mental and motor function of very low birth weight children at six years of age. *Neuropediatrics* 1997; **28**: 149–54.

35. Volpe JJ. Brain injury in the premature infant – from pathogenesis to prevention. *Brain Dev* 1997; **19**: 519–34.

36. Olsén P, Vainionpää L, Pääkkö E, *et al.* Psychological findings in preterm children related to neurological status and magnetic resonance imaging. *Pediatrics* 1998; **102**: 329–36.

37. Krägeloh-Mann I, Toft P, Lunding J, *et al.* Brain lesions in preterms – origin, consequences, and compensation. *Acta Paediatr* 1999; **88**: 897–908.

38. Stewart AL, Rifkin L, Amess PN, *et al.* Brain structure and neurocognitive and behavioural function in adolescents who were born very preterm. *Lancet* 1999; **353**: 1653–7.

39. Ancel PY, Livinec F, Larroque B, *et al.*; Epipage Study Group. Cerebral palsy among very preterm children in relation to gestational age and neonatal ultrasound abnormalities: the EPIPAGE cohort study. *Pediatrics* 2006; **117**: 828–35.

40. Flodmark O, Lupton B, Li D, *et al.* MR imaging of periventricular leukomalacia in childhood. *AJR Am J Roentgenol* 1989; **152**: 583–90.

41. Krägeloh-Mann I, Petersen D, Hagberg G, *et al.* Bilateral spastic cerebral palsy – MRI pathology and origin. Analysis from a representative series of 56 cases. *Dev Med Child Neurol* 1995; **38**: 379–97.

42. Krägeloh-Mann I, Horber V. The role of magnetic resonance imaging in elucidating the pathogenesis of cerebral palsy: a systematic review. *Dev Med Child Neurol*, 2007; **49**: 144–51.

43. De Vries LS, Groenendaal F, van Haastert I, *et al.* Asymmetrical myelination of the posterior limb of the internal capsule in infants with periventricular haemorrhagic infarction: an early predictor of hemiplegia. *Neuropediatrics* 1999; **30**: 314–19.

44. Staudt M, Pavlova M, Böhm S, Grodd W, Krägeloh-Mann I. Pyramidal tract damage correlates with motor dysfunction in bilateral periventricular leukomalacia (PVL). *Neuropediatrics* 2003; **34**: 182–8.

45. Koeda T, Takeshita K. Visuo-perceptual impairment and cerebral lesions in spastic diplegia with preterm birth. *Brain Dev* 1992; **14**: 239–44.

46. Peterson BS, Vohr B, Staib LH, *et al.* Regional brain volume abnormalities and long-term cognitive outcome in preterm infants. *JAMA* 2000; **284**: 1939–47.

47. Gunn A, Cory E, Atkinson J, *et al.* Dorsal and ventral stream sensitivity in normal development and hemiplegia. *Neuroreport* 2002; **13**: 843–7.

48. Pavlova M, Sokolov A, Birbaumer N, Krägeloh-Mann I. Biological motion processing in adolescents with early periventricular brain damage. *Neuropsychologia* 2006; **44**: 586–93.

Imaging the preterm brain

Terrie E. Inder, Russell K. Lawrence, and Jeffrey J. Neil

Introduction

The three major neuroimaging modalities used in the evaluation of the premature infant brain are cranial ultrasound (CUS), computed tomography (CT), and magnetic resonance imaging (MRI) – each of which has relative strengths and weaknesses. In this chapter, we will compare and contrast these methods with specific regard to their clinical utility in the evaluation of brain injury and altered brain development in the premature infant. A major focus of this chapter will be on MRI, since there have been many recent advances in the application of this methodology in the premature infant.

Due to the high incidence of neurodevelopmental disability in the premature infant, this patient population has a clear need for accurate and reliable neuroimaging. Imaging of the brain of the premature infant has at least two major aims. Firstly, to accurately define the nature of cerebral injury in this population for research purposes; and secondly, to determine the imaging features that most accurately predict adverse neurodevelopmental outcome. In addition to defining direct cerebral injury, recently developed neuroimaging techniques are now providing insight into alterations in structural and functional brain maturation associated with premature birth.

Five to 15% of prematurely born children develop cerebral palsy (CP), with an additional 30–50% displaying impaired academic achievement and/or behavioral disorders requiring additional educational resources [1–6]. To understand and apply potentially beneficial neuroprotective strategies in the neonatal intensive care unit (NICU), it is necessary to first establish the nature, timing, and location of the cerebral lesions predisposing premature infants to these long-term neurodevelopmental difficulties. In addition, accurate prognostic information before discharge from the hospital would be of high clinical utility by assisting in defining the need for continuing intervention strategies, such as physical therapy. With current conventional neuroimaging techniques, severely abnormal findings are moderately accurate for predicting an adverse outcome, particularly in relation to motor outcomes such as CP. However, there is less of a relationship between the findings of these conventional techniques and cognitive outcome in the premature infant, even when images are obtained later in life (e.g., see [7]). Newer MRI methods, including quantitative volumetric measurements and diffusion tensor imaging, may offer higher sensitivity to more subtle anatomic alterations. Thus, they have the potential to provide a better understanding of the anatomic substrate for the increased susceptibility for cognitive difficulties in this high-risk population.

There are several well-defined forms of cerebral injury with proven diagnostic significance that are routinely detected in the premature infant with current neuroimaging technologies. The most common form of cerebral injury currently detected with conventional neuroimaging, particularly CUS, is intraventricular hemorrhage (IVH) with an incidence of approximately 20% for all grades of IVH. The complications associated with IVH include posthemorrhagic hydrocephalus, periventricular hemorrhagic infarction [8], and an increased incidence of periventricular leukomalacia (PVL) [9–12]. Another common neuropathology is isolated PVL. This consists of necrosis of the white matter in a characteristic distribution dorsal and lateral to the external angles of the lateral ventricles, involving particularly the centrum semiovale (frontal horn and body), optic radiation (trigone and occipital horn), and acoustic radiation (temporal horn) [9]. The incidence of PVL varies in relation to its method of detection,

Neurodevelopmental Outcomes of Preterm Birth, ed. Chiara Nosarti, Robin M. Murray, and Maureen Hack. Published by Cambridge University Press. © Cambridge University Press 2010.

which will be discussed further. In autopsy studies of premature infants, it was found to differ between medical centers, ranging from 25% to 75%. Other major forms of neuropathology in the premature infant, less common than PVL, include selective neuronal injury and focal cerebral ischemic lesions.

Cranial ultrasound

Background

Ultrasound relies on the reflection of ultrasound waves from tissue to provide images. Its greatest advantage lies in its portability, as it is possible to image infants without moving them from the NICU. Cranial ultrasound images show the outline of the cerebral ventricles clearly, as the ventricles appear echolucent or dark as compared to adjacent white matter. Cranial ultrasound also has high sensitivity for detection of hemorrhage, which appears echogenic or bright. Thus, CUS is very useful for detection of intracranial hemorrhage and associated posthemorrhagic hydrocephalus. Cranial ultrasound is also used for detection of PVL, and a characteristic progression of imaging features has been described [9]. During the first week following injury, there are echogenic foci in the periventricular white matter due to local necrosis with congestion and/or hemorrhage. This is followed, during the ensuing one through three weeks, by the appearance of echolucent cysts, which correlates with cyst formation due to tissue dissolution. By two to three months, ventriculomegaly appears, often with disappearance of the cysts.

One of the disadvantages of CUS is that it provides relatively poor contrast for lesions of the brain parenchyma. Acute stroke, for example, can be difficult to detect with CUS as compared with CT and MRI [13]. In addition, since CUS images are typically obtained through the anterior fontanel, there is a limited field of view which does not "see" the cerebral convexities. Further, image detail in the posterior fossa, which is relatively far from the transducer, is often poor. This can be overcome by imaging through the posterior fontanel, which should be encouraged as a standard of practice. Acquisition and interpretation of CUS images are also more operator-dependent than CT or MRI, and quality can vary markedly from medical center to medical center. Finally, assessment of increased echodensity is subjective, though this could potentially be overcome by comparing the echodensity of the region of possible abnormality with that of a standard structure, such as the choroid plexus.

Correlation of image findings with outcome

Cranial ultrasound studies have been available for evaluation of premature infants for nearly 30 years. There is a relatively large literature describing associations between CUS findings and outcomes. Comparison of these studies is complicated by a variety of factors, some of the more prominent of which are differences in: (a) the timing and frequency of the head ultrasound studies obtained, (b) the technical quality of the ultrasound equipment used, (c) the technical skills of the ultrasonographers, and (d) the duration of time for which subjects were in clinical follow-up (more subtle neurodevelopmental abnormalities are not readily detected at younger ages). Nevertheless, the majority of studies suggest that 30–60% of premature infants who develop CP had lesions detected by CUS during the perinatal period (e.g., [14–17]). More recent studies include that of Vohr and coworkers [18], who reported the outcomes from extremely low birth weight infants born between 1993 and 1998 in the National Institute of Child Health and Human Development (NICHD) Neonatal Research Network. There was no specific CUS protocol in this study, which is recognized to limit the capability of CUS. After adjusting for numerous confounding variables, the authors found that cystic PVL (odds ratio [OR] = 10.5, 95% confidence interval [CI] = 7.2–15.2) and grade 3 or 4 IVH (OR = 2.4, 95% CI = 1.8–3.1) were strongly associated with moderate to severe CP. In the larger EPIPAGE study [19], infants 22–32 weeks' gestational age (GA) born in nine French regions during 1997 were followed to 2 years of age. Cranial ultrasound was obtained more frequently with one to three scans in the first two weeks, then every one to two weeks. White matter abnormalities, defined as prolonged echodensity, ventricular dilatation, or intraparenchymal hemorrhage or cyst, were associated with CP. Nearly 20% of children (n = 344) had a history of white matter abnormalities (18% of the total follow-up group), which was associated with a 25% risk of CP compared with 4% CP rate in the no abnormality group. Similar data were reported in the EPICure study for infants 20–26 weeks' GA born in 1995 where severe CUS abnormalities, defined as parenchymal hemorrhage, cystic changes, or ventricular dilatation on the last CUS, were associated with CP (OR = 4.95, 95% CI = 2.25–10.85), and severe motor disability (OR = 7.15, 95% CI = 2.73–18.74) [20].

A recently published study by DeVries *et al.* suggests that CUS may be more sensitive than previously believed [21]. In this study, preterm children underwent CUS studies weekly up to and including a scan at 40 weeks' postmenstrual age (PMA) (the latter scan was typically done as an outpatient). Children were followed for two years and evaluated for CP and cognitive difficulties. Ninety-two percent of children with CP had abnormalities found on CUS studies. These abnormalities were major (IVH with ventricular dilatation, hemorrhagic periventricular infarction, cystic PVL, subcortical leukomalacia, and basal ganglia lesions) in 83% and minor in 17%. Notably, CUS abnormalities were first detected after 28 days of life in 29% of infants with major abnormalities. Their data give a specificity of 95%, sensitivity of 76%, and positive predictive value of 48% for CUS detection of CP in infants ≤ 32 weeks' GA. Similar values were obtained for infants between 33 and 36 weeks' GA. The high sensitivity for CUS in this study as compared with the rest of the literature may be related to the fact that infants were scanned more regularly and for a longer period of time than in typical CUS studies. It is also possible that a high level of technical competence contributed to the high sensitivity, as Wheater and Rennie, performing weekly CUS studies and assessing children for CP at age 18 months, found CUS abnormalities in only 56% of children with CP [16].

Studies of later childhood outcomes have also found associations between severely abnormal CUS findings and neurodevelopmental sequelae [22]. Severe cognitive impairment also was related to PVL and/or ventricular enlargement [23], but the association was not significant after controlling for differences in motor ability and perinatal factors. In the Victorian Infant Cohort Study (VICS), follow-up at 8 years of age [24] demonstrated a linear relationship between increasing grade of IVH and rates of CP and neurosensory disability.

While the studies described above address the detection of motor disability (CP), studies have also been done to evaluate the sensitivity of CUS to cognitive disabilities. In general, CUS seems relatively insensitive for predicting children who will go on to have cognitive difficulties, particularly subtle ones [18–24].

Guidelines for the use of CUS

The frequency and duration for which CUS studies should be obtained in premature infants remains an area of controversy. It has been suggested that clinically stable premature infants do not need repeat screening CUS if they have two normal studies ≥ 7 days apart, though infants < 25 weeks' GA require an additional CUS study at the time of discharge [25]. The Quality Standards Subcommittee of the American Academy of Neurology and the Practice Committee of the Child Neurology Society recommend that infants be scanned at 7–14 days of age and again at 36–40 weeks' PMA [26]. In light of the findings of DeVries et al. [21] and the EPIPAGE study [19], which were not available at the time the practice parameter was developed, it seems likely that CUS is more sensitive for detecting injury if studies are obtained more frequently. Further, the window for the appearance of injury is longer than previously believed. As a result, it would be reasonable to obtain weekly CUS studies from birth to 32 weeks' PMA and a final study between 36 and 40 weeks' PMA. This guideline applies, of course, to clinically stable infants. Infants with clinical deterioration or alteration in neurological state may require more frequent imaging.

As noted above, CUS is also very useful for evaluating ventricular size. Posthemorrhagic ventricular dilatation (PHVD) is a relatively common complication of IVH and should be carefully monitored for following the detection of grade 2 or higher IVH. The incidence of adverse neurodevelopmental outcome following PHVD is high, and there is an increasing trend to earlier and more aggressive therapy for this condition to improve outcome [27,28]. At present, CUS images are typically evaluated qualitatively for ventricular size. While this strategy has proven useful, it would appear more informative to evaluate ventricular size in a quantitative fashion, based on established norms (e.g., [29]). Further, the occipital horn is the first and the frontal horn is the last to enlarge following IVH [30]. Thus, measurement of the thalamo-occipital dimension of the ventricle [29], via the posterior fontanel, is the earliest and most sensitive indicator of ventriculomegaly. Frequent CUS monitoring of the ventricular dimensions, particularly in the acute period, may assist in assessing the infant's course and determining the need for intervention with ventricular drainage. It may also guide the frequency and volume of cerebrospinal fluid (CSF) drainage necessary to decrease ventricular size.

Finally, there may be concerns over the reliability of the reporting of CUS. A recent retrospective analysis of CUS data assessed inter-observer reliability between two central readers, and accuracy of local compared with central readers (regarded as the "gold standards") [31]. The level of agreement between central readers was high for major CUS findings, such as grade 3 or 4 IVH and degree of ventriculomegaly (kappa = 0.84 and 0.75, respectively), but poor for lower grade IVH (kappa = 0.4) and for PVL alone. The sensitivity of local reader interpretation was also excellent for grade 3 or 4 IVH (88–92%), but was poor for grade 1 or 2 IVH (48–68%). These results, similar to the few previous large analyses in the literature [32–34], raise significant concerns about the validity of interpretations about mild to moderate hemorrhage by CUS. Thus, CUS may be a better predictive instrument with optimal and detailed protocols performed by highly skilled hands.

Computed tomography

Background

Computed tomography has been available for approximately 30 years. The method is based on passing an X-ray beam (ionizing radiation) through the sample at a series of different angles. Based on the attenuation of these beams, an image can be constructed using a method known as filtered back projection. Contrast in CT images is dependent on differing degrees of attenuation of X-rays by various structures. Bone, for example, causes a high degree of attenuation, and appears bright on CT images. Cerebrospinal fluid, on the other hand, causes a low degree of attenuation, appearing dark. Computed tomography provides excellent views of bone and is also very sensitive for the detection of hemorrhage, which appears bright. It allows differentiation of white and gray matter, though the contrast between these two types of tissue is relatively low in comparison with MRI. While it does not suffer the field-of-view difficulties associated with CUS, structures in the posterior fossa are relatively poorly demonstrated on CT because of non-uniform attenuation of X-ray energy by the bone at the base of the skull (beam-hardening artifact). Computed tomography scans usually require that the infant be removed from the ICU, which is a disadvantage as compared with CUS. On the other hand, the scan time is shorter than that of a typical MRI study. Further, the infant is more readily accessible while in the scanner, in the event of an emergency, than for an MR scan, though there is a trend in MR magnet design towards more open magnet configurations which provide better patient access.

A further issue for CT is the exposure of the infant brain to ionizing radiation. There are two main areas of concern related to this exposure – firstly, the risk of future malignancy and secondly, cognitive impairment. The adverse impact of cranial irradiation on brain and cognitive development following radiation treatment of brain tumors has been clearly shown and is dose related. However, the threshold value for the effect is not known. Recently, Hall et al. [35] suggested that even low doses of ionizing radiation, similar to those delivered by CT scans, may adversely affect brain and cognitive development. They found significant reductions in scores on tests for learning ability and cognitive reasoning for individuals who were exposed to > 100 mGy ionizing radiation for the treatment of cutaneous hemangioma before age 18 months. In a study of 20 000 Israeli children treated with cranial irradiation for tinea capitis, Ron et al. found poorer cognitive performance in irradiated children as compared with controls [36]. Currently, it is unclear what long-term effects, if any, low doses of cranial irradiation, such as those delivered during a cranial CT scan, may have when administered during infancy, a phase of rapid brain development. In relation to the risk of subsequent malignancy, a 0.1% risk of lifetime fatal malignancy from a head CT at age 12 months has been estimated [37]. However, the risk of tumor may be significantly greater with exposure at a younger age. The risk of development of brain tumor was found to be tenfold higher in infants exposed to cranial irradiation under 5 months of age in comparison to over 7 months of age [38]. While extrapolation of findings from cranial irradiation of children to head CT studies of premature infants must be regarded cautiously, the studies raise concerns about exposure to ionizing radiation during infancy. Further research would be necessary to accurately define the nature of any risk associated with CT scanning of the infant brain. Until such data are available, it is reasonable to restrict the use of this neuroimaging technique to selected settings in which the information obtained from the imaging study is clearly of immediate benefit to the patient.

Computed tomography scanning of the premature infant has been employed for detection of both hemorrhage and PVL. Although it is likely no more sensitive than CUS for detecting cystic PVL during the perinatal period, findings of reduced volume of periventricular white matter and ventriculomegaly with irregular outline of the lateral ventricles have been described in older children with clinical findings consistent with PVL (i.e., spastic diplegia) [39]. Computed tomography can also be used to detect stroke, though image contrast for non-hemorrhagic stroke is weak [40], particularly in comparison with MRI.

Correlation of image findings with outcome

There are relatively few studies correlating CT findings with outcome, and the majority of them are from the mid 1980s. In general, the correlations have not been especially strong. For example, there was no relationship found between neonatal CT and clinical outcome at age 18 months in a study of 145 children [41]. However, in a series of 45 infants imaged at 40 weeks' PMA, the finding of ventriculomegaly correlated with the presence of learning disabilities at school age [42].

Guidelines for the use of CT

Computed tomography scanning has not been demonstrated to add in the evaluation of the brain of the premature infant. Correlations between CT findings and outcome are weak, and similar information can be gleaned from CUS studies. In addition, the concerns regarding exposure to ionizing radiation must be considered. CT has a role in the rapid evaluation of the newborn infant with traumatic head injury following delivery in consideration of urgent neurosurgical intervention, but this situation is rarely encountered in preterm infants.

Magnetic resonance imaging
Background

Over the last several years the demand for MRI in neonates has increased. While relatively expensive, MRI offers several advantages when compared to other imaging modalities. Unlike CT, it does not involve ionizing radiation, making it relatively safer. It also offers a rich variety of tissue contrasts, providing tissue characterization superior to both CT and CUS. Preliminary studies suggest that MRI is more sensitive to subtle tissue injury than either CT or CUS [43–44]. However, MRI can also reflect a similar neuropathology as that of CUS, but gives the opportunity for additional information (Fig. 4.1). In addition, MRI can define alterations in cerebral development, including both global and regional reductions in cerebral growth. An understanding of alterations in the sequence of normal cerebral development, combined with or independent of cerebral injury, will likely render a greater understanding of the impact of preterm birth and neonatal intensive care therapies.

The signal from which MR images are derived arises from the ^{1}H atoms of water ([1]H$_2$O). The high concentration of ^{1}H in water provides a strong signal from which to obtain images. Other nuclei, such as [23]Na and ^{31}P, also provide MR signal, but their concentrations in the brain are on the order of tens of mM – roughly 10 000 times less than that of ^{1}H in water. While signals from these nuclei are detectable by MR spectroscopy, for which signal is obtained from a relatively large volume of brain, they are not strong enough to be used to obtain images of high spatial resolution. Though MR spectroscopy has been applied to evaluation of the neonate brain and has proven to have prognostic value in ischemic cerebral injury [45,46], this review will not cover MR spectroscopy in any detail. There is a need for greater systematic studies combining MR spectroscopy alongside the techniques reviewed in this chapter.

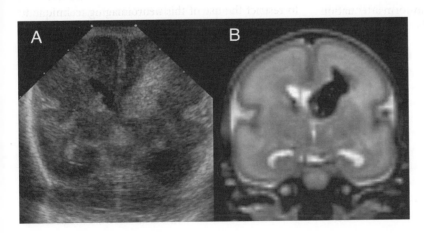

Fig. 4.1. Cranial ultrasound (A) and MRI (B) obtained within the same week in a preterm infant with grade 4 IVH. Note the similarity in the nature and extent of hemorrhage present on both imaging modalities. However, note that CUS has limitations in the visualization of the cortical neuronal boundaries.

Conventional MRI

Image contrast obtained in MR images is primarily the result of the different MR properties for the ¹H atoms of water residing in the different parts of the brain. Depending on the image acquisition conditions (or acquisition parameters), images with a variety of contrasts can be obtained. Two common forms of contrast are based on the T1 and T2 MRI characteristics of water (T1 and T2 represent different MR relaxation time constants, which will simply be referred to as "T1" and "T2" for this discussion). The T1 and T2 values differ for water in the tissue types of CSF, white matter, and gray matter, providing contrast for the images. For example, water in CSF has a relatively long T1, and thus appears dark on T1-weighted images. In T2 images, on the other hand, water in CSF looks bright relative to brain tissue. It can sometimes be difficult to distinguish injured brain from adjacent CSF-containing spaces on T2-weighted images. This is because both injured tissue and CSF appear bright. One means of compensating for this is the use of fluid-attenuated inversion recovery (FLAIR) imaging. In this case, an additional radio-frequency (RF) pulse is applied during image acquisition, serving to eliminate signal from CSF, making it appear dark on an otherwise T2-weighted image. In current clinical practice, T1-weighted, T2-weighted, and FLAIR images are usually obtained.

Diffusion MRI

Magnetic resonance images can also be obtained in which contrast is dependent on water displacement (diffusion-weighted imaging or DWI). With this method, water displacements on the order of 10 µm can be detected. The physical constant characterizing this water motion is called the "apparent" diffusion coefficient (ADC) in recognition of the fact that water displacements in tissue are influenced by factors other than simple Brownian motion, such as restrictions due to cell membranes. While one might not expect tissue water displacements to be especially useful for image contrast, diffusion-based MRI provides remarkably rich information about cerebral structure and its disruption. For example, water ADC values decrease within minutes after a variety of forms of tissue injury, including stroke [47]. As a result, diffusion-based MR images provide one of the earliest indicators of tissue injury, showing changes many hours to days before abnormalities are detectable with other forms of imaging.

There are a confusing variety of ways of obtaining and displaying diffusion images, including diffusion-weighted images and parametric maps. Typical diffusion-weighted images also contain contrast related to T2-weighting, an effect known as "T2 shine through" [48]. This effect is eliminated in parametric maps in which image intensity is directly related to quantitative ADC values (in units of $\mu m^2/ms$), simplifying image interpretation. It is worth noting that parametric maps and diffusion-weighted images often have opposite image intensity conventions – areas of low ADC values appear dark on parametric maps, but bright on diffusion-weighted images. When evaluating ADC image sets, one approach is to first assess CSF which, being almost pure water, has a high ADC value relative to brain. If CSF appears bright in the image set, then tissue with high ADC values will appear bright also. Conversely, if CSF appears dark, then tissue with high ADC values will also appear dark. In general, one is typically looking for areas of acute injury which have low ADC. These areas are most conspicuous on images displayed so that areas of low ADC are bright (i.e., CSF is dark).

Another form of contrast available with diffusion imaging is based on diffusion anisotropy. Anisotropy refers to the condition in which water ADC values differ depending upon the direction along which they are measured. In myelinated white matter, for example, water molecular displacements are smaller perpendicular to fibers than parallel to them because motion perpendicular to fibers requires passing through or around layers of myelin membrane, whereas motion parallel to them does not. Thus, water apparent diffusion in mature white matter is highly anisotropic. In this manner, diffusion imaging characterizes tissue microstructure. Two parameters related to diffusion anisotropy are particularly useful for microstructural characterization: the degree of anisotropy of water motion (e.g., relative anisotropy or RA) and the direction along which water apparent diffusion is greatest (the direction of the major eigenvector of the diffusion tensor). Relative anisotropy values approach zero for CSF, for which diffusion is isotropic and ADC values are equal in all directions. RA values are relatively high for myelinated white matter, for which ADC values are on the order of three times smaller for diffusion perpendicular to fibers as compared with parallel to them. For white matter, the direction along which water ADC values are greatest represents the primary orientation of myelinated fibers with an image voxel (remember that water displacements are greatest parallel to fibers). This information can be used for a form of "tract tracing" in which neural connections can be inferred [49]. For gray matter, the direction along which water ADC values are greatest reflects the radial organization of developing cortex [50]. Please also refer to Chapter 8 for further discussion on diffusion tensor imaging studies.

Volumetric measurements through MRI

Magnetic resonance imaging can be used to measure cerebral volumes. Images of different contrasts, such as T1-, T2-, and proton density-weighted, are analyzed to classify tissue as CSF, gray matter, or white matter in a process referred to as "segmentation" (Fig. 4.2). The number of image elements, or voxels, corresponding to each class can be summed to compute volumes in units of cm³. This can be achieved manually by outlining cerebral structures in each image or by semi- or fully automated techniques. There is not yet a consensus as to the optimal means of obtaining and comparing these volumes. While the techniques have proven useful to measure total intracranial volumes for tissue types, it is also desirable to evaluate volumes on a regional basis because injuries affecting cerebral volumes may preferentially affect some brain areas. One approach is to apply arbitrary boundaries for regions, similar to lines for latitude and longitude on a map [51]. Though this approach is fairly simple and relatively straightforward to implement, it tends to group brain regions of disparate function and physiology, such as brainstem and temporal lobe, in the same volume. It also may miss volume abnormalities that involve small brain regions that cross the border of adjacent areas chosen for analysis. A more sophisticated approach consists of applying statistical methods to compare the volume of the brain of interest with that of a "standard" brain on a voxel-by-voxel basis [52]. This method provides parametric maps of the regions for which volumes are statistically different, similar to the maps generated for functional MRI studies. There is also no agreement on how these volumes should be normalized. For example, should gray matter be expressed as an absolute volume (cm³), as a percentage of total brain volume, or as a percentage of intracranial volume? It might also be useful to express brain volumes in relation to PMA. Though the uncritical application of the volumetric approach has been unfavorably likened to phrenology [53], identification of areas of volume abnormality is an important step in identifying the anatomical substrate of brain injury in premature infants.

Brain metrics

While volumetric approaches hold much promise in the research setting, their integration into clinical care remains limited because of their complexity. Generating volumetric measurements is typically not fully automated and may require hours of operator input. Brain metrics, or the simple measurement of different anatomic regions of the brain from conventional MR images, offers a simple alternative technique for quantifying regional abnormalities. Using measurements obtained from fetal MRIs as a reference [54,55], clinicians can take simple, one-dimensional measurements of specific areas of the brain

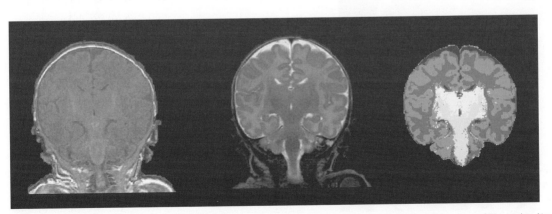

Fig. 4.2. An example of image segmentation for quantitative volumetric analysis. The image on the left is a coronal T1-weighted image. The image in the center is the corresponding T2-weighted image. The image on the right is the segmentation map derived from these MR images. Blue represents CSF, gray is gray matter, red is unmyelinated white matter, white is basal ganglia and thalamus, and yellow is myelinated white matter. This map can be used to determine relative volumes (in cm³) of these different tissue types. See plate section for color version.

(frontal lobes, cerebellum, sulcal distance) for comparison to gestational norms [56]. The measurement of simple brain metrics can be easily taught to a radiologist, neonatologist, or neurologist with minimal training and obtained using widely available image viewing packages. The application of these metrics in a large group of preterm (at term-equivalent PMA) and term control infants demonstrated that the bifrontal, biparietal (Fig. 4.3), and transverse cerebellar diameters were reduced (−11.6 %; 95% confidence interval[CI] = −13.8% to −9.3%; −12%, −14% to −9.8% and −8.7%, −10.5% to −7% respectively) and the left ventricle diameter was increased (+22.3%; 2.9% to 41.6%) in preterm infants (p< 0.01). The biparietal diameter was weakly related to immaturity at birth, although the most striking difference was observed between preterm and term infants (Fig. 4.3). Although one may wonder if this narrowing in biparietal diameter is related to the preterm scaphocephalic head shape, there was no difference in the fronto-occipital measures suggesting no narrowing but lengthening in the head shape. In comparison to tissue-segmented brain volumes, there were strong correlations between the bifrontal and biparietal measures and total brain tissue volume, while the size of the ventricles and interhemispheric measure correlated with CSF volume. Intra-observer reliability was high (interclass correction [ICC] > 0.7), while inter-observer agreement was acceptable for tissue measures (ICC > 0.6), but lower for fluid measures (ICC < 0.4) Thus, simple brain metrics at term-equivalent age showed smaller brain diameters and increased ventricle size in preterm infants when compared with full-term infants. These measures represent a reliable and easily applicable method to quantify brain growth and assess brain atrophy in this at-risk population.

Surface-based analyses of cerebral cortex

In adults, studies of cortical folding patterns and their variability across individuals and groups have been greatly aided by surface-based approaches. Surface-based analysis (cortical cartography) offers inherent advantages in terms of visualization (easier visualization of cortex buried in sulci), quantitative analysis (determination of cortical surface area), and comparison across individuals (surface-based registration as an alternative to conventional volume-based registration) [57–61]. Semiautomated methods for segmentation, surface-based analysis, and visualization have been critical to the success of these efforts. The power of this approach has been demonstrated in a recent study of Williams syndrome [62], which revealed 33 statistically significant cortical folding abnormalities compared to control subjects. Moreover, quantitative

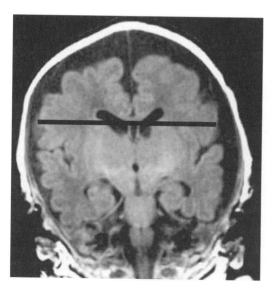

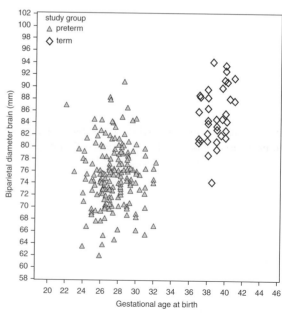

Fig. 4.3. Biparietal diameter on a coronal T1-weighted MR image of a preterm infant at term equivalent. The graph demonstrates the biparietal diameter (*y*-axis) against the gestational age at birth demonstrating a major difference in the diameter between preterm infants and term-born infants.

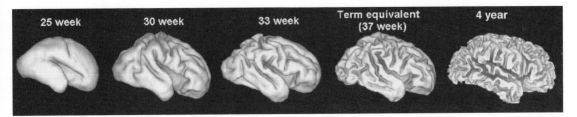

Fig. 4.4. Surface-based renderings of preterm infants from 25 weeks through 37 weeks. The majority of cortical folding is apparent by 37 weeks, particularly in comparison to later childhood at 4 years. This emphasizes the enormous changes in cortical morphometry occurring in the neonatal intensive care unit.

analyses of shape characteristics indicate that surface-based methods have diagnostic utility at the level of individual subjects. Folding abnormalities are also being explored in autistic spectrum disorder (ASD) using this approach.

In a similar manner, norms for sulcal and gyral development for infants from 30 to 40 weeks' PMA have been developed (Fig. 4.4). They have been used to identify unique features of altered cortical folding in premature infants with intrauterine growth restriction [63,64]. These studies illustrate the power of this approach in defining alterations of cerebral cortical development.

Functional MRI

Functional MRI (fMRI) offers a novel way to bridge the gap between injury seen on MRI in the preterm population and the deficiencies seen in neurodevelopmental follow-up. This imaging technique can be used to detect neural activation through its sensitivity to local oxyhemoglobin and deoxyhemoglobin levels. Neural activation is associated with a local reduction in deoxyhemoglobin level, which leads to an increase in signal intensity in the blood-oxygenation-level-dependent (BOLD) imaging method used for fMRI. This method is commonly used in studies in which the subjects are asked to perform a task. The BOLD images obtained with the subject resting and performing the task are subtracted to identify regions of activation associated with the task. Clearly, such an experimental paradigm is impractical for infants. However, a modification of fMRI, known as "functional connectivity" MRI (fcMRI), is applicable to infants. With this approach, spontaneous fluctuations in the BOLD signal during the resting state are measured. It has been shown that these spontaneous fluctuations have similar phases for regions of brain that are functionally connected [65]. In essence, this method shows neural networks. For example, if a seed point is placed in the leg motor

area, fcMRI shows a connection to the contralateral leg motor area, which is known to be connected via the corpus callosum. While fMRI during task activation has been studied in preterm infants at term and during childhood (review [66], see also Chapter 7), fcMRI offers great potential for the study of developing neural systems in the preterm population due to the fact that there is no need for cooperation with any task-related activity.

Practical issues

Obtaining an MRI in the preterm infant in a safe manner is a unique challenge to both the neonatology and radiology staff. Compared to ultrasound, MRI has the disadvantage of requiring that the infant be transported from the NICU to the scanner for study. The risk to the infant associated with transport out of the NICU has been ameliorated by the availability of MR-compatible, purpose-built transport isolettes. These devices include an MRI-compatible ventilator, support equipment for the infant, and the RF coil necessary for MR studies. The entire isolette can be placed in the MRI scanner for imaging. Once placed in such an isolette in the NICU, an infant can be taken to the scanner and left undisturbed until he/she returns to the NICU after the scan. These isolettes are now commercially available.

While many centers perform MRI studies with sedation, our center has a long experience in obtaining quality MRI in unsedated infants [67]. It is important to allow prep time in the NICU prior to taking the infant to the scanner. Infants should be fed between 30 and 45 minutes prior to the scan. The MRI-compatible pulse-oximetry probe should then be placed with confirmed adequate signal prior to wrapping. Ear protection (Minimuffs, Natus, San Carlos, CA) should also be placed to minimize distraction from noise. Patients are then wrapped snugly in 1–2 sheets and a vac-fix device, placed in the transport isolette, and allowed to settle for a period of time. Using this approach, infants are often sleeping by the time the transport team arrives at the MRI scanner, resulting in quality scans with very little motion artifact.

MRI findings and neurodevelopmental outcome

Magnetic resonance imaging of the premature infant brain has been available for approximately 20 years and remains an area of active research. The earliest studies used conventional MR imaging and focused on studies obtained after discharge from the hospital on patients for whom PVL had been diagnosed by CUS during the perinatal period. Areas of abnormal signal intensity in periventricular white matter, ventriculomegaly, varying degrees of cerebral atrophy, thinning of the corpus callosum, and delayed myelination have been described in children as old as 5 years [68,69]. These findings are common in prematurely born children [70,71] and suggest that MRI can be used to detect the sequelae of PVL in older children. However, MRI abnormalities consistent with PVL detected in prematurely born children at ages 8 [72] and 15–17 years [7] show only moderate correlation with cognitive and motor deficits. In contrast, abnormalities of visual pathways detected on MR images obtained in late infancy show strong correlation with visual impairment [73].

Conventional MRI studies obtained at term equivalent, near the time of discharge of the premature infant from the hospital, have prognostic significance. The presence of parenchymal lesions gave a sensitivity of 100% and specificity of 79% for motor abnormality in a study of 51 infants, 11 of whom had neurological deficits at follow-up [74]. The parenchymal lesions consisted of hemorrhage, changes consistent with PVL, infarction, and reduction in white matter volume. In a study of 167 very preterm infants (≤ 30 weeks' GA) moderate to severe cerebral white matter injury on term-equivalent MRI, whether cystic or diffuse in nature, was strongly predictive of cognitive delay (odds ratio[OR] = 3.6, 95% CI = 1.5–8.7), motor delay (OR = 10.3, 95% CI = 3.5–30.8), cerebral palsy (OR = 9.6; 95% CI = 3.2–28.3), and neurosensory impairment (OR = 4.2, 95% CI = 1.6–11.3) at 2 years of age [75]. In this study white matter injury was quantified from a composite scoring system compiling white matter signal abnormalities, periventricular white matter volume, presence of cystic abnormalities, ventricular dilatation, or thinning of the corpus callosum.

The clinical significance of more subtle white matter abnormalities such as diffuse excessive high signal intensities (DEHSI) remains more controversial. These high signal intensity lesions of the white matter extend from the immediate periventricular region into the adjacent periventricular and subcortical regions and are commonly detected on T2-weighted fast spin echo imaging. Diffuse excessive high signal intensities are present in the majority of preterm infants imaged at term equivalent while being absent in healthy term controls. Debate exists as to whether they represent a delayed form of maturation, or true pathology. Recent studies have shown that these white matter lesions correspond to diffuse quantitative abnormalities in diffusion measurements throughout the white matter implicating either axonal or oligodendrocyte injury [76,77]. Several studies have now linked these lesions with reduced developmental quotients at 18–24 months [78,79].

There has also been focus on abnormalities of the posterior limb of the internal capsule (PLIC) and outcome. Abnormal signal intensity in the PLIC on conventional imaging in term infants following hypoxic-ischemic injury correlates with adverse neurodevelopmental outcome [80]. In preterm infants with IVH and unilateral hemorrhagic parenchymal involvement, signal abnormalities in the PLIC on MRI studies obtained at term equivalent strongly predicted future hemiplegia [81]. Abnormalities of diffusion parameters of the PLIC also correlate with outcome. In term infants with hypoxic-ischemic encephalopathy, low values for ADC [82] predict poor outcome. For preterm infants imaged at term equivalent, low values for diffusion anisotropy [83] correlate with adverse outcome. It is likely that changes in the MRI properties of the PLIC reflect the effects of Wallerian degeneration of the corticospinal motor system as a consequence of gray and/or white matter injury [84,85].

Abnormalities in ADC are associated with adverse neurodevelopmental outcome. In a study of 12 term infants with hypoxic-ischemic encephalopathy, the presence of white matter abnormalities on diffusion imaging correlated with adverse outcome in infants followed for up to 11 months [86].

While the evaluation of ADC values is useful for detecting injury, measures of diffusion anisotropy have the potential to provide additional information regarding tissue microstructure. As noted above, diffusion anisotropy is present in both white and gray matter. For white matter, anisotropy values are relatively low until myelination takes place. For gray matter, diffusion anisotropy values are highest during early development and decrease during maturation. This is due to the radial organization of developing cortex which diminishes steadily up to term. To date, there have been relatively few studies of anisotropy in the injured premature brain. One small study found that decreases in fractional anisotropy (FA) over the internal capsule and the occipital white matter correlated with poor motor outcome by neurodevelopmental evaluation at 2 years' corrected GA [87]. Furthermore, alterations in white matter anisotropy have been described in infants with PVL and those who go on to develop spastic CP. In one provocative study Als *at al.* demonstrated that institution of the Newborn Individualized Developmental Care and Assessment Program (NIDCAP) program in a small cohort of patients resulted in increased RA in the internal capsule along with improved behavioral testing compared to premature controls at 9 months' corrected GA [88]. This demonstrates the potential for application of anisotropy measures as a biomarker to evaluate the short-term impact of potential neurological-based interventions. Anisotropy measures also show promise for providing prognostic information and likely will soon be integrated into clinical practice.

Magnetic resonance images can also be evaluated for tissue volumes. In general, prematurity and white matter injury are associated with reduced brain tissue and increased CSF volumes. Studies of former premature infants when they reach adolescence show reductions in overall brain volume and gray matter volume with an increase in lateral ventricular volume [89]. The presence of signal abnormalities in white matter of former premature infants evaluated at the age of 15 years was associated with reduced white matter volume [90]. Further, increased lateral ventricular size in this population is associated with cognitive and motor deficits [91]. The volumes of sensorimotor and midtemporal cortices were associated positively with full-scale, verbal, and performance IQ scores [92]. Thus, alterations in cerebral volumes have significant clinical correlates (see also Chapters 5 and 6).

Fewer studies have been obtained in which volumes are reported for premature infants imaged at term-equivalent PMA, and there are not yet any published studies that include clinical follow-up. Nevertheless, a variety of MRI abnormalities have been described. In infants with prior evidence of PVL by either CUS or MRI, there is a marked reduction in cerebral cortical gray matter volume as compared with either preterm infants without PVL or term control infants. This change is associated with a significant decrease in total myelinated white matter volume and an apparent compensatory increase in total CSF volume [93]. Further, studies indicate that gyral development is markedly immature in infants with evidence of white matter injury [94]. Thus, while there has been a strong focus on white matter injury in premature infants, these studies provide evidence for abnormalities in the development of cortical gray matter. It is not yet known whether these gray matter changes are a consequence of white matter injury or occur independently.

Functional MRI has been used to compare sensory, language, memory, and executive function between premature infants and term controls in subjects ranging from term-equivalent PMA to early adolescence. The technology, currently only used in a research context, offers fascinating clues as to how the premature brain adapts its neural networks following injury in order to maximize neurodevelopmental functioning. Studies have shown that premature infants studied at age 12 years have different patterns of activation when compared to their term counterparts in aspects of language processing, though they do not show any associated differences in performance scores [95]. Rushe *et al.* [96] studied six preterm infants with known corpus callosal thinning and compared their phonological processing skills at 16 years of age with six term controls. Their hypothesis was that the children with a history of corpus callosal thinning would display incomplete lateralization of language function to the left hemisphere. The BOLD signal response did indeed differ between the two groups, with activation in the left peristriate cortex, left cerebellum and right precuneus regions being reduced in the preterm infants along with an apparently compensatory increase in activation in the right precentral gyrus and superior frontal cortex. Despite these differences, there was no difference in the task performance score between the two groups. These variations in brain functional networks are not isolated to language function. Nosarti *et al.* [97] found similar alterations in activation in a population of preterm males tested at age 16 years compared to term controls in executive function tasks such as attention and inhibition. Again, despite these differences on imaging, both the preterm and term controls tested similarly in respect to overall graded task performance. These studies suggest the development of compensatory neural networks in response to injury in the premature brain that seem to preserve overall function through plasticity. In the future, fMRI may provide the key to understanding why some preterm infants are able to compensate for environmental stresses and preserve overall function while others develop significant neurodevelopmental delay (see also Chapter 7 for further discussion on fMRI studies).

Guidelines for the use of MRI

The use of MRI to evaluate the brain of premature infants is still a moving target in the sense that advanced diffusion, fcMRI, and volumetric methods are still under active investigation. However, MRI clearly has a role to play in evaluating premature infants today. When establishing MRI protocols for infants, it is important to note that brain water content is higher for infant brain than for older children, and T1 and T2 are consequently greater. Thus, it is critically important that the image acquisition parameters be optimized for greatest gray/white contrast-to-noise ratio for newborn infants and not simply taken from protocols employed for imaging older children. For evaluation of acute injury, diffusion images are particularly useful, as they show injury early as local decreases in ADC. For infants who have reached term-equivalent PMA, it is useful to obtain T1-weighted, T2-weighted, T2*-weighted (sensitive to hemorrhage) and diffusion images to evaluate the PLIC, as abnormalities in this region are strongly correlated with hemiparesis. In addition, modern MRI systems typically provide diffusion anisotropy maps which provide information regarding white matter integrity in other brain areas.

References

1. Hack M, Flannery DJ, Schluchter M, *et al*. Outcomes in young adulthood for very-low-birth-weight infants. *N Engl J Med* 2002; **346**(3): 149–57.

2. Hack M, Taylor HG, Klein N, Mercuri-Minich N. Functional limitations and special health care needs of 10- to 14-year-old children weighing less than 750 grams at birth. *Pediatrics* 2000; **106**(3): 554–60.

3. Hack M, Fanaroff AA. Outcomes of children of extremely low birthweight and gestational age in the 1990's. *Early Hum Dev* 1999; **53**(3): 193–218.

4. Saigal S, Szatmari P, Rosenbaum P, Campbell D, King S. Cognitive abilities and school performance of extremely low birth weight children and matched term control children at age 8 years: a regional study. *J Pediatr* 1991; **118**(5): 751–60.

5. Whitaker AH, Van Rossem R, Feldman JF, *et al*. Psychiatric outcomes in low-birth-weight children at age 6 years: relation to neonatal cranial ultrasound abnormalities. *Arch Gen Psychiatry* 1997; **54**(9): 847–56.

6. Whitfield MF, Grunau RV, Holsti L. Extremely premature (< or = 800 g) schoolchildren: multiple areas of hidden disability. *Arch Dis Child Fetal Neonatal Ed* 1997; **77**(2): F85–90.

7. Cooke RW, Abernethy LJ. Cranial magnetic resonance imaging and school performance in very low birth weight infants in adolescence. *Arch Dis Child Fetal Neonatal Ed* 1999; **81**(2): F116–21.

8. Guzzetta F, Shackelford GD, Volpe S, Perlman JM, Volpe JJ. Periventricular intraparenchymal echodensities in the premature newborn: critical determinant of neurological outcome. *Pediatrics* 1986; **78**(6): 995–1006.

9. Volpe JJ. *Neurology of the Newborn*, 4th edn. Philadelphia, PA: W.B. Saunders Company; 2001.

10. Armstrong DL, Sauls CD, Goddard-Finegold J. Neuropathologic findings in short-term survivors of intraventricular hemorrhage. *Am J Dis Child* 1987; **141**(6): 617–21.

11. Takashima S, Mito T, Houdou S, Ando Y. Relationship between periventricular hemorrhage, leukomalacia and brainstem lesions in prematurely born infants. *Brain Dev* 1989; **11**(2): 121–4.

12. Leviton A, Gilles F. Ventriculomegaly, delayed myelination, white matter hypoplasia, and "periventricular" leukomalacia: how are they related? *Pediatr Neurol* 1996; **15**(2): 127–36.

13. Golomb MR, Dick PT, MacGregor DL, Armstrong DC, DeVeber GA. Cranial ultrasonography has a low sensitivity for detecting arterial ischemic stroke in term neonates. *J Child Neurol* 2003; **18**(2): 98–103.

14. Stewart A, Kirkbride V. Very preterm infants at fourteen years: relationship with neonatal ultrasound brain scans and neurodevelopmental status at one year. *Acta Paediatr Suppl* 1996; **416**: 44–7.

15. O'Shea TM, Klinepeter KL, Dillard RG. Prenatal events and the risk of cerebral palsy in very low birth weight infants. *Am J Epidemiol* 1998; **147**(4): 362–9.

16. Wheater M, Rennie JM. Perinatal infection is an important risk factor for cerebral palsy in very-low-birthweight infants. *Dev Med Child Neurol* 2000; **42**(6): 364–7.

17. Nelson KB, Grether JK, Dambrosia JM, *et al*. Neonatal cytokines and cerebral palsy in very preterm infants. *Pediatr Res* 2003; **53**(4): 600–7.

18. Vohr BR, Wright LL, Poole WK, *et al*. NICHD Neonatal Research Network Follow-up Study (Neurodevelopmental outcomes of extremely low birth

weight infants < 32 weeks' gestation between 1993–1998). *Pediatrics* 2005; **116**(2): 635–43.

19. Ancel P-Y, Livinec F, Larroque B, *et al.* Cerebral palsy among very preterm children in relation to gestational age and neonatal ultrasound abnormalities: The EPIPAGE Cohort Study. *Pediatrics* 2006; **117**(3): 828–35.

20. Wood NS, Costeloe K, Gibson AT, *et al.* The EPICure study: associations and antecedents of neurological and developmental disability at 30 months of age following extremely preterm birth. *Arch Dis Child Fetal Neonatal Ed* 2005; **90**(2): F134–40.

21. De Vries LS, Van Haastert IL, Rademaker KJ, Koopman C, Groenendaal F. Ultrasound abnormalities preceding cerebral palsy in high-risk preterm infants. *J Pediatr* 2004; **144**(6): 815–20.

22. Pinto-Martin JA, Whitaker AH, Felman JF, *et al.* Relation of cranial ultrasound abnormalities in low-birthweight infants to motor or cognitive performance at 2, 6, and 9 years. *Dev Med Child Neurol* 1999; **41**(12): 826–33.

23. Whitaker AH, Feldman JF, Van Rossem R, *et al.* Neonatal cranial ultrasound abnormalities in low birth weight infants: relation to cognitive outcomes at six years of age. *Pediatrics* 1996; **98**(4 pt 1): 719–29.

24. Sherlock RL, Anderson PJ, Doyle LW, *et al.* Neurodevelopmental sequelae of intraventricular hemorrhage at 8 years of age in a regional cohort of ELBW/very preterm infants. *Early Hum Dev* 2005; **81**(11): 909–16.

25. Nwafor-Anene VN, DeCristofaro JD, Baumgart S. Serial head ultrasound studies in preterm infants: how many normal studies does one infant need to exclude significant abnormalities? *J Perinatol* 2003; **23**(2): 104–10.

26. Ment LR, Bada HS, Barnes P, *et al.* Practice parameter: neuroimaging of the neonate: report of the Quality Standards Subcommittee of the American Academy of Neurology and the Practice Committee of the Child Neurology Society. *Neurology* 2002; **58**(12): 1726–38.

27. Whitelaw A, Pople I, Cherian S, Evans D, Thoresen M. Phase 1 trial of prevention of hydrocephalus after intraventricular hemorrhage in newborn infants by drainage, irrigation, and fibrinolytic therapy. *Pediatrics* 2003; **111**(4 Pt 1): 759–65.

28. Whitelaw A, Cherian S, Thoresen M, Pople I. Posthaemorrhagic ventricular dilatation: new mechanisms and new treatment. *Acta Paediatr Suppl* 2004; **93**(444): 11–14.

29. Davies MW, Swaminathan M, Chuang SL, Betheras FR. Reference ranges for the linear dimensions of the intracranial ventricles in preterm neonates. *Arch Dis Child Fetal Neonatal Ed* 2000; **82**(3): F218–23.

30. Allan WC, Holt PJ, Sawyer LR, Tito AM, Meade SK. Ventricular dilation after neonatal periventricular-intraventricular hemorrhage. Natural history and therapeutic implications. *Am J Dis Child* 1982; **136**(7): 589–93.

31. Hintz SR, Slovis T, Bulas D, *et al.* Interobserver reliability and accuracy of cranial ultrasound interpretation in premature infants. *J Pediatr* 2007; **150**(6): 592–6.

32. O'Shea, Volberg F, Dillard RG. Reliability of interpretation of cranial ultrasound examinations of very low-birthweight neonates. *Dev Med Child Neurol* 1993; **35**(2): 97–101.

33. Pinto JA, Paneth N, Kazam E, *et al.* Interobserver variability in neonatal cranial ultrasonography. *Paediatr Perinat Epidemiol* 1988; **2**(1): 43–58.

34. Corbett SS, Rosenfeld CR, Laptook AR, *et al.* Intraobserver and interobserver reliability in assessment of neonatal cranial ultrasounds. *Early Hum Dev* 1991; **27**(1–2): 9–17.

35. Hall P, Adami HO, Trichopoulos D, *et al.* Effect of low doses of ionising radiation in infancy on cognitive function in adulthood: Swedish population based cohort study. *BMJ* 2004; **328**(7430): 19.

36. Ron E, Modan B, Floro S, Harkedar I, Gurewitz R. Mental function following scalp irradiation during childhood. *Am J Epidemiol* 1982; **116**(1): 149–60.

37. Brenner DJ, Doll R, Goodhead DT, *et al.* Cancer risks attributable to low doses of ionizing radiation: assessing what we really know. *Proc Natl Acad Sci U S A* 2003; **100**(24): 13761–6.

38. Karlsson P, Holmberg E, Lundell M, *et al.* Intracranial tumors after exposure to ionizing radiation during infancy: a pooled analysis of two Swedish cohorts of 28,008 infants with skin hemangioma. *Radiat Res* 1998; **150**(3): 357–64.

39. Flodmark O, Roland E, Hill A, Whitfield M. Radiologic diagnosis of periventricular leukomalacia. *Acta Radiol Suppl* 1986; **369**: 664–6.

40. De Vries LS, Regev R, Connell JA, Bydder GM, Dubowitz LM. Localized cerebral infarction in the premature infant: an ultrasound diagnosis correlated with computed tomography and magnetic resonance imaging. *Pediatrics* 1988; **81**(1): 36–40.

41. Fitzhardinge PM, Flodmark O, Fitz CR, Ashby S. The prognostic value of computed tomography of the brain in asphyxiated premature infants. *J Pediatr* 1982; **100**(3): 476–81.

42. Ishida A, Nakajima W, Arai H, *et al.* Cranial computed tomography scans of premature babies predict their eventual learning disabilities. *Pediatr Neurol* 1997; **16**(4): 319–22.

43. Inder T, Anderson N, Spencer C, Wells S, Volpe J. White matter injury in the premature infant: a comparison

between serial cranial ultrasound and MRI at term. *AJNR Am J Neuroradiol* 2003: **24**(5): 805–9.

44. Miller SP, Cozzio CC, Goldstein RB, *et al.* Comparing the diagnosis of white matter injury in premature newborns with serial MR imaging and transfontanel ultrasonography findings. *AJNR Am J Neuroradiol* 2003; **24**(8): 1661–9.

45. Roth SC, Edwards AD, Cady EB, *et al.* Relation between cerebral oxidative metabolism following birth asphyxia, and neurodevelopmental outcome and brain growth at one year. *Dev Med Child Neurol* 1992; **34**(4): 285–95.

46. Penrice J, Cady EB, Lorek A, *et al.* Proton magnetic resonance spectroscopy of the brain in normal preterm and term infants, and early changes after perinatal hypoxia-ischemia. *Pediatr Res* 1996; **40**(1): 6–14.

47. Moseley ME, Cohen Y, Mintorovitch J, *et al.* Early detection of regional cerebral ischemia in cats: Comparison of diffusion- and T2-weighted MRI and spectroscopy. *Magn Reson Med* 1990; **14**(2): 330–46.

48. Burdette JH, Elster AD, Ricci PE. Acute cerebral infarction: quantification of spin-density and T2 shine-through phenomena on diffusion-weighted MR images. *Radiology* 1999; **212**(2): 333–9.

49. Mori S, van Zijl PC. Fiber tracking: principles and strategies – a technical review. *NMR Biomed* 2002; **15**(7–8): 468–80.

50. McKinstry RC, Mathur A, Miller JP, *et al.* Radial organization of developing human cerebral cortex revealed by non-invasive water diffusion anisotropy MRI. *Cereb Cortex* 2002; **12**(12): 1237–43.

51. Peterson BS, Vohr B, Staib LH, *et al.* Regional brain volume abnormalities and long-term cognitive outcome in preterm infants. *JAMA* 2000; **284**(15): 1939–47.

52. Sowell ER, Thompson PM, Holmes CJ, *et al.* Localizing age-related changes in brain structure between childhood and adolescence using statistical parametric mapping. *Neuroimage* 1999; **9**(6 Pt 1): 587–97.

53. Mink JW, McKinstry RC. Volumetric MRI in autism: can high-tech craniometry provide neurobiological insights? *Neurology* 2002; **59**(2): 158–9.

54. Garel C. The role of MRI in the evaluation of the fetal brain with an emphasis on biometry, gyration and parenchyma. *Pediatr Radiol* 2004; **34**(9): 694–9. Epub 2004 Jul 28. Review.

55. Garel C. *MRI of the Fetal Brain.* Berlin, New York: Springer; 2004.

56. Nguyen The Tich S, Anderson PJ, Shimony JS, *et al.* A novel quantitative simple brain metric using MR imaging for preterm infants. *AJNR AM J Neuroradiol* 2009; **30**(1): 125–31.

57. Drury HA, Van Essen DC, Anderson CH, *et al.* Computerized mappings of the cerebral cortex: a multiresolution flattening method and a surface-based coordinate system. *J Cogn Neurosci* 1996; **8**(1): 1–28.

58. Fischl B, Sereno MI, Dale AM. Cortical surface-based analysis. II: Inflation, flattening, and a surface-based coordinate system. *Neuroimage* 1999; **9**(2): 195–207.

59. Van Essen DC. Towards a quantitative, probabilistic neuroanatomy of cerebral cortex. *Cortex* 2004; **40**(1): 211–12.

60. Toga AW, Thompson PM, Sowell ER. Mapping brain maturation. *Trends Neurosci* 2006; **29**(3): 148–59.

61. Van Essen DC. A Population-Average, Landmark- and Surface-based (PALS) atlas of human cerebral cortex. *Neuroimage* 2005; **28**(3): 635–62.

62. Van Essen DC, Dierker D, Snyder AZ, *et al.* Symmetry of cortical folding abnormalities in Williams syndrome revealed by surface-based analyses. *J Neurosci* 2006; **26**(20): 5470–83.

63. Dubois J, Benders M, Borradori-Tolsa C, *et al.* Primary cortical folding in the human newborn: an early marker of later functional development *Brain* 2008; **131** (pt 8): 2028–41.

64. Dubois J, Benders M, Cachia A, *et al.* Mapping the early cortical folding process in the preterm newborn brain *Cereb Cortex* 2008; **18**(6): 1444–54.

65. Fair DA, Cohen AL, Dosenbach NU, *et al.* The maturing architecture of the brain's default network. *Proc Natl Acad Sci U S A* 2008; **105**(10): 4028–32.

66. Ment LR, Constable RT. Injury and recovery in the developing brain: evidence from functional MRI studies of prematurely born children. *Nat Clin Pract Neurol* 2007; **3**(10): 558–71.

67. Mathur AM, Neil JJ, McKinstry RC, Inder TE. Transport, monitoring, and successful brain MR imaging in unsedated neonates. *Pediatr Radiol* 2008; **38**(3): 260–4.

68. De Vries LS, Connell JA, Dubowitz LM, *et al.* Neurological, electrophysiological and MRI abnormalities in infants with extensive cystic leukomalacia. *Neuropediatrics* 1987; **18**(2): 61–6.

69. Flodmark O, Lupton B, Li D, *et al.* MR imaging of periventricular leukomalacia in childhood. *AJR Am J Roentgenol* 1989; **152**(3): 583–90.

70. Barkovich AJ, Truwit CL. Brain damage from perinatal asphyxia: correlation of MR findings with gestational age. *AJNR Am J Neuroradiol* 1990; **11**(6): 1087–96.

71. Truwit CL, Barkovich AJ, Koch TK, Ferriero DM. Cerebral palsy: MR findings in 40 patients. *AJNR Am J Neuroradiol* 1992; **13**(1): 67–78.

72. Olsén P, Pääkkö E, Vainionpää L, Pythinen J, Jarvelin M-J. Magnetic resonance imaging of periventricular leukomalacia and its clinical correlation in children. *Ann Neurol* 1997; **41**(6): 754–61.

73. Lanzi G, Fazzi E, Uggetti C, *et al.* Cerebral visual impairment in periventricular leukomalacia. *Neuropediatrics* 1998; **29**(3): 145–50.

74. Valkama AM, Pääkkö EL, Vainionpää LK, *et al.* Magnetic resonance imaging at term and neuromotor outcome in preterm infants. *Acta Paediatr* 2000; **89**(3): 348–55.

75. Woodward LJ, Anderson PJ, Austin NC, Howard K, Inder TE. Neonatal MRI to predict neurodevelopmental outcomes in preterm infants. *N Engl J Med* 2006; **355**(7): 685–94

76. Counsell SJ, Allsop JM, Harrison MC, *et al.* Diffusion-weighted imaging of the brain in preterm infants with focal and diffuse white matter abnormality. *Pediatrics* 2003; **112**(1 Pt 1): 1–7.

77. Counsell SJ, Shen Y, Boardman JP, *et al.* Axial and radial diffusivity in preterm infants who have diffuse white matter changes on magnetic resonance imaging at term-equivalent age. *Pediatrics* 2006; **117**(2): 376–86.

78. Dyet LE, Kennea N, Counsell SJ, *et al.* Natural history of brain lesions in extremely preterm infants studied with serial magnetic resonance imaging from birth and neurodevelopmental assessment. *Pediatrics* 2006; **118**(2): 536–48.

79. Domizio S, Barbante E, Puglielli C, *et al.* Excessively high magnetic resonance signal in preterm infants and neuropsychobehavioural follow-up at 2 years. *Int J Immunopathol Pharmacol* 2005; **18**(2): 365–75.

80. Rutherford MA, Pennock JM, Counsell SJ, *et al.* Abnormal magnetic resonance signal in the internal capsule predicts poor neurodevelopmental outcome in infants with hypoxic-ischemic encephalopathy. *Pediatrics* 1998; **102**(2 Pt 1): 323–8.

81. De Vries LS, Groenendaal F, van Haastert IC, *et al.* Asymmetrical myelination of the posterior limb of the internal capsule in infants with periventricular haemorrhagic infarction: an early predictor of hemiplegia. *Neuropediatrics* 1999; **30**(6): 314–19.

82. Hunt RW, Neil JJ, Coleman LT, Kean MJ, Inder TE. Apparent diffusion coefficient in the posterior limb of the internal capsule predicts outcome following perinatal asphyxia. *Pediatrics* 2004; **114**(4): 999–1003.

83. Arzoumanian Y, Mirmiran M, Barnes PD, *et al.* Diffusion tensor brain imaging findings at term-equivalent age may predict neurologic abnormalities in low birth weight preterm infants. *AJNR Am J Neuroradiol* 2003; **24**(8): 1646–53.

84. Mazumdar A, Mukherjee P, Miller JH, Malde H, McKinstry RC. Diffusion-weighted imaging of acute corticospinal tract injury preceding Wallerian degeneration in the maturing human brain. *AJNR Am J Neuroradiol* 2003; **24**(6): 1057–66.

85. Neil JJ, Inder TE. Detection of wallerian degeneration in a newborn by diffusion magnetic resonance imaging (MRI). *J Child Neurol* 2006; **21**(2): 115–18.

86. Johnson AJ, Lee BC, Lin W. Echoplanar diffusion-weighted imaging in neonates and infants with suspected hypoxic-ischemic injury: correlation with patient outcome. *AJR Am J Roentgenol* 1999; **172**(1): 219–26.

87. Drobyshevsky A, Bregman J, Storey P, *et al.* Serial diffusion tensor imaging detects white matter changes that correlate with motor outcome in premature infants. *Dev Neurosci* 2007; **29**(4–5): 289–301.

88. Als H, Duffy FH, McAnulty GB, *et al.* Early experience alters brain function and structure. *Pediatrics* 2004; **113**(4): 846–51

89. Nosarti C, Al-Asady MH, Frangou S, *et al.* Adolescents who were born very preterm have decreased brain volumes. *Brain* 2002; **125**(Pt 7): 1616–23.

90. Panigrahy A, Barnes PD, Robertson RL, *et al.* Volumetric brain differences in children with periventricular T2-signal hyperintensities: a grouping by gestational age at birth. *AJR Am J Roentgenol* 2001; **177**(3): 695–702.

91. Melhem ER, Hoon AH, Jr., Ferrucci JT, Jr., *et al.* Periventricular leukomalacia: relationship between lateral ventricular volume on brain MR images and severity of cognitive and motor impairment. *Radiology* 2000; **214**(1): 199–204.

92. Petersen BS, Vohr B, Staib LH, *et al.* Regional brain volume abnormalities and long term cognitive outcome in preterm infants. *JAMA* 2000; **284**(15): 1939–47.

93. Inder TE, Huppi PS, Warfield S, *et al.* Periventricular white matter injury in the premature infant is followed by reduced cerebral cortical gray matter volume at term. *Ann Neurol* 1999; **46**(5): 755–60.

94. Inder TE, Wells SJ, Mogridge NB, Spencer C, Volpe JJ. Defining the nature of the cerebral abnormalities in the premature infant: a qualitative magnetic resonance imaging study. *J Pediatr* 2003; **143**(2): 171–9.

95. Ment LR, Peterson BS, Meltzer JA, *et al.* A functional magnetic resonance imaging study of the long-term influences of early indomethacin exposure on language processing in the brains of prematurely born children. *Pediatrics* 2006; **118**(3): 961–70

96. Rushe TM, Temple CM, Rifkin L, *et al.* Lateralisation of language function in young adults born very preterm. *Arch Dis Child Fetal Neonatal Ed* 2004; **89**(2): F112–18.

97. Nosarti C, Rubia K, Smith AB, *et al.* Altered functional neuroanatomy of response inhibition in adolescent males who were born very preterm. *Dev Med Child Neurol* 2006; **48**(4): 265–71.

Structural magnetic resonance imaging

Richard W. I. Cooke

Introduction

It has been long recognized that the survivors of very preterm birth and very low birth weight (VLBW) have a relatively high prevalence of major neurodevelopmental sequelae in childhood years. Early major motor problems such as cerebral palsy and later cognitive, behavioral, and minor motor impairments have all been extensively described [1]. While cranial ultrasound examination immediately after birth has been demonstrated to be successful in predicting major motor difficulties at school age with some accuracy, it has proved much less useful in studying the origins of lesser impairments, and is of little value outside the neonatal period (see also Chapters 3 and 4). The increasing use of magnetic resonance imaging (MRI) of the head, as a research tool in childhood during the last two decades, together with long-term follow-up and assessments, has considerably increased our understanding of brain development after preterm birth.

Whilst early use of MRI often necessitated long acquisition times, more powerful magnetic fields in modern scanners have enabled, at least in older children, more rapid imaging to be achieved with minimal or no sedation. In addition, more recent techniques such as diffusion-weighted imaging, functional MRI, vascular MRI, and tractometry have greatly increased the types of information that can be obtained.

Published studies have concentrated on area or volume measurements of whole brain and specific areas of the brain such as the caudate nucleus, cerebellum, hippocampus, or cortical regions, and correlated these with behavioral, cognitive or motor outcomes. Others have looked at the long-term effects of neonatal management on later outcomes and MRI appearances. Examples of this are postnatal corticosteroid therapy, indomethacin, and so-called developmental care. A few studies have used MRI to look at longitudinal brain growth in relation to neurodevelopmental outcome, and these are described in detail in Chapter 6.

Quantitative MRI of the preterm brain

Total brain size and gross anatomical subdivisions

Mean fronto-occipital head circumference is generally smaller in ex-preterm individuals in childhood when compared with their term-born peers, and is reflected in lower IQ scores [2]. As head circumference is strongly related to brain volume, it is not surprising that MRI studies of cross-sectional area or total brain volume have shown a lower mean brain size in children born preterm compared to controls. Peterson *et al.* in 2000 published values for regional brain volumes in 25 8-year-old preterm children and 39 term controls [3]. The preterm children had been born weighing between 600 and 1250 g, and were part of a cohort recruited to an intraventricular hemorrhage prevention trial. Significant differences, mostly reductions, in regional brain volumes were seen between preterm children and controls for most regions examined. For some regions, these differences were dissimilar for right and left sides of the brain. For example, reductions of 11.2% (left) and 12.6% (right) were seen for the premotor region, 14.6% (left) and 14.3% (right) for the sensorimotor region, but 7.4% (left) and 10.2% (right) for the mid temporal region. The authors concluded that preterm birth was associated with a regionally specific and long-term reduction in brain volumes.

A similar study of 73 preterm individuals and 33 term controls, aged between 7.3 and 11.4 years, examined gray and white matter volumes separately in several cortical regions [4]. The cohort of preterm infants, of birth weights 600–1250 g, had been drawn from the same follow-up programme as the previous study.

Neurodevelopmental Outcomes of Preterm Birth, ed. Chiara Nosarti, Robin M. Murray, and Maureen Hack. Published by Cambridge University Press. © Cambridge University Press 2010.

Magnetic resonance imaging showed disproportionately enlarged parietal and frontal gray matter, as well as reduced temporal and subcortical gray matter volumes. Parietal and frontal gray matter volumes were lower in those preterm infants who were the most premature or had suffered intraventricular hemorrhage in the neonatal period. Although statistically significant, the overall changes were small; +2.2% in the frontal, +4.5% in the parietal, and −4.5% in the temporal lobe volumes. The authors concluded that preterm birth may be associated with disorganized cortical development, possibly involving disrupted synaptic pruning and neural migration.

In addition to reduction in overall cortical tissue with particular vulnerability in the temporal lobe, cortical gyrification index in very preterm-born control children at 8 years was significantly increased in the temporal lobe bilaterally compared with term controls [5]. These findings are consistent with studies of cortical surface area in preterm infants, reporting significant associations with brain volumes and reduced values compared to controls [6,7].

Structural brain differences seem to persist into adolescence and in a study of 87 VLBW individuals at 15–17 years, both coronal and transverse cross-sectional areas of the brain were smaller when compared with term controls. These differences averaged 7% in coronal and 12% in transverse sections [2]. A similar study using volumetric analysis in 72 very preterm 14- to 15-year-old children showed broadly similar findings, in that an average decrease of 6% in whole brain, and nearly 11.8% in cortical gray matter, was observed [8].

Cerebral asymmetry has been long recognized, and extends to individual lobes, other cortical subdivisions, and the brain as a whole. It can be observed as early as 20 weeks of gestation. This generally results in a larger right frontal lobe and a larger left occipital lobe in normative samples. Diminished or reversed asymmetry has been observed in autism and adult-onset schizophrenia [9]. To test whether such a change in normal asymmetry occurred following preterm birth, Lancefield *et al.* examined 61 14-year-olds who had been born at less than 33 weeks' gestation and a term control group [10]. They estimated cerebral regional volumes, and computed asymmetry indices, controlling for confounding variables. No significant differences were found, suggesting that preterm birth is unlikely to cause deviation in the development of normal fronto-occipital asymmetry.

The sex of the preterm infant appears to influence the degree of this reduction of brain size. When gray and white matter volumes were estimated at 8 years in 65 very preterm children compared with term controls, significant reduction in both gray and white matter were seen [11]. The reduction in white matter seen was, however, only significant in the males. Reduction in white matter volumes correlated with lower birth weight in both males and females, whereas gray matter volume was reduced only in girls who had suffered intraventricular hemorrhage. Results from the same group investigating a sample of 12-year-old children with no evidence of intraventricular hemorrhage or cystic periventricular leukomalacia on neonatal ultrasound, showed significantly lower white matter volumes in cingulum, corpus callosum, corticospinal tract, prefrontal cortex, and superior and inferior longitudinal fasciculi in preterm boys only compared to controls. Gray matter volumes in prefrontal cortex, basal ganglia, and temporal lobe were also significantly reduced in preterm boys only [12]. These findings suggest that the sex of a preterm infant influences the response to perinatal adversity. There is some evidence that boys who were born with a VLBW are at increased risk of developing neurodevelopmental morbidity compared to girls [13], although the cellular and molecular mechanisms underpinning these findings have yet to be established.

With improved quantitative MRI methods more detailed studies of specific brain regions have been made.

The lateral cerebral ventricles

Enlargement of the lateral ventricles is frequently seen in preterm infants in the early neonatal period, and is usually associated with intraventricular hemorrhage. In the majority of cases it is transient and probably related to a temporary disturbance in the reabsorbtion of cerebrospinal fluid. A few infants develop permanent hydrocephaly, but a much larger number develop a generalized ventricular enlargement in early infancy which in most cases persists into later childhood. Kesler *et al.* reported a mean ventricular volume of 15 cm³ in their preterm group compared with 7.5 cm³ in controls at 7–14 years of age [4].

Increased cerebral ventricular size has been also reported in preterm adolescent samples. Stewart *et al.* observed a 44% incidence of ventricular enlargement in a comparable cohort of 72 preterm (less than 33 weeks) survivors at 14 years of age [14], while 28% of a group of VLBW infants imaged at 15–17 years were reported as having ventricular enlargement [2]. In both cases, the diagnosis of ventricular enlargement was made by qualitative observation rather than measurement. Nosarti *et al.* reporting on a subset of the Stewart *et al.*'s 1999 cohort, again in adolescence, showed a mean increase of 42% in mean ventricular volumes over term controls (22.39 vs. 9.46 cm³) [8]. When sub-regions of the ventricle were considered, however, no group differences were observed for the frontal horns, but there were significant differences for the midbody, temporal, and occipital horns [3]. Peterson *et al.* later describe similar findings in their preterm cohort scanned near term [15]. The enlargement of the ventricles in these studies is assumed to be mainly due to loss of subcortical tissue, the greater degree of enlargement in the posterior body and occipital horns corresponding with a greater degree of subcortical loss in those regions [4]. This loss is probably associated with diffuse periventricular leukomalacia which is prevalent in this region of the brain in the neonatal period.

Cerebellum

Until recently, despite its importance in motor coordination, the cerebellum has been measured rather less often with MRI than other regions of the preterm brain. Mean volumes of 117.1 cm³ at 8 years have been reported in preterm-born children compared with 125.5 cm³ in term controls, a reduction of 6.7% [3]. Allin *et al.* also reported similar values in adolescence, a mean cerebellar volume of 135 cm³ in preterm-born individuals compared with 147 cm³ in controls, a difference of 8% [16].

Recent studies in the neonatal period using serial MRI measurements have shown that the rate of growth from 28 weeks to term in the mean cerebellar volume is 177% compared with 107% for mean brain volume [17]. This rate of growth was seriously affected by preterm birth and associated brain lesions, even in the absence of direct cerebellar injury, and the authors suggest that the long-term disabilities seen in many children born preterm may be attributable to impaired cerebellar development. Argyropoulou *et al.* have shown that very preterm infants at term equivalent and with periventricular leukomalacia have a very much reduced mean cerebellar volume of 68.2 cm³ compared with 100.6 cm³ in term controls [18]. It is therefore likely that altered cerebellar development starts from the time of preterm birth, although at term-equivalent age in the absence of white matter damage cerebellar volumes do not seem to be decreased in preterm-born infants [19].

In adolescence, differences in cerebellar subdivisions are still evident. Allin *et al.* [16] measured midline and lateral cerebellar volumes from 67 very preterm children at 14–15 years and compared them with 50 full-term controls at the same age. They found that the volumes of the vermis and lateral lobes were reduced in the preterm group even after controlling for overall reduced brain volume. The reduction in lateral cerebellar volumes was associated with reduced cerebral white matter volumes and with tests of executive, visuospatial, and language function. Reductions in the volumes of the vermis were less strongly related to cognitive function.

Corpus callosum

The corpus callosum is the largest white matter structure in the brain and connects the right and left cerebral hemispheres. Much of the interhemispheric communication of the brain is conducted across the corpus callosum. Because of its position relative to the lateral ventricles, particularly the posterior area of the splenium, it is very vulnerable to injury through periventricular leukomalacia [20].

Descriptive studies of the MRI appearances of the corpus callosum in children born very prematurely emphasize the frequency and extent of lesions, which appear to be greater when preterm birth is accompanied by other medical complications. Rademaker *et al.* [21] studied 7–8-year-old preterm-born children (weight < 1500 g) and controls; a subgroup of the preterm children had a diagnosis of cerebral palsy. The mean total cross-sectional callosal area was significantly smaller in preterm-born individuals compared with their term-born peers. The preterm children with cerebral palsy had significantly smaller mean callosal areas compared with the preterm children without cerebral palsy. However, the preterm children without cerebral palsy had significantly smaller body, posterior, and total callosal areas compared with controls [21].

Growth rates of corpus callosum length and height have been studied with serial MRI following very preterm birth. Anderson *et al.* [22] reported that corpus callosum growth rates were normal for the first 2 weeks of life after preterm birth (gestations of 23–33 weeks), but slower thereafter. Slowing of corpus callosum growth below expected reference range was consistently detectable by age 6 weeks for 96% of the preterm-born infants. A small percentage of infants (15%) showed some improvement in growth rate after 6 weeks, but only individuals born after 28 weeks [22].

In adolescence, callosal alterations in very preterm-born samples have been reported. In one investigation, 26 out of 72 (36%) preterm children had thinning of the corpus callosum [14] and in another 15 out of 87 (17%) [2]. The middle and posterior callosal sections seem to be particularly affected. Reductions in the cross-sectional area of the anterior, middle, and posterior thirds of the corpus callosum in preterm adolescents compared to controls have been reported as amounting to 16%, 19%, and 19%, respectively [2]. Another study with ex-preterm adolescents reported a 7.5% decrease in callosal surface-area, after adjusting for total white matter volume; an 11.6% decrease in mid-posterior, and a 14.7% decrease in the posterior callosal quarters. Loss of thickness of the corpus callosum has been reported as being associated with other white matter lesions and particularly ventriculomegaly [2,23].

Work with diffusion tensor imaging in a group of 11-year-old children born prematurely without evidence of major periventricular leukomalacia used computed fractional anisotropy and coherence to compare the white matter integrity with that of control children [24]. The preterm children were chosen as they had been identified as having attention deficit disorder at follow-up. Measures of fractional anisotropy suggested that white matter integrity in the preterm group was poorer in the posterior corpus callosum and within regions of both the anterior and posterior internal capsule on either side. Calculation of a coherence measure showed no difference between preterm individuals and controls, suggesting that the lower anisotropy in the preterm children was not likely to be due to disorganization of the white matter fibers, but rather impaired myelination, reduced number of axons, or poor axonal growth. The authors concluded that these results were compatible with previous similar studies in newborn preterm children, and indicate that, at least in those preterm children with attention deficits, these changes are not compensated for before 11 years of age.

Caudate nucleus

The head and body of the caudate nucleus form part of the floor of the anterior horn of the lateral cerebral ventricle, whilst the tail curving back on itself forms the roof of the inferior horn. Although thought to be involved in higher order motor control, it has been shown more recently to be involved in learning and memory, through its connections with other cortical regions, including the temporal lobe [25]. Because of its periventricular location, the caudate nucleus is thought to be at risk of damage in preterm neonates

[26]. Injury to the caudate nucleus may occur following cerebral hemorrhage and perinatal asphyxia [27]. Paneth et al. described basal ganglia necrosis in 17% of preterm infants examined post-mortem [28].

Cooke and Abernethy [2] measured the mid-coronal and mid-transverse cross-sectional areas of the right and left caudate nuclei in very preterm adolescents at 15–17 years. Caudate areas were 17–20% smaller in the coronal section and 6–10% in the transverse sections; R/L ratios and ratios of caudate to total cross-sectional areas of the brains were similar in preterm adolescents and controls suggesting that the reduction in caudate size in the preterm individuals was of the same order as the reduction in total brain size. When the same cohort was examined using volume measurements, significant differences were again seen [29]. Preterm individuals had a mean right caudate volume of $3.7\,cm^3$ and left of $3.6\,cm^3$ (−16.5% and −15% compared to controls). Right/left caudate ratios did not differ significantly. Similar results were seen in a more recent study with preterm adolescents of a similar age, but from another birth cohort [30]. Mean caudate volumes of $4.6\,cm^3$ (right) and $4.5\,cm^3$ (left) were estimated (−4% and −7% compared to controls), although these findings were not statistically significant. The differences between the studies are likely to be methodological.

Hippocampus

The hippocampus is located in the medial temporal lobe and forms part of the limbic system, and is involved in memory and spatial navigation. There is limited evidence that the hippocampus may change in size with time, increasing with use, or decreasing in size after adverse experiences such as war or sexual abuse.

Because of its complex shape, it is difficult to measure the volume of the hippocampus precisely. A number of studies have estimated mean hippocampal volumes in preterm children and term controls at school age [3,8,31,32]. Volumes varied between 2.6 and $3.7\,cm^3$ on the right, and 2.5 and $3.5\,cm^3$ on the left. Differences between preterm individuals and controls were between 0 and −17%, but mostly exceeded −10%. The varied nature of the gestation, age, sex, and history of these groups, together with technical differences in the studies, makes general conclusions difficult to draw. It does appear, however, that the hippocampus in common with many other parts of the brain is reduced in size in preterm children. Hippocampal injury is likely to be caused by hypoxic-ischemic damage [33].

Qualitative MRI of the preterm brain

Apart from quantitative differences in size related to abnormal growth and development of the brain of those born preterm, a high prevalence of focal lesions and qualitative differences has been described from MRI in these children. These lesions include cerebral atrophy, porencephaly, periventricular leukomalacia, and thinning of the corpus callosum. More subtle differences in signal from white matter can be used to estimate the extent of myelination in the absence of focal lesions.

Focal lesions

Olsén *et al.* reported MRI findings in 42 preterm children at 8 years and matched term controls. Periventricular leukomalacia was seen in 32% of the preterm individuals but none of the controls [34].

Stewart *et al.* [14] examined 72 preterm children at 14–15 years and 21 term controls. They concluded that only 17 preterm adolescents were normal on MRI, 15 equivocal, and 40 abnormal. The equivocal cases included scans showing ventricular dilatation, thinning of the corpus callosum, reduced white matter volume, and change in white matter signal. A similar proportion of the control children had equivocal findings also. Of the 40 preterm adolescents with definitely abnormal scans, 36 had evidence of white matter abnormalities, compared with only 1 of the term controls (relative risk = 11.7, 95% CI = 1.7–79.8). It was noted that the MRI scans had detected more abnormalities than had cranial ultrasonography in the neonatal period (40 vs. 31 of 72). This was considered hardly surprising bearing in mind the relatively crude techniques in use at the time the initial study was performed, in the late 1970s and early 1980s. Nevertheless, more recent studies with better developed ultrasound equipment mirror these findings with 70% agreement only in the severest group, and much poorer correspondence with lesser lesions [35]. More subtle white matter lesions were only detected on MRI, and this probably explained the tighter correlation between MRI findings and neurodevelopmental outcome.

A similar cohort of preterm children from about the same time period showed 37 out of 87 (42.5%) infants to have abnormalities on their MRI scans at 15–17 years [2]. In addition to the usual T1 and T2 sequences used, axial fluid-attenuated inversion recovery (FLAIR) was used to detect areas of periventricular leukomalacia. Periventricular leukomalacia was recognized by a characteristic triad of abnormalities; abnormally high signal within the periventricular white matter on T2-weighted and FLAIR images, loss of periventricular white matter, particularly in the periatrial regions, and compensatory focal ventricular enlargement adjacent to regions of abnormal signal intensity. The majority of the lesions seen were periventricular leukomalacia, ventricular dilatation, and thinning of the corpus callosum. None of the term controls had an MRI abnormality.

Qualitative differences

T2 relaxation times have been widely used to investigate regions of interest in epilepsy, such as the temporal lobe and hippocampus. The duration of the T2 relaxation in milliseconds correlates with the density of water in the tissue and so acts as a surrogate measure for myelination, the longer the T2 relaxation time the less extensive is myelination. Isaacs *et al.* [32] measured T2 times in the right and left hippocampus in 11 preterm adolescents (< 30 weeks of gestation). Values of 104 ms were found in both preterm individuals and controls. A similar study of 103 7-year-old premature children examined T2 relaxation times in the right and left hippocampus and right and left cortical white matter [36]. Mean values of between 116 and 119 ms were seen in the hippocampus in various subgroups, but no significant group differences were observed. When the T2 times for the cortex were examined, mean values of 89–93 ms were seen, with significantly higher values in those with minor motor impairment. Children with major motor impairment were not included in the cohort.

A newer technique, magnetization transfer ratio (MTR), enables a semiquantitative tissue characterization using the phenomenon of saturation transfer between immobile macromolecular protons and mobile water protons. The efficacy of transferring the magnetization is quantified by the MTR. Xydis and colleagues have used MTR to study the progress of myelination in the normal preterm newborn, and in preterm infants with periventricular leukomalacia [37,38]. One hundred and twenty-five premature infants with ages from newborn to 26 months were studied with the technique, after conventional MRI had showed them to be free from obvious abnormalities, and early neurodevelopmental follow-up had proved normal at 1–2 years. Areas measured included the corpus callosum, cortical white matter, and the basal ganglia. The MTR was highly age related for all parts of the brain studied. The most rapid changes occurred between birth and 6 months, corrected postnatal age, with much slower increases after that. The pattern of increase was monoexponential, although the actual rates of increase varied between different areas. For example, the corpus callosum achieved its final value later than the cortical white and gray matter. When 28 preterm children with known periventricular leukomalacia were studied using MTR at ages ranging from birth to 8 years, marked changes in myelination were seen. The thalamus and caudate nuclei followed a different trajectory from normal, and the splenium of the corpus callosum reached a final value lower than normal at an earlier age than normal. The cortical white matter and genu of the corpus callosum reached a normal level, but earlier than seen in preterm children without periventricular leukomalacia. The authors concluded that although an apparent early arrest and deficiency in myelination is seen in the splenium, an accelerated myelination in unaffected white matter in preterm children with periventricular leukomalacia might suggest a process of compensatory reorganization.

Diffusion tensor imaging

Although conventional MRI is able to show remarkably detailed anatomy of the brain, it is unable to indicate much about individual white matter tracts. Damage to these is thought to be behind many major and minor neurological deficits in children born preterm. Diffusion tensor imaging (DTI) is an advanced imaging technique which can spatially map white matter tracts. From the fact that the preferential direction of water diffusion within the white matter of the brain occurs along the axons, this technique identifies white matter and indicates the direction of the fiber bundles within.

In a pilot study of two 6-year-old premature boys with spastic quadriplegia, known to be secondary to periventricular leukomalacia, and two normal controls, Hoon et al. used DTI to produce maps of the white matter tracts in the cerebral hemispheres [39]. The authors were surprised to find more prominent abnormalities in white matter fiber tracts projecting to and from occipital and parietal lobes, rather than in the anterior and middle parts of the posterior limb of the internal capsule, which normally contain the descending corticospinal tract. They suggested that white matter projections to or from the sensory cortex, rather than classical pyramidal motor tracts, may play an important role in the pathophysiology of motor disability in some preterm children with periventricular leukomalacia.

Most recently, a larger study of 34 15-year-old preterm individuals and 47 age-matched controls compared fractional anisotropy findings from DTI with tests of behavior, motor, and cognitive functions [40]. The preterm cohort had areas of significant difference in fractional anisotropy which corresponded to areas commonly observed to be involved in periventricular leukomalacia. These were internal and external capsule; corpus callosum; and the superior, middle superior, and inferior fasciculus. Significantly lower values for fractional anisotropy in these areas were variously related to the neurodevelopmental and psychological measures used. Please refer to Chapter 8 for a comprehensive review of DTI studies in very preterm/VLBW samples.

Neurodevelopmental outcomes and MRI in childhood

Many authors have correlated neurodevelopmental outcomes of preterm children with MRI appearances and measurements in childhood. Caution is needed in the interpretation of such associations, as many may not be directly causal, but simply both resulting from prematurity itself and the associated neurodevelopmental complications (see also Chapter 12 for other methodological considerations). The outcomes most studied are major motor outcomes such as cerebral palsy, cognitive measures such as developmental quotient (DQ) or IQ, minor motor impairment, behavioral problems, such as attention deficit disorder, and sensory deficits. It should be noted that some studies of later outcomes have excluded children with major deficits not attending mainstream schools, and so are not representative of preterm children as a whole.

Major motor deficits

A recent systematic review of papers describing MRI appearances in children with cerebral palsy found that 90% of those who were born preterm had evidence of periventricular white matter lesions [41] (see also Chapters 3 and 4). These lesions were in the majority of cases periventricular leukomalacia or the result of periventricular hemorrhage. Of those with white matter damage on MRI, 84% had spastic diplegia. A retrospective study of 50 very preterm infants presenting in childhood with cerebral palsy showed a wide variety of appearances from normality to decreased white matter volume without gliosis, periventricular leukomalacia, and a thin corpus callosum [42]. Thirty-two of the children had cerebellar abnormalities which included destruction of major portions of the vermis and hemispheres, and focal or unilateral loss of cerebellar tissue. This high level of cerebellar injury had not previously been reported, and was attributed to a vascular insult. The cortical pattern of white matter loss, particularly in the periventricular areas, was thought to relate to the susceptibility of pro-oligodendrocytes in the very preterm infant to injury from cytokines and oxygen-derived free radicals, leading to later myelination problems.

Kwong et al. in a relatively large MRI study of preterm and term infants with spastic cerebral palsy, aged between 1 and 16 years, divided the lesions seen into "preterm-type" and "term-type" brain injuries [43]. The preterm-type consisted of periventricular leukomalacia and posthemorrhagic porencephaly, whilst the term-type included basal ganglia lesions, multicystic encephalomalacia, middle cerebral artery infarcts, subcortical leukomalacia, and border-zone infarcts. Term-type lesions were only seen in term and near-term infants with cerebral palsy, but preterm-types were seen in both preterm groups and term. Almost a third of children with the preterm-type of injury were born at term, suggesting that the insult causing the cerebral palsy in these children occurred well before birth.

In a similar, but larger, European study, white matter damage of immaturity again predominated, being noted in 42.5% of all cases, and 71.3% of those with spastic diplegia [44]. Twenty-five percent of the cases with white matter damage of immaturity were born at or near term, again suggesting that the lesions seen related to insults occurring some time before birth. Focal infarcts, basal ganglia damage, and subcortical damage were again practically confined to term infants with cerebral palsy. Hayakawa et al. examined only children with spastic diplegia [45]. They also showed a high frequency (90.7%) of periventricular leukomalacia in the preterm infants, while 55% of the term infants had normal or minimal changes on MRI. This suggests that the etiology of spastic diplegia may be different in term when compared with preterm children. Most infants with diplegia showed significant reductions in the sagittal cross-sectional area of the corpus callosum when compared with normal controls. The severity of the motor defect correlated well with the extent of the involvement of the corpus callosum, thus, this area appears to be a sensitive marker site for the assessment of the overall extent of white matter injury in these children.

Cognitive deficits

Cognitive deficits have been extensively described in very preterm infants, whether or not they have additional motor deficits such as cerebral palsy, and when standardized tests are used, a mean difference of up to −1 standard deviation is often reported. Fedrizzi et al. reporting on 30 preterm children with spastic diplegia showed the usual significant difference between the near normal verbal IQ and poorer performance IQ [46]. Periventricular leukomalacia was observed in all the children on MRI, and the severity of the ventricular dilatation, white matter reduction, optic radiation involvement, and thinning of the corpus callosum correlated significantly with the Wechsler full-scale and performance IQ, but not the verbal IQ (median scores 84, 69, 97 respectively).

Where a group of 221 preterm 8-year-olds were tested with developmental assessment and MRI, IQ could be compared with MRI appearances [35]. The MRI scans were reported as normal, mildly abnormal (mild gliosis, ventricular enlargement, or corpus callosum thinning), or severely abnormal (extensive gliosis or marked ventricular enlargement). Significant differences were seen with mean IQ of 104 in the normal, 100 in the mildly affected, and 91 in the severely affected group.

Volumetric analysis has shown significant correlations between regional brain volumes and the Wechsler IQ scores [3]. The cohort of very preterm infants was largely free of major motor deficits. The highest correlations were seen for the full-scale IQ scores and ranged from 0.4 to 0.6 for various cerebral regions and the cerebellum. Correlations of 0.4–0.5 were seen for cross-sectional areas of the various regions of the corpus callosum. Broadly similar correlations were seen between the verbal IQ and performance IQ scores for the regions measured. Another study showed that reading recognition scores in preterm children aged 8 years were significantly negatively correlated with left temporal gyrification index and left temporal lobe gray matter volume [5].

Volumetric studies of the cerebellum at 15 years show significant correlations between cognitive test scores and cerebellar volume [16]. Full-scale Wechsler IQ and subsets of the Kaufman Assessment Battery for Children (Kaufman-ABC) at 8 years were significantly correlated with cerebellar volume at 15 years, as was reading age at 15 years. The authors concluded that the lower volumes seen represented a disruption of cerebellar development caused by preterm birth, and that this provided further evidence of the role of the cerebellum in cognition. Interestingly, cerebellar volumes were not significantly related to motor deficits, possibly because of functional compensation during later development.

The hippocampus and caudate volumes have been also correlated with cognitive ability. The right caudate and left hippocampus and hippocampal volume ratio have all been shown to be significantly lower in preterm children with an IQ of less than 85 [29]. In a subsequent larger cohort of preterm children, selected geographically, the same authors showed a highly significant reduction in right and left caudate volumes in those with IQ below 80 [31]. Correlations between volumes and IQ scores were between 0.28 and 0.37. When T2 relaxation times were measured in the hippocampus and cortical white matter in the same cohort, significant correlations were only seen for the right hippocampus, which were lost when only cases without visible cerebral lesions on MRI were considered [36].

Although IQ is thought to remain relatively stable in the normal population with age, a decline has been described in preterm individuals over time. Isaacs *et al.* measured IQ in a cohort of preterm 8-year-olds who were free of obvious neurological signs, and then remeasured IQ together with MRI in adolescence [47]. A decline in both mean verbal and performance IQ was seen. About 50% of the MRI scans were normal, and the presence of visible abnormalities in the remainder did not seem to relate to IQ. The use of voxel-based morphometry showed the full IQ scores to be related to areas in the parietal and temporal lobes. Decline in verbal IQ over time was associated with frontal and temporal lobe measurements, and decline in performance IQ with the occipital and temporal lobes (including the hippocampus).

Verbal IQ and verbal fluency in adolescence has been compared with sagittal cross-sectional area of the corpus callosum on MRI [23]. Verbal IQ was significantly correlated with the area of the mid-posterior corpus callosum, and verbal fluency with total and posterior corpus callosum area. The authors suggested that this finding indicates a role for the corpus callosum in higher-order cognitive processes. However, when the sexes were considered apart, only boys, IQ and verbal fluency was significantly associated with the corpus callosum measurements. This is a significantly different finding to other authors where both sexes appear to have been affected [3,46]. This may relate to differences in cohort selection and size, and the cognitive tests chosen.

Minor motor impairments

In addition to cerebral palsy and cognitive delay, many children born preterm show minor motor impairments at school age [1]. Of the most immature children, up to a third may be affected. The condition has been variously described as clumsiness, minimal brain dysfunction, dyspraxia, and developmental coordination disorder. It is often, but not invariably, associated with visuospatial or perceptual difficulties. Because of the coordination problems, some investigators have looked for evidence of cerebellar damage in preterm children, but several other brain lesions have been demonstrated on MRI in children showing minor motor problems. Measurements of cerebellar volume have not been shown to correlate with evidence of minor neurological abnormality or poor upper limb coordination at 14–15 years [16]. This may reflect a degree of functional compensation which could have occurred between preterm birth and 14 years. T2 relaxometry measurements have shown significantly longer times from the cortical white matter in preterm-born children with minor motor impairments [36]. This may reflect a general delay or defect in cerebral myelination as a cause for minor motor impairment.

Abnormalities of the corpus callosum have been frequently described in preterm individuals, as described in a previous section of this chapter. Thinning of the corpus callosum, particularly in the posterior part, has been significantly associated with Movement ABC scores. Children with obvious thinning on sagittal MRI views had a median impairment score of 20 compared with 7.75 for those without thinning. Cross-sectional area studies have shown a significant inverse association between the total impairment score on the Movement ABC and the area of the corpus callosum. For the whole corpus callosum this was −3.3 mm² per score point. Although the association existed all over the corpus callosum, it was most pronounced in the posterior part [21]. Again, using the Movement ABC, Rademaker *et al.* showed similar median impairment scores of 5.25 and 5.0 for preterms with normal or mildly abnormal MRI scans, but 15.75 for the severely abnormal scans [35]. The mildly abnormal group did contain infants with corpus callosum thinning, but no quantitative measures of this were made.

Visuo-perceptual function

In association with the difficulties already described, preterm-born individuals also often show spatial and visuo-perceptual problems when performing simple tasks.

61

Koeda and Takeshita examined visuo-perceptual impairment in preterm children with spastic diplegia using the Frostig developmental test of visual perception and cranial MRI. All the subjects had cerebral lesions on MRI, and the volume of the peritrigonal white matter of the parietal and occipital lobes was significantly correlated with the degree of visuo-perceptual impairment [48].

A more recent study of preterm adolescents, free of visible lesions on conventional MRI scans, used voxel-based morphometric analysis of cortical MRI [49]. Among other psychological testing, the children were administered the Benton Judgment of Line Orientation test. This measures the ability to estimate the angular relationships between line segments. In adults, scores of between 15 and 18 represent a mild to moderate deficit. No standards for adolescents exist, so the group scores were converted to z-scores and a Deficit group (more than −2) and a No Deficit group (−0.5 or higher) were created. The No Deficit group had a mean raw score of 17.3 and the Deficit group a score of 26.8, a highly significant difference. When statistical parametric maps of the Deficit and No Deficit groups were compared, a highly significant difference was seen in gray matter in the area of the right ventral extrastriate cortex. This is the area previously identified as associated with line orientation. A corresponding area in the left cortex showed similar changes, but they did not reach statistical significance. The study also showed local increases in white matter. The etiology of this, if real, is difficult to explain, as in general this group tend to show loss of white matter, and gray matter loss has been suggested to be secondary to that. A similar study by the same authors in a group of preterm adolescents examined the neural correlates of calculation difficulty, a common problem in preterm children [50]. The Wechsler Objective Numeric Dimensions test, and Wechsler Intelligence scales for Children were used, and the difference between the actual numeracy score and that predicted from the general IQ were determined. The Deficit group was selected as having a higher than expected difference, and had a mean discrepancy of −12.7 points, compared to the control No Deficit group with a mean discrepancy of −4.7. Magnetic resonance imaging statistical parametric maps showed a highly significant difference between the two groups with the controls having higher gray matter probability in the area of the left intraparietal sulcus, an area previously implicated in mathematical functioning.

Rademaker *et al.* examined the relationship between the areas of parts of the corpus callosum and the standardized results from the Beery Developmental Test of Visual Motor Integration (VMI), in a cohort of preterm children at 7–8 years [21]. They hypothesized that since the splenium of the corpus callosum receives fibers from both the primary and secondary visual cortex, a reduction in the cross-sectional area of the splenium might be associated with poorer performance in the VMI. They actually found evidence for a significant, although weak, association between all areas of the corpus callosum and the VMI scores. The association was however strongest for the posterior part, and persisted when adjusted for gestational age at birth, birth weight, and total cerebral area.

Reduced lateral cerebellar volume, but not the volume of the vermis, has also been shown to correlate with reduced visuospatial function in adolescence [51]. There was, however, an associated general reduction of cerebral white matter volume.

Most recently, studies on preterm children at 6–7 years, using a wide variety of auditory and visual cognitive function, showed significant deficits on both auditory and visual tests of attention and attentional control, tests of location memory, block construction, and other visuocognitive and visuomotor tests [52]. Verbal IQ again was generally near normal. Although general IQ accounted for most of the variance in the tests, significant deficits in spatial motor attention and executive function tests together with MRI findings accounted for the rest. The authors concluded that the deficits seen in the preterm child were related to networks involving the cortical dorsal stream and its connections to parietal, frontal, and hippocampal areas.

Visual impairment

Preterm children, particularly those with periventricular leukomalacia, have a high prevalence of visual impairments. These may include low acuity, crowding, visual field defects, and ocular motility disturbances [53]. Cognitive tests often show an uneven profile with better performance on verbal compared to visuospatial tasks. In these children, visual impairment is complicated by their visual perceptual difficulties, which accounts for why their visual handicap is often greater than would be expected from their visual acuities and strabismus alone.

Early MRI studies showed that in the preterm child visual impairment, especially poor visual acuity, was more frequent among infants with evidence of direct damage to the visual pathways [54]. However, this was not an invariable finding, and the authors concluded that a variety of visual problems could arise from preterm cerebral insults, the nature and severity of which could not be predicted by MRI. Others since have not agreed with this conclusion. Lanzi *et al.* found that MRI findings did in the main correlate with visual acuity [55]. They examined preterm children with periventricular leukomalacia, and tested them with Teller Acuity Cards and a full ophthalmic examination. Visual acuity correlated well with the degree of loss of peritrigonal white matter, and the extent of calcarine atrophy. Others have described a variety of lesions in the optic radiation and the posterior visual pathways and cortex [56]. Thalamic atrophy has also been described alongside damage to the optic radiations [57].

Volumetric techniques have also been used to study visual problems preterm following birth. Thirty-five percent of a cohort of preterm children had abnormal oculomotor control, including abnormal saccadic movements, smooth pursuit, or strabismus [58]. When compared with preterm individuals without visual problems, these infants had significantly smaller inferior occipital region brain tissue volumes bilaterally. The mean difference was $5.7\,cm^3$ and remained statistically significant after adjustment for intracranial volume. Within the occipital region, the most significant reduction was in the cortical gray matter, and the largest effect on visual problems was on saccadic eye movements.

Attention deficit

Attention deficit, usually in association with hyperactivity, is mostly described in boys born at term. Familial, social, and perinatal factors predominate. In the preterm child, the incidence of attention deficit has been found to be about equal in boys and girls, and tends to comprise more inattention than hyperactivity [1]. Early MRI studies showed a variety of inconsistent findings, such as differences in caudate size and dominance. Gender, handedness, body size and developmental stage may all have contributed to these differences. Stewart *et al.* describing an early preterm cohort, reported Rutter questionnaire scores and MRI appearances at 14–15 years [14]. A score of over 12 was considered abnormal and was seen in 27.5% of those with clearly abnormal MRI scans, as against 11.7% of preterm adolescents with normal scans and 4.7% in term controls. The behaviors described by the Rutter questionnaire include others than just attention deficit.

In a volumetric morphological MRI study of preterm children, attention deficit was recorded using Connor's Hyperactivity scale [29]. Right and left hippocampi, but not caudate nuclei, were both smaller in children with attention deficit, a difference of nearly 12%.

A more recent study on the same cohort as Stewart *et al.*, but using volumetric MRI methods, examined caudate volumes [30]. The authors investigated caudate volume in relation to a hyperactivity score derived from the Rutter Parents' Scale questionnaire, and scores on a social adjustment scale, which covers peer relationships, the ability to function outside the nuclear family (e.g., school performance and adaptation), and the capacity to form intimate social ties across two different age periods (middle/late childhood [5–11 years] and adolescence [12–16 years]). High hyperactivity scores were seen more frequently in the preterm-born adolescents compared to controls, and in the preterm group more often in boys than in girls. In the preterm boys only, the left caudate volume was negatively correlated with the hyperactivity score ($r = -0.43$, $p = 0.018$), and social adjustment score in childhood ($r = -0.40$, $p = 0.028$).

The differences found between these studies may reflect differences in technique, or more likely population selection. They may simply be markers of abnormal brain maturation subsequent to perinatal injury, or poor postnatal growth.

Effects of early management on brain MRI in childhood

The very preterm infant suffers a range of perinatal insults due to immaturity and illness which affect later brain appearances and development. Periventricular hemorrhage and infarction, and periventricular leukomalacia have already been referred to, along with more subtle effects such as reduced brain volume and delayed myelination. In addition to these influences, therapeutic and other management has the potential to alter subsequent brain development, and several of these have been studied.

Corticosteroids

Chronic lung disease (CLD) following survival from neonatal surfactant deficiency disease is a common sequela of very preterm birth. It is associated with considerable later morbidity both respiratory and in terms of growth and neurodevelopment. A number of randomized controlled trials were performed to test the effect of various corticosteroids on the prophylaxis and treatment of CLD. Some of the studies showed at least short-term benefits, but later follow-up studies indicated that there may be an increased risk of subsequent cerebral palsy, especially where early and high doses were used. This effect was thought to relate to impaired cortical growth produced in the main by dexamethasone. Later studies utilized hydrocortisone in the hope that the effect on brain growth would be less. Two follow-up studies with MRI of preterm children treated for CLD with hydrocortisone have been published.

Lodygensky *et al.* studied 60 preterm children at a mean age of 8 years together with term controls [59]. Twenty-five of the preterm children had received treatment with hydrocortisone in the neonatal period. A starting dose of 5 mg/kg per day tapering over a minimum of three weeks was used. The children were assessed with quantitative MRI techniques and the Wechsler Intelligence Scales for Children–Revised (WISC-R). Automatic image segmentation was used to determine the tissue volumes of cerebral gray and white matter and cerebrospinal fluid. The volume of the hippocampus was also determined, but manually. Cerebral gray matter was reduced in the two preterm groups compared with term controls, and the volume of cerebrospinal fluid was increased. Total hippocampal volume was reduced in the preterm children compared with term controls, and this effect was more marked in boys. The IQ scores were lower in the preterm group, but remained within normal limits. No effects of the hydrocortisone treatment were noted, in that IQ and brain volumes did not differ significantly between preterm children who had hydrocortisone and those who did not.

Another very similar study looked at 62 preterm children treated with the same dosage schedule of hydrocortisone, and 164 untreated preterm controls [60]. Subscales of the WISC-R, the VMI, a Word Memory Test, and the Movement ABC were used together with conventional MRI of the head. The groups were not matched as the treated infants were younger, lighter, and sicker in the neonatal period than the untreated controls. After adjustments for gestation, birth weight, sex, use of ventilation, and growth restriction were made, no significant differences in any of the tests or MRI appearances were noted between the groups. These two studies appear to show that a weak corticosteroid at modest doses may be used to manage CLD without subsequent serious neurodevelopmental or MRI abnormalities.

Indomethacin

Indomethacin has been used for many years in the management of the persistent ductus arteriosus in preterm infants. Following randomized controlled trials, it has also been used prophylactically, immediately after birth, to prevent problems with later patent ductus arteriosus (PDA) and also reduce major periventricular hemorrhage. Nevertheless, follow-up studies have not shown a reduction in major neurodevelopmental problems at 2 years of age. One follow-up study has particularly examined the possible effects of exposure to indomethacin on later language development and processing [61]. Preterm subjects from a randomized controlled trial of indomethacin prophylaxis had MRI scans and fMRI at age 8 years at the time of their neurodevelopmental assessments. Preterm children exposed to indomethacin and those not exposed were compared with term controls on an functional MRI (fMRI) passive language task. Intelligence quotient and vocabulary tests were also applied. Neural activity was assessed during both phonological and semantic processing in the fMRI protocol. The cognitive assessments showed as expected lower scores in the preterm children compared to the controls. Preterm males not exposed to indomethacin tended to have lower vocabulary scores. During phonological processing, a significant treatment-by-gender effect was demonstrated in three brain regions; the left inferior parietal lobule, the left inferior frontal gyrus (Broca's area), and the right dorsolateral prefrontal cortex. The authors concluded that their study showed a differential effect of indomethacin exposure in early life on the subsequent development of neural systems that serve language functioning in male and female preterm infants. Please refer to Chapter 11 for further results from the International Indomethacin Trial.

Non-cerebral malformations and brain MRI

Prematurity and low birth weight are both known to be associated with congenital malformations. It is not clear whether this association is causal, or whether both the malformation and prematurity or low birth weight are the result of other factors operating during early development. There are no published studies of cerebral MRI in children born preterm, but a recent study of children born at 36 weeks' gestation or more with congenital heart disease showed frequent abnormalities related to white matter [62]. Forty-one infants were studied soon after birth and before surgery for their malformations. The malformations included transposition of the great arteries and other single ventricle pathologies. Infants were studied using MRI, but also magnetic resonance spectroscopy (MRS) and DTI. Magnetic resonance imaging was then repeated after cardiac surgery. Forty-one percent of infants with transposition and 17% of those with other malformations had signs of white matter injury before surgery. This varied from stroke to intraventricular hemorrhage. Additional white matter injury was seen after surgery. Changes in the MRS and DTI measurements provided further evidence for white matter injury. The patterns of injury seen were not those of hypoxia-ischemia in the term newborn, but more like the changes that were seen in preterm newborns. This white matter vulnerability may be due to impaired brain development occurring in utero and related to circulatory abnormalities associated with congenital cardiac malformations.

Conclusion

Magnetic resonance imaging studies in children born preterm have broadly shown either signs of earlier damage, mainly to white matter, or disordered growth which has mostly occurred after birth. Periventricular leukomalacia and other white matter damage is strongly associated with motor problems such as cerebral palsy and dyspraxia. Poor growth results in smaller brains overall, but also a greater volume reduction in structures such as the caudate nucleus and the corpus callosum. Reduction in brain size is associated with poorer cognitive performance and behavioral difficulties at school age. The reduction in brain volume is not only due to a reduction in white matter volume, as a reduction in gray matter volume is also often seen. Failure of later brain growth may reflect early injury such as damage to preoligodendrocytes in association with infection, hypoxia, hemorrhage, or circulatory disorders; or poor nutritional status in the early weeks and months after preterm birth. Future studies should involve the use of longitudinal studies of brain growth, and the use of newer techniques such as DTI tractography to investigate the effects of injury and growth on subsequent brain development.

References

1. Foulder-Hughes LA Cooke RW. Motor, cognitive, and behavioural disorders in children born very preterm. *Dev Med Child Neurol* 2003; **45**: 97–103.

2. Cooke RW Abernethy LJ. Cranial magnetic resonance imaging and school performance in very low birth weight infants in adolescence. *Arch Dis Child Fetal Neonatal Ed* 1999; **81**: F116–21.

3. Peterson B S, Vohr B, Staib L H, *et al*. Regional brain volume abnormalities and long-term cognitive outcome in preterm infants. *JAMA* 2000; **284**: 1939–47.

4. Kesler SR, Ment LR, Vohr B, *et al*. Volumetric analysis of regional cerebral development in preterm children. *Pediatr Neurol* 2004; **31**: 318–25.

5. Kesler SR, Vohr B, Schneider KC, *et al*. Increased temporal lobe gyrification in preterm children. *Neuropsychologia* 2006; **44**: 445–3.

6. Ajayi-Obe M, Saeed N, Cowan FM, Rutherford MA, Edwards AD. Reduced development of cerebral cortex in extremely preterm infants. *Lancet* 2000; **356**: 1162–3.

7. Kapellou O, Counsell SJ, Kennea N, *et al*. Abnormal cortical development after premature birth shown by altered allometric scaling of brain growth. *PLoS Med* 2006; **3**: e265.

8. Nosarti C, Al Asady MH, Frangou S, *et al*. Adolescents who were born very preterm have decreased brain volumes. *Brain* 2002; **125**: 1616–23.

9. Szeszko PR, Gunning-Dixon F, Ashtari M, *et al*. Reversed cerebellar asymmetry in men with first-episode schizophrenia. *Biol Psychiatry* 2003; **53**: 450–9.26.

10. Lancefield K, Nosarti C, Rifkin L, *et al*. Cerebral asymmetry in 14 year olds born very preterm. *Brain Res* 2006; **1093**: 33–40.

11. Reiss AL, Kesler SR, Vohr B, *et al*. Sex differences in cerebral volumes of 8-year-olds born preterm. *J. Pediatr* 2004; **145**: 242–9.

12. Kesler SR, Reiss AL, Vohr B, *et al*. Brain volume reductions within multiple cognitive systems in male preterm children at age twelve. *J Pediatr* 2008; **152**: 513–20, 520.el.

13. du Plessis AJ, VolpeJJ. Perinatal brain injury in the preterm and term newborn. *Curr Opin Neurol* 2002; **15**: 151–7.

14. Stewart AL, Rifkin L, Amess PN. Brain structure and neurocognitive and behavioural function in adolescents who were born very preterm. *Lancet* 1999; **353**: 1653–7.

15. Peterson BS, Anderson AW, Ehrenkranz R, *et al*. Regional brain volumes and their later neurodevelopmental correlates in term and preterm infants. *Pediatrics* 2003; **111**: 939–48.

16. Allin M, Matsumoto H, Santhouse AM, *et al*. Cognitive and motor function and the size of the cerebellum in adolescents born very pre-term. *Brain* 2001; **124**: 60–6.

17. Limperopoulos C, Soul JS, Gauvreau K, *et al*. Late gestation cerebellar growth is rapid and impeded by premature birth. *Pediatrics* 2005; **115**: 688–95.

18. Argyropoulou MI, Xydis V, Drougia A, *et al*. MRI measurements of the pons and cerebellum in children born preterm; associations with the severity of periventricular leukomalacia and perinatal risk factors. *Neuroradiology*, 2003; **45**: 730–4.

19. Srinivasan L, Allsop J, Counsell SJ, *et al*. Smaller cerebellar volumes in very preterm infants at term-equivalent age are associated with the presence

of supratentorial lesions. *AJNR Am J Neuroradiol,* 27: 573–9.

20. Flodmark O, Lupton B, Li D, *et al.* MR imaging of periventricular leukomalacia in childhood. *AJR Am J Roentgenol* 1989; 152: 583–90.

21. Rademaker KJ, Lam JN, Van Haastert IC, *et al.* Larger corpus callosum size with better motor performance in prematurely born children. *Semin Perinatol* 2004; 28: 279–87.

22. Anderson NG, Laurent I, Woodward LJ, Inder TE. Detection of impaired growth of the corpus callosum in premature infants. *Pediatrics* 2006; 118: 951–60.

23. Nosarti C, Rushe TM, Woodruff PW, *et al.* Corpus callosum size and very preterm birth: relationship to neuropsychological outcome. *Brain* 2004; 127: 2080–9.

24. Nagy Z, Westerberg H, Skare S, *et al.* Preterm children have disturbances of white matter at 11 years of age as shown by diffusion tensor imaging. *Pediatr Res*, 2003; 54: 672–9.

25. Calabresi P, De Murtas M, Bernardi G. The neostriatum beyond the motor function: experimental and clinical evidence. *Neuroscience* 1997; 78: 39–60.

26. Mutch L, Leyland A, McGee A. Patterns of neuropsychological function in a low-birthweight population. *Dev Med Child Neurol* 1993; 35: 943–56.

27. Volpe JJ. Intracranial hemorrhage. In: *Neurology of the Newborn*, 4th edn. Philadelphia, PA: W.B. Saunders Company. 2001; 397–496.

28. Paneth N, Rudelli R, Kazam E, Monte W. *Brain Damage in the Preterm Infant*. Cambridge, UK: Mac Keith Press/Cambridge University Press; 1994.

29. Abernethy LJ, Palaniappan M, Cooke RW. Quantitative magnetic resonance imaging of the brain in survivors of very low birth weight. *Arch Dis Child* 2002; 87: 279–83.

30. Nosarti C, Allin M, Frangou S, Rifkin L, Murray R. Decreased caudate volume is associated with hyperactivity in adolescents born very preterm. *Biol Psychiatry* 2005; 13: 339.

31. Abernethy LJ, Cooke RW, Foulder-Hughes L. Caudate and hippocampal volumes, intelligence, and motor impairment in 7-year-old children who were born preterm. *Pediatr Res* 2004; 55: 884–93.

32. Isaacs EB, Lucas A, Chong WK, *et al.* Hippocampal volume and everyday memory in children of very low birth weight. *Pediatr Res* 2000; 47: 713–20.

33. Kuchna I. Quantitative studies of human newborns' hippocampal pyramidal cells after perinatal hypoxia. *Folia Neuropathol* 1994; 32: 9–16.

34. Olsén P, Pääkkö, E, Vainionpää, L, Pyhtinen J, Jarvelin MR. Magnetic resonance imaging of periventricular leukomalacia and its clinical correlation in children. *Ann Neurol* 1997; 41: 754–61.

35. Rademaker KJ, Uiterwaal CS, Beek FJ, *et al.* Neonatal cranial ultrasound versus MRI and neurodevelopmental outcome at school age in children born preterm. *Arch Dis Child Fetal Neonatal Ed* 2005; 90: F489–93.

36. Abernethy LJ, Klafkowski G, Foulder-Hughes L, Cooke RW. Magnetic resonance imaging and T2 relaxometry of cerebral white matter and hippocampus in children born preterm. *Pediatr Res* 2003; 54: 868–74.

37. Xydis V, Astrakas L, Zikou A, *et al.* Magnetization transfer ratio in the brain of preterm subjects: age-related changes during the first 2 years of life. *Eur Radiol* 2006; 16: 215–20.

38. Xydis V, Astrakas L, Drougia A, *et al.* Myelination process in preterm subjects with periventricular leucomalacia assessed by magnetization transfer ratio. *Pediatr Radiol* 2006; 36: 934–9.

39. Hoon AH, Jr., Lawrie W T, Jr., Melhem ER, *et al.* Diffusion tensor imaging of periventricular leukomalacia shows affected sensory cortex white matter pathways. *Neurology* 2002; 59: 752–6.

40. Skranes J, Vangberg TR, Kulseng S, *et al.* Clinical findings and white matter abnormalities seen on diffusion tensor imaging in adolescents with very low birth weight. *Brain* 2007;130: 654–66.

41. Krägeloh-Mann I, Horber V. The role of magnetic resonance imaging in elucidating the pathogenesis of cerebral palsy: a systematic review. *Dev Med Child Neurol* 2007; 49: 144–51.

42. Bodensteiner JB, Johnsen SD. Magnetic resonance imaging (MRI) findings in children surviving extremely premature delivery and extremely low birthweight with cerebral palsy. *J Child Neurol* 2006; 21: 743–7.

43. Kwong KL, Wong YC, Fong CM, Wong SN, So KT. Magnetic resonance imaging in 122 children with spastic cerebral palsy. *Pediatr Neurol* 2004; 31: 172–6.

44. Bax M, Tydeman C, Flodmark O. Clinical and MRI correlates of cerebral palsy: the European Cerebral Palsy Study. *JAMA* 2006; 296: 1602–8.

45. Hayakawa K, Kanda T, Hashimoto K, *et al.* MR imaging of spastic diplegia. The importance of corpus callosum. *Acta Radiol* 1996; 37: 830–6.

46. Fedrizzi E, Inverno M, Bruzzone MG, *et al.* MRI features of cerebral lesions and cognitive functions in preterm spastic diplegic children. *Pediatr Neurol* 1996; 15: 207–12.

47. Isaacs EB, Edmonds CJ, Chong WK, *et al.* Brain morphometry and IQ measurements in preterm children. *Brain* 2004; 127: 2595–607.

48. Koeda T, Takeshita K. Visuo-perceptual impairment and cerebral lesions in spastic diplegia with preterm birth. *Brain Dev* 1992; 14: 239–44.

49. Isaacs EB, Edmonds CJ, Chong WK, Lucas A, Gadian DG. Cortical anomalies associated with visuospatial processing deficits. *Ann Neurol* 2003; **53**: 768–73.

50. Isaacs EB, Edmonds CJ, Lucas A, Gadian DG. Calculation difficulties in children of very low birthweight: a neural correlate. *Brain* 2001; **124**: 1701–7.

51. Allin MP, Salaria S, Nosarti C. *et al.* Vermis and lateral lobes of the cerebellum in adolescents born very preterm. *Neuroreport* 2005; **16**: 1821–4.

52. Atkinson J. Braddick O. Visual and visuocognitive development in children born very prematurely. *Prog Brain Res* 2007; **164**: 123–49.

53. Jacobson L, Ek U, Fernell E, Flodmark O, Broberger U. Visual impairment in preterm children with periventricular leukomalacia – visual, cognitive and neuropaediatric characteristics related to cerebral imaging. *Dev Med Child Neurol* 1996; **38**: 724–35.

54. Pike MG, Holmstrom G, de Vries LS, *et al.* Patterns of visual impairment associated with lesions of the preterm infant brain. *Dev Med Child Neurol* 1994; **36**: 849–62.

55. Lanzi G, Fazzi E, Uggetti C, *et al.* Cerebral visual impairment in periventricular leukomalacia. *Neuropediatrics* 1998; **29**: 145–50.

56. Jacobson L, Lundin S, Flodmark O, Ellstrom KG. Periventricular leukomalacia causes visual impairment in preterm children. A study on the aetiologies of visual impairment in a population-based group of preterm children born 1989–95 in the county of Varmland, Sweden. *Acta Ophthalmol Scand* 1998; **76**: 593–8.

57. Ricci D, Anker S, Cowan F, *et al.* Thalamic atrophy in infants with PVL and cerebral visual impairment. *Early Hum Dev* 2006; **82**: 591–5.

58. Shah DK, Guinane C, August P, *et al.* Reduced occipital regional volumes at term predict impaired visual function in early childhood in very low birth weight infants. *Invest Ophthalmol Vis Sci* 2006; **47**: 3366–73.

59. Lodygensky GA, Rademaker K, Zimine S, *et al.* Structural and functional brain development after hydrocortisone treatment for neonatal chronic lung disease. *Pediatrics* 2005; **116**: 1–7.

60. Rademaker KJ, Uiterwaal CS, Groenendaal F, *et al.* Neonatal hydrocortisone treatment: neurodevelopmental outcome and MRI at school age in preterm-born children. *J Pediatr* 2007; **150**: 351–7.

61. Ment LR, Peterson BS, Meltzer JA, *et al.* A functional magnetic resonance imaging study of the long-term influences of early indomethacin exposure on language processing in the brains of prematurely born children. *Pediatrics* 2006; **118**: 961–70.

62. Miller SP, McQuillen PS, Hamrick S, *et al.* Abnormal brain development in newborns with congenital heart disease. *N Engl J Med* 2007; **357**: 1928–38.

Chapter 6

Magnetic resonance imaging findings from adolescence to adulthood

Matthew P. G. Allin, Muriel Walshe, and Chiara Nosarti

Introduction

As has been demonstrated elsewhere in this volume, preterm birth and/or low birth weight is common, possibly increasing and associated with adverse consequences [1]. Magnetic resonance imaging (MRI) studies in childhood have done an excellent job of relating the cognitive, behavioral, and academic problems faced by preterm and low birth weight individuals to underlying alterations of brain structure, as described in Chapter 5. However, a largely unanswered question is what happens to these individuals, and to their brains, as they grow up. This lack of information is not because preterm researchers have been idle, of course, but rather because the phenomenon of widespread survival after short gestation is historically quite recent. As cohorts of prematurely born people are now becoming adults, there is now a pressing need to determine their adult outcomes. Do impairments become attenuated, persist, or worsen? How are the usual processes of development and maturation altered by preexisting structural brain abnormalities? Is neural plasticity part of the problem, as well as a potential solution? What happens to the ageing preterm brain? Many of these questions are yet to be addressed, but in this chapter we will describe some imaging studies that are starting to bridge the gap between adolescence and adulthood. In this, we will be helped considerably by recent studies which have used MRI techniques to investigate normal adolescent brain development, and which will give us a baseline for understanding changes in the preterm brain. In writing this chapter we have tried to avoid repetition with Chapter 5, which took us through MRI findings up to age 14, and instead to concentrate on studies that have directly assessed brain structure in preterm and low birth weight adults, and those which have followed longitudinal brain development from adolescence to adulthood.

Adult MRI findings

As explained in Chapters 4 and 5, there are two broad analysis strategies for structural MRI data – region-of-interest (ROI) and computational morphometry, also known as voxel-based morphometry (VBM). There is a relative paucity of MRI studies in preterm and low birth weight adults, however, Fearon et al. [2] studied a group of 33 very low birth weight (VLBW; < 1500 g) adults (mean age 23 years), along with 18 normal birth weight controls. This was an ROI study, including the volume of the following structures/regions: whole brain; cortical gray matter; ventricular system; corpus callosum; hippocampus. They found that VLBW adults had significantly larger ventricles and smaller corpora callosa than controls, but there were no group differences in the other brain volumes that they measured [2]. Of course, this analysis was not comprehensive – many structures of potential interest were omitted (the cerebellum, for example, or the caudate nucleus), which is an inherent limitation of ROI methods. The results of this study indicate that at least some of the common brain structural abnormalities noted in premature cohorts in childhood and adolescence persist into adulthood.

In a related paper from our group, we used VBM to examine these same VLBW and normal birth weight comparison groups [3]. Consistent with the ROI analysis of Fearon et al. [2], we found enlarged lateral ventricular volume in the VLBW group. We also found an increased ratio of gray matter to white matter in the VLBW subjects, indicative of a more subtle alteration in brain structure. This was confirmed and extended by the group maps, which showed spatially extensive areas of altered gray and white matter distribution. This indicated that the brains of the VLBW participants had undergone considerable reorganization of cortical and subcortical structure.

Neurodevelopmental Outcomes of Preterm Birth, ed. Chiara Nosarti, Robin M. Murray, and Maureen Hack. Published by Cambridge University Press. © Cambridge University Press 2010.

It thus seems clear that brain structural alterations are indeed present in adulthood in those who were born VLBW. The nature of the differences suggests that the brains of these individuals had undergone widespread changes in structure, which would be compatible with plastic reorganization of structure in response to early brain lesions. Such an interpretation would be consistent with Thomas and Karmiloff-Smith[4], who argue persuasively that developmental brain disorders are qualitatively different from disorders arising from *de novo* brain lesions in adulthood. A brain that has developed with a preexisting lesion is likely to have developed alterations in its functional and connectional anatomy that affect multiple systems.

These two linked studies of VLBW outcome may not be generalizable to the preterm and VLBW cohorts of today. The majority of the participants were born in the era just preceding many neonatal intensive care innovations that are currently commonplace (see Chapter 2). However, a recently published study has extended these findings in a group of individuals born very preterm (VPT – i.e., before 33 weeks' gestation) in mid-adolescence at age 14–15 years. The study of Nosarti et al. [5] analyzed structural brain MRI in a large cohort of 218 VPT and 128 term-born control individuals. This was a VBM study, and the results were again consistent with widespread differences in the architecture of the brains of the VPT group. More specifically, there were areas of gray matter reduction in temporal, frontal, and occipital cortex, the cuneus (parietal cortex), fusiform gyrus, insula, cerebellum, caudate, and putamen in the VPT group. There were also areas in which the VPT group had relatively more gray matter than term-born controls. These areas included parts of the frontal and temporal lobes, the cingulate and fusiform gyri, and parts of the cerebellum. Patterns of white matter increase and decrease were also observed, with white matter being decreased in VPT-born individuals relative to controls in the brainstem, internal capsule, temporal and frontal regions, and long association pathways. By contrast, white matter was relatively increased in the VPT group in temporal, frontal, and parietal regions. The changes in different regions were associated with each other, suggesting that abnormalities in one area affected the development of other brain systems and regions [5]. This complexity of structural changes suggests that a large amount of plastic remodeling of the brain has occurred in the VPT group. In this case it would be reasonable to suggest that the neural architecture underlying cognition and behavior could be altered in this group. This alteration of structure might account for the fact that cognitive impairments have been reported in an array of domains in VPT individuals [6,7]. The gray and white matter changes found by Nosarti et al [5] were related to the severity of neonatal brain injury (based on ultrasound appearances), and to gestational age in the VPT group. Thus it seems likely that the degree of plastic reorganization that occurs is directly related to the severity of the early lesion. Kapellou et al. looked at serial MRI scans in preterm infants, and in particular looked at the way their brain volume and surface area scaled together over time. They found that slower rates of growth of cortical surface area in relation to brain volume were associated with poorer outcome. They interpret the reduced growth as being due to diminished connectivity in white matter [8].

The paper of Nosarti et al [5] went further than just examining structural differences, however. This VPT group had lower performance on language and executive function tests, and this was related to gray and white matter changes. Several possible explanations suggest themselves: (1) possibly the plastic changes that allow function to be broadly spared in VPT individuals are incomplete; (2) perhaps the altered brain architecture that results from plasticity is less efficient; (3) perhaps plastic reorganization results in some brain areas carrying out more tasks than they would otherwise have done, leaving fewer processing resources to cope with cognitive demands.

There is some functional MRI (fMRI) evidence that neural networks are altered in individuals born VPT (see Chapter 7). For example, judging visual and auditory information across the midline recruits different areas in VPT individuals than term-born controls [9]. This may relate to the abnormality of the corpus callosum, which is a common finding in VPT groups [10–12]. Another example could be given by fMRI of VPT-born adolescents during challenges with motor response inhibition processing. Nosarti et al.[13] observed hyperactivation in VPT individuals compared to controls predominantly in right prefrontal areas during successful response inhibition, which were hypothesized as representing alternative response pathways, compensating for a possible dysfunction of frontal-striatal-cerebellar circuitry, which underlies this type of task. For more on fMRI in the preterm brain see Chapter 7.

Development from adolescence into adulthood

"Everything is the way it is because of how it got that way," wrote D'Arcy Wentworth Thompson in his book *On Growth and Form* [14]. Our evidence so far suggests that VPT and VLBW adult brains are constituted rather differently to the brains of those born at term. The nature of the alterations suggests a diffuse reorganization that would be compatible with alterations of development, or interactions of developmental processes with an early "static" lesion. Is there any direct evidence that neurodevelopment is altered in VPT individuals? And what specific processes are altered? We have been carrying out a longitudinal imaging study of VPT adolescents to try to answer these questions, and will set out some of the early results below.

Adolescence

Why study brain development in adolescence? It is a truism to say that adolescence is a period of great changes in social, cognitive, and behavioral function. It is a period during which there are many brain changes, enabling individuals make the transition from childhood to adulthood and take on adult roles, responsibilities, and abilities [15]. There is disagreement about when adolescence starts and ends – and we propose not to get involved in this debate here. Instead, we shall (perhaps over-inclusively) take adolescence to be the period of transition to adulthood, running roughly from the mid-teens to the early twenties. Adolescence is also of interest because it is the time when "adult" psychiatric disorders tend to make their first appearance – particularly schizophrenia, but also depression and anxiety [16]. Adults with schizophrenia have a higher rate of what are known as "obstetric complications," including preterm birth and low birth weight [17]. One influential hypothesis about the aetiology of schizophrenia (the "neurodevelopmental hypothesis") postulates that there is an interaction between adolescent brain development and an early (pre- or perinatal) brain lesion that increases the risk of developing the disorder (for a recent review, see [18]).

Recently, the extent and nature of some of the developmental brain changes happening in adolescence have started to be demonstrated in healthy volunteers. These studies have provided a clear story of how the brain develops, and how different areas do so at different rates and different times. These background studies are reviewed briefly below.

Longitudinal studies of adolescent brain development in healthy volunteers

One of the initially surprising things about brain development is how protracted it is. The processes of neurogenesis, neural migration, and axonal outgrowth produce, during fetal life, a brain possessing around 100 billion neurons [19]. By the time of birth, around half of these will have been lost through apoptosis [20]. After birth there is overproduction of synapses, which are then "pruned" from middle childhood, through adolescence depending on the region considered. Most studies have focused on neurons of the cerebral cortex, and as a result we now know quite a lot about the developmental trajectory of this structure. On the other hand, the developmental trajectories of other tissues, structures, and cell-types of the brain have been rather neglected – so we know rather less about the developmental trajectories of glial cells, white matter (reliant on a particular kind of glial cell – the oligodendrocyte), and "subcortical" structures such as the cerebellum, basal ganglia, and thalamus.

The use of MRI, of course, lends itself to studying development because it allows serial measurements to be made in a way that post-mortem and animal studies cannot. One of the first developmental MRI studies was performed by Giedd and colleagues [21], which demonstrated that changes in gray matter volumes during development are not linear. Sowell *et al.* [22] extended these observations, demonstrating that gray matter generally increases as individuals pass from childhood into adolescence, and then subsequently decreases, possibly reflecting synaptogenesis and subsequent pruning. The peak of gray matter volume is reached in different lobes at different ages. Boys and girls differ in the age at which this occurs (gray matter peaks in boys between 1 and 2 years earlier than in girls). The order of maturation of different lobes is interesting – with primary motor and sensory cortices maturing first, and "association" cortices (such as temporal and prefrontal cortices) maturing later [23]. Since association cortices are important for "higher" cognitive functions this pattern has face-validity. Thus during adolescence one would expect to see reduction in gray matter volume in frontal and temporal areas. In an elegant recent study, Shaw *et al.* [24] demonstrated that developmental changes in cerebral cortex related to the Brodmann cortical architecture – areas with a more complex laminar organization were later-maturing.

The cellular basis for this reduction is not yet known, but the best guesses are: (1) ongoing pruning of synapses that were overproduced in childhood; (2) ongoing myelination in white matter axons that penetrate the gray matter of the cortex. Other potential explanations include changes in the size of neurons or glia, or reductions in the amounts of dendrites, or alterations of vasculature. Currently, the available data do not allow us to distinguish between these hypotheses – which are not mutually exclusive.

White matter follows a different trajectory to gray matter, and the majority of authors believe that it shows a generally linear increase from childhood, through adolescence and into adulthood. Thus, white matter volume increases during adolescence, as does fractional anisotropy (a diffusion property of white matter revealed by diffusion tensor MRI [DT-MRI]) [25]. The most likely explanation for this is ongoing myelination by oligodendrocytes. Myelination is not the only possible cellular correlate of these MRI changes, however. Other possibilities include changes in cell membranes, changes in the regularity of axonal bundle, so that their "tortuosity" is reduced [25], the growth of new axons (which may occur over short distances [26]), and changes in axonal diameter.

Brain development between adolescence and young adulthood in a VPT cohort

Truly longitudinal studies are difficult and expensive to perform. Our own research, on the University College Hospital London (UCHL) cohort which has been described earlier (Chapter 5), has tried in a limited way to give a longitudinal developmental perspective on adolescent brain development. The experimental design was simple: we took VPT individuals and controls who had already received an MRI brain scan at 14 years (the *adolescent* assessment), and scanned them again using an identical protocol at 19 years (the *young adult* assessment). We thus have data from two time points in the two groups, and can look at brain changes in young people who are just entering adult life. We found interesting, unexpected and functionally relevant alterations in growth patterns in the VPT group in two structures: the cerebellum and the corpus callosum.

It may be useful here to re-cap our findings in relation to these two structures in VPT adolescents (age 14). The cerebellum was reduced in volume [27], particularly in the lateral lobes [28] – and this was associated with poorer cognitive function on a variety of domains. This was consistent with the growing realization among neuroscientists that the cerebellum does more than co-ordinate the motor system, but is also involved in cognition – see Schmahmann and Sherman's [29] paper on the "cerebellar cognitive-affective syndrome" for further details. Abnormalities of the corpus callosum are readily observed on MRI in VPT individuals – and seem particularly to affect the rear portion (the splenium). Nosarti *et al* [11] showed that the cross-sectional area of the corpus callosum is reduced in VPT adolescents, and furthermore that this is associated with reduced verbal performance (in boys, but not girls).

As far as we are aware, only one other study looked at longitudinal changes in ex-preterm children between the ages of 8 and 12. Results showed brain volume increases of 2–3% which were similar to changes observed in controls. During the same time period ex-preterm children showed a smaller decrease in cerebral gray matter compared to controls (2.5% vs. 9.5%, respectively), and a smaller increase in cerebral white matter volumes (> 26% vs. 10%, respectively) [30].

Changes in the cerebellum

Between adolescence and young adulthood (14–19 years) the cerebellum decreased in size by about 3% in the VPT group [31]. In the term comparison group it did not change. This cerebellar decrease appeared to have some "real world" consequences too – it was associated with reduced "well-being" as assessed by the 12-item General Health Questionnaire (GHQ). Cerebellar shrinkage was associated with worse GHQ ratings of: concentration; feeling useful; confidence; decision-making capacity; and feelings of worthlessness.

Changes in the corpus callosum

By contrast, the corpus callosum was growing in both VPT and term groups between adolescence and young adulthood. In the term group, it grew by about 3%, which would be consistent with longitudinal studies of corpus callosum growth in healthy volunteers [32,33]. In the VPT group there was also growth, but to a much greater extent – corpus callosum grew by 13% in this group between adolescence and young adulthood. As with the cerebellum, this growth had functional consequences, as it was associated with cognitive outcome (the greater the growth, the higher the IQ scores at age 19). Total white matter volume increased in both groups, and total gray matter volume decreased [31], consistent with the developmental models of Gogtay *et al.* [23] – but growth trajectories of the cerebellum and corpus callosum deviated from those of our control group.

What could the cellular correlates of this growth be? Axonal and dendritic outgrowth do occur in adults – for example in the case of peripheral sensory deafferentation. After amputation of a limb, for example, there is reorganization of cortical circuits, with cortical axons growing over distances of up to 1 cm. This axonal growth into adjacent cortical territory is associated with phantom limb pain [34]. There is no evidence to suggest that long-range white matter axons are formed *de novo* in adult life, however, and it seems likely that developmental changes in white matter volume represent myelination rather than growth of new axons.

What is the significance of these developmental alterations?

These alterations of developmental trajectory are interesting, and deserve further comment. There are several possible explanations for them. Firstly, it is possible that they represent developmental delays. For example, if we had scanned our control group earlier, say between 10 and 14, we might have seen similar growth changes. In other words, the VPT subjects are undergoing a normal developmental process, but it has been delayed. Unfortunately, normative data do not exist for cerebellar development over this time. Fortunately, however, corpus callosum development has been more studied. Giedd *et al.* [33] found the relationship between age and corpus callosum size to be linear, which would not support developmental delay as the underlying cause of the pattern that we have described. However, this study is not truly longitudinal, but cross-sectional (it was a group of individuals spanning the age range, each of whom was scanned only once). Pujol *et al.* [32] did have a longitudinal component to their study. They found that corpus callosum size increases were greatest between 15 and 20 years in healthy volunteers. Again, this does not back up the developmental delay theory, as that would require healthy volunteers to have a pronounced growth spurt in the corpus callosum some time before their fourteenth birthday, for which there is currently no evidence.

So, on balance, it appears more likely that the changes in the VPT brain between adolescence and adulthood represent a phenomenon that is specific to this group. (Of course, other neurodevelopmental conditions might also be associated with non-linear growth patterns in adolescence, but this is simply not known as yet.) What, then, could these changes represent?

We shall take the cerebellar changes first. Although we did not segment the cerebellum into gray and white matter, it seems likely that the cerebellar volume decreases represent gray matter loss rather than white matter loss. As we have seen, the developmental trajectory of white matter is for it to increase in volume with age – a relationship that was also true for the total white matter volume in the VPT group. Our VPT group experienced similar levels of overall white matter growth between adolescence and adulthood to the term comparison group, making it more likely that the cerebellar changes are within the gray matter compartment.

One possible explanation for the developmental vulnerability of the cerebellum after preterm birth is that the protracted postnatal development of the cerebellum renders it vulnerable to insult [35]. Cerebellar granule cells continue to differentiate and migrate into position until after birth, unlike cerebral cortical neurons (which are all in position prenatally) [36], and are therefore particularly susceptible to hypoxia-ischemia around the time of VPT birth [37,38]. Hypoxic injury to granule cells in the cerebellum might result in reduced numbers of this cell type, or reductions in the extent of their arborization and dendritic contacts. This could have knock-on effects on the development of other cell types and functional cellular complexes in the cerebellum [39].

Around the time of adolescence, a cerebellum which has developed abnormally in this way may have difficulty performing the increasing number and complexity of computational tasks that are required of it. This might explain the functional deficit, and associated mental health consequences described above, but the processes that bring about adolescent atrophy of the cerebellum are still unclear.

An alternative possibility is that individuals born VPT are less likely, either through temperament, cognitive impairment, or social circumstances, to be exposed to "learning experiences" which would ordinarily have stimulated cerebellar development. Some evidence suggests that VPT and VLBW adults have altered personality styles – with less extraversion [40], greater aversion to taking risks [41], reduced fun-seeking, and increased behavioral inhibition [42]. Individuals who restrict their environments in this way may have less need for cerebellar input, and the cerebellar decrement that we observed could simply be the normal physiological consequence of living a quiet life.

The changes in the corpus callosum, however, would tend to contradict this environmental-restriction hypothesis. White matter has been shown to be responsive to environmental demands. For example, learning to play a musical instrument appears to be correlated with white matter structure in the corpus callosum, corona radiata, and internal capsule [43]. Similarly, Bengtsson *et al.* found that playing the piano had developmentally specific effects on cerebral white matter [44]. It is hard to envisage a developmental or plastic process that would reduce one element (the cerebellum) while greatly increasing another (interhemispheric connectivity).

White matter is, as other chapters have discussed, another tissue that is particularly vulnerable in VPT and VLBW groups. This has been related to the vulnerability of developmentally immature oligodendrocyte precursors (which will eventually go on to form all the central nervous system myelin) [45]. White matter lesions, and reduced white matter volume, are well-known findings in VPT and VLBW individuals, and are reviewed in Chapter 8. It is not immediately clear how oligodendrocyte pathology around the time of premature birth is related to corpus callosum growth in adolescence, however.

A tentative developmental model of cerebellar and callosal changes

One possible explanation which is compatible with these observations – for which we should emphasize, there is no direct evidence currently – is that the callosal changes represent a plastic response to a primarily cerebellar deficit. In this model, a damaged cerebellum fails to cope adequately with the cognitive and social demands of the adolescent–adult transition. This is detrimental, and is associated with poorer mental health, as we have seen [31]. The corpus callosum growth represents myelination of interhemispheric connections in a plastic response, which enables some of the effects of the cerebellar deficit to be mitigated. In particular, it allows cognitive function to be relatively spared (remember that callosal growth in the VPT group was associated with better cognitive function). Thus the changes that we have observed in the VPT brain in adolescence could be an instantiation of a plastic response that compensates for a developmental deficit. This model is at the moment incomplete – we do not have information on the development of other white matter pathways, for example, but it could perhaps be of use in formulating hypotheses about brain development that could be tested in animal models, in fMRI studies, and in future further longitudinal studies.

Conclusion

We have demonstrated non-linearities of growth of cerebellum and corpus callosum in VPT adolescents. We currently do not know whether these non-linearities persist into adulthood, and what their longer-term functional consequences may be. We have recently reported increased psychiatric morbidity in VPT adults [46] – it is not clear whether this relates to altered neurodevelopment. Will such functional problems worsen in adulthood? Again, we don't know. If we can identify potential "sensitive periods" – such as the adolescent surge in corpus callosum – we may be able to plan cognitive, behavioral, or even pharmacological interventions to target them, making using of the new information that is available about the genetics and function of oligodendrocytes [47].

Another possible future concern is development into old age. If ageing can be said to be a process, how is it altered in individuals who have developmentally different brains? For example, are individuals who suffered perinatal brain injuries at increased risk of dementia? This is a possibility, since such individuals may have reduced brain volumes and cognitive deficits in adulthood. On the other hand, it has been suggested that breakdown of myelin is involved in the pathogenesis of Alzheimer's disease [48]. If this is so, could the adolescent surge of white matter growth in preterm adolescents actually be protective against later dementia? Clearly, it will be essential to follow up preterm birth cohorts across the lifespan to answer these questions. Whatever else, it is becoming clear that brain development does not cease in childhood – it may not be too late to teach old brains new tricks.

References

1. Guyer B, Hoyert DL, Martin JA, *et al.* Annual summary of vital statistics – 1998. *Pediatrics* 1999; **104**: 1229–46.

2. Fearon P, O'Connell P, Frangou S, *et al.* Brain volumes in adult survivors of very low birth weight: a sibling-controlled study. *Pediatrics* 2004; **114**: 367–71.

3. Allin M, Henderson M, Suckling J, *et al.* Effects of very low birthweight on brain structure in adulthood. *Dev Med Child Neurol* 2004; **46**: 46–53.

4. Thomas M, Karmiloff-Smith A. Are developmental disorders like cases of adult brain damage? Implications from connectionist modelling. *Behav Brain Sci* 2002; **25**: 727–50.

5. Nosarti C, Giouroukou E, Healy E, *et al.* Grey and white matter distribution in very preterm adolescents mediates neurodevelopmental outcome. *Brain* 2008; **131**: 205–17.

6. Botting N, Powls A, Cooke RW, Marlow N. Cognitive and educational outcome of very-low-birthweight children in early adolescence. *Dev Med Child Neurol* 1998; **40**: 652–60.

7. O'Brien F, Roth S, Stewart A, *et al.* The neurodevelopmental progress of infants less than 33 weeks into adolescence. *Arch Dis Child* 2004; **89**: 207–11.

8. Kapellou O, Counsell SJ, Kennea N, *et al.* Abnormal cortical development after premature birth shown by altered allometric scaling of brain growth. *PLoS Med* 2006; **3**: e265.

9. Santhouse AM, Ffytche DH, Howard RJ, *et al.* The functional significance of perinatal corpus callosum damage: an fMRI study in young adults. *Brain* 2002; **125**: 1782–92.

10. Stewart AL, Rifkin L, Amess PN, *et al.* Brain structure and neurocognitive and behavioural function in adolescents who were born very preterm. *Lancet* 1999; **353**: 1653–7.

11. Nosarti C, Rushe TM, Woodruff PW, *et al.* Corpus callosum size and very preterm birth: relationship to neuropsychological outcome. *Brain* 2004; **127**: 2080–9.

12. Allin M, Nosarti C, Narberhaus A, *et al.* Growth of the corpus callosum in adolescents born preterm. *Arch Pediatr Adolesc Med* 2007; **161**: 1183–9.

13. Nosarti C, Rubia K, Smith A, *et al.* Altered functional neuroanatomy of response inhibition in adolescent males who were born very preterm. *Dev Med Child Neuro* 2006; **48**: 265–71.

14. Thompson DW. *On Growth and Form.* Douer reprint of 1942 2nd edn. (1st edn., 1917); 1992.

15. Blakemore SJ. The social brain in adolescence. *Nat Rev Neurosci* 2008; **9**: 267–77.

16. Patton GC, Coffey C, Carlin JB, Olsson CA, Morley R. Prematurity at birth and adolescent depressive disorder. *Br J Psychiatry* 2004; **184**: 446–7.

17. Cannon M, Jones PB, Murray RM. Obstetric complications and schizophrenia: historical and meta-analytic review. *Am J Psychiatry* 2002; **159**: 1080–92.

18. Murray RM, Lappin J, Di FM. Schizophrenia: from developmental deviance to dopamine dysregulation. *Eur Neuropsychopharmacol* 2008; **18** Suppl 3: S129–34.

19. Rapoport JL, Gogtay N. Brain neuroplasticity in healthy, hyperactive and psychotic children: insights from neuroimaging. *Neuropsychopharmacology* 2008; **33**: 181–97.

20. Rabinowicz T, de Courten-Myers GM, Petetot JM, Xi G, de los Reyes RE. Human cortex development: estimates of neuronal numbers indicate major loss late during gestation. *J Neuropathol Exp Neurol* 1996; **55**: 320–8.

21. Giedd JN, Blumenthal J, Jeffries NO, *et al.* Brain development during childhood and adolescence: a longitudinal MRI study. *Nat Neurosci* 1999; **2**: 861–3.

22. Sowell ER, Thompson PM, Tessner KD, Toga AW. Mapping continued brain growth and gray matter density reduction in dorsal frontal cortex: Inverse relationships during postadolescent brain maturation. *J Neurosci* 2001; **21**: 8819–29.

23. Gogtay N, Giedd JN, Lusk L, *et al.* Dynamic mapping of human cortical development during childhood through early adulthood. *Proc Natl Acad Sci USA* 2004; **101**: 8174–9.

24. Shaw P, Kabani NJ, Lerch JP, *et al.* Neurodevelopmental trajectories of the human cerebral cortex. *J Neurosci* 2008; **28**: 3586–94.

25. Ashtari M, Cervellione KL, Hasan KM, *et al.* White matter development during late adolescence in healthy males: a cross-sectional diffusion tensor imaging study. *Neuroimage* 2007; **35**: 501–10.

26. Chklovskii DB, Koulakov AA. Maps in the brain: what can we learn from them? *Annu Rev Neurosci* 2004; **27**: 369–92.

27. Allin MPG, Matsumoto H, Santhouse AM, *et al.* Cognitive and motor function and the size of the cerebellum in adolescents born very preterm. *Brain* 2001; **124**: 60–6.

28. Allin MPG, Salaina S, Nosarti C, *et al.* Vermis and lateral lobes of the cerebellum in adolescents born very preterm. *Neuroreport* 2005; **16**: 1821–4.

29. Schmahmann JD, Sherman JC. The cerebellar cognitive affective syndrome. *Brain* 1998; **121**(Pt 4): 561–79.

30. Ment LR, Kesler S, Vohr B, *et al.* Longitudinal brain volume changes in preterm and term control subjects during late childhood and adolescence. *Pediatrics* 2009; **123**: 503–11.

31. Parker J, Mitchell A, Kalpakidou A, *et al.* Cerebellar growth and behavioural & neuropsychological outcome in preterm adolescents. *Brain* 2008; **131**: 1344–51.

32. Pujol J, Vendrell P, Junque C, Marti-Vilalta JL, Capdevila A. When does human brain development end? Evidence of corpus callosum growth up to adulthood. *Ann Neurol* 1993; **34**: 71–5.

33. Giedd JN, Rumsey JM, Castellanos FX, *et al.* A quantitative MRI study of the corpus callosum in children and adolescents. *Brain Res Dev Brain Res* 1996; **91**: 274–80.

34. Pons TP, Garraghty PE, Ommaya AK, *et al.* Massive cortical reorganization after sensory deafferentiation in adult macaques. *Science* 1991; **252**: 1857–60.

35. Wang VY, Zoghbi HY. Genetic regulation of cerebellar development. *Nat Rev Neurosci* 2001; **2**: 484–91.

36. Rakic P. Pre- and post-developmental neurogenesis in primates. *Clin Neurosci Res* 2002; **2**: 29–39.

37. Sohma O, Mito T, Mizuguchi M, Takashima S. The prenatal age critical for the development of the pontosubicular necrosis. *Acta Neuropathol* 1995; **90**: 7–10.

38. Johnston MV. Selective vulnerability in the neonatal brain. *Ann Neurol* 1998; **44**: 155–6.

39. Leiner HC, Leiner AL, Dow RS. Cognitive and language functions of the human cerebellum. *Trends Neurosci* 1993; **16**: 444–7.

40. Allin M, Rooney M, Cuddy M, *et al*. Personality in young adults who are born preterm. *Pediatrics* 2006; **117**: 309–16.

41. Hack M, Cartar L, Schluchter M, Klein N, Forrest CB. Self-perceived health, functioning and well-being of very low birth weight infants at age 20 years. *J Pediatr* 2007; **151**: 635–41, 641.el–2.

42. Pykälä R, Räikkönen K, Feldt K, *et al*. Blood pressure responses to psychosocial stress in young adults with very low birth weight: Helsinki study of very low birth weight adults. *Pediatrics* 2009; **123**: 731–4.

43. Schmithorst VJ, Wilke M. Differences in white matter architecture between musicians and non-musicians: a diffusion tensor imaging study. *Neurosci Lett* 2002; **321**: 57–60.

44. Bengtsson SL, Nagy Z, Skare S, *et al*. Extensive piano practicing has regionally specific effects on white matter development. *Nat Neurosci* 2005; **8:** 1148–50.

45. Back SA, Luo NL, Borenstein NS, *et al*. Late oligodendrocyte progenitors coincide with the developmental window of vulnerability for human perinatal white matter injury. *J Neurosci* 2001; **21**: 1302–12.

46. Walshe M, Rifkin L, Rooney M, *et al*. Psychiatric disorder in young adults born very preterm: role of family history. *Eur Psychiatry* 2008; **23**: 527–31.

47. Dugas JC, Tai YC, Speed TP, Ngai J, Barres BA. Functional genomic analysis of oligodendrocyte differentiation. *J Neurosci* 2006; **26**: 10967–83.

48. Bartzokis G. Age-related myelin breakdown: a developmental model of cognitive decline and Alzheimer's disease. *Neurobiol Aging* 2004; **25**: 5–18.

Functional neuroimaging following very preterm birth

Chiara Nosarti and Larry Rifkin

…we must not search for the physiological substratum of mental activity in this or that part of the brain but we have to regard it as the outcome of processes spread widely over the brain.

(De Watteville, quoted in [1], p. 17)

Introduction

Mortality among very preterm (VPT) (e.g., < 33 completed weeks of gestation) and very low birth weight (VLBW) (e.g., < 1500 g) infants has significantly decreased in recent decades, particularly among the least mature individuals [2]. Very low birth weight infants are either born prematurely or are small for gestational age or both [3]. Therefore, VPT and VLBW individuals share several characteristics.

Alterations in key structural brain regions which have been reported in VPT and VLBW populations [4–9] may result in functional brain changes in distributed systems, underlying the long-term cognitive and behavioral sequelae often reported in these groups [9–13]. Functional neuroimaging investigations in VPT and VLBW individuals can therefore enhance the understanding of the mechanisms underlying the development of a variety of cognitive and behavioral problems in high-risk individuals, as well as the pathways to competent adaptation despite exposure to perinatal conditions of adversity.

Recent developments of functional neuroimaging techniques, based on measures of blood oxygenation and flow, have allowed the in vivo monitoring of metabolic changes in key brain structures and the neuroanatomical substrates of complex cognitive processes, providing new opportunities to advance the understanding of brain organization. In this chapter we will focus on investigations which have studied VPT and VLBW individuals with functional neuroimaging during different stages of development. The often observed long-term alterations in patterns of task-specific neuronal activity can be studied in relation to human cerebral plasticity, defined as reorganization of distributed patterns of neuronal activity that, at least partly, compensates for varying degrees of structural brain changes, possibly following early injury. Functional neuroimaging techniques provide information about functional segregation and neural organization; however, they supply no information about cell cytoarchitectural structure, such as neuronal packing or cell morphometry, which may be responsible for the observed plastic processes. Therefore, neuroimaging methods are used to study neuronal interactions and activity at the level of large-scale neuronal populations.

This chapter will be structured as follows: after a brief description of the basic principles of widely used functional neuroimaging techniques, we will summarize the results of published functional neuroimaging studies and discuss them in relation to methodological considerations and issues related to data interpretation.

Basic principles of functional neuroimaging techniques

Functional magnetic resonance imaging (fMRI)

Functional MRI is a relatively new technique that can be used to map changes in brain hemodynamics that correspond to mental operations. During a typical experiment, several images of the brain are repeatedly acquired, while participants are presented with specific stimuli or are required to complete a task. Functional MRI provides measures of the neural activity detected by a blood-oxygen-level-dependent (BOLD) signal [14], which refers to the increase in blood flow to the local blood vessels that accompanies neural activity in the brain.

Neurodevelopmental Outcomes of Preterm Birth, ed. Chiara Nosarti, Robin M. Murray, and Maureen Hack. Published by Cambridge University Press. © Cambridge University Press 2010.

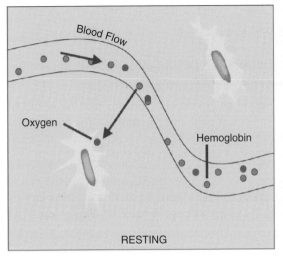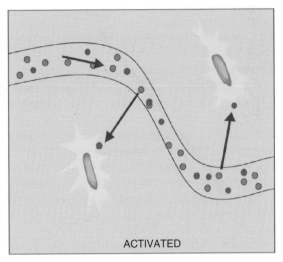

Fig. 7.1. Blood-oxygen-level-dependent contrast in magnetic resonance images: upon metabolic activation, oxygen is extracted by the cells, thereby increasing the level of deoxyhemoglobin in the blood. This is compensated for by an increase in blood flow in the vicinity of the active cells, leading to an increase in oxyhemoglobin and an increase in signal. See plate section for color version.

The blood contains oxygen required by metabolic processes, and a protein called hemoglobin, oxygen can bind to. When an oxygen molecule binds to hemoglobin, it is regarded as being oxyhemoglobin, and when no oxygen is bound, it is labeled deoxyhemoglobin. These molecules are diamagnetic, i.e., weakly repulsed from a magnetic field, and paramagnetic, i.e., attracted to externally applied magnetic fields, respectively. The presence of deoxyhemoglobin in the blood causes a susceptibility difference between the blood and its surrounding tissue, which results in color change in those voxels containing vessels of interest, caused by a dephasing of the MR proton signal [15]. As oxyhemoglobin is diamagnetic and is not associated with such dephasing, changes in oxygenation in the blood are detected as the signal changes [16]. Upon metabolic activation, oxygen is extracted by the cells, thereby increasing the level of deoxyhemoglobin in the blood. This is compensated for by an increase in blood flow in the vicinity of the active cells, leading to an increase in oxyhemoglobin and an increase in signal (Fig. 7.1). The term "hemodynamic response" to a stimulus refers to the changes in blood flow that accompany the time course for the BOLD signal changes, which is delayed from the onset of the neural activity by a few seconds.

The physiological basis of the fMRI signal has been investigated by simultaneously recording intracortical neural signals and BOLD responses [17]. Results demonstrated that the BOLD signal is closely associated with local field potentials, which mostly measure the input and processing of neuronal information within a region, rather than the output signal sent out to other brain regions.

Positron emission tomography (PET) and single photon emission computed tomography (SPECT)

Positron emission tomography and SPECT neuroimaging techniques involve the use of radioactive nuclides either from natural or synthetic sources, and hence are considered to be invasive. The use of a radiopharmaceutical substance introduced into the bloodstream is used as a tracer to study its absorption in selective brain region(s).

Single photon emission computed tomography is used to measure regional cerebral blood flow (rCBF). The radiopharmaceutical substance used in SPECT emanates gamma rays, as opposed to positron emitters employed in PET. A variety of radiotracers can be used, according to the variables of interest: i.e., I-123–3-quinuclidinyl 4-isodobenzilate, a neurotransmitter agonist, can be used for studying receptors; Xe-133 can be used for rCBF measurements. The SPECT radioisotopes have often long half lives, which range from a few hours to a few days; this helps to keep their cost low. In fact, the low cost of SPECT represents its main advantage as a brain imaging technique over either PET or fMRI. However, SPECT is inferior to the other

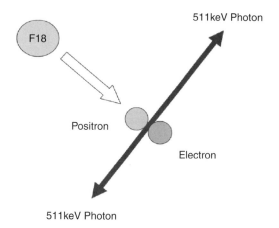

Fig. 7.2. A positron emitter, [18F]-fluorodeoxyglucose, travels a short distance before colliding with an electron. The annihilation of the two particles creates photon pairs with energy 511 keV.

mentioned neuroimaging modalities in terms of both spatial and temporal resolution, sensitivity, and quantification capability.

Positron emission tomography is a measure of regional cerebral perfusion, oxygen extraction fraction, oxygen consumption, and blood volume requiring the synthesis of [15O]-water-containing radiotracing compounds. The use of more stable isotopes such as [18F]-fluorodeoxyglucose has been used to image the neonatal brain [18].

Positron emission tomography has a superior spatial resolution and greater sensitivity compared to SPECT. Unlike fMRI, where the BOLD signal has no absolute interpretation, the signal measured can be quantified (e.g., ml blood/100 g of tissue per minute). In PET, molecules of biological interest are labeled with a positron emitter before being introduced into the bloodstream. Subsequently, the positron travels a short distance before colliding with an electron. The annihilation of the two particles creates photon pairs with energy 511 keV (Fig. 7.2). A tomographic reconstruction algorithm applied to the acquired data provides a three-dimensional distribution of positron emitter absolute concentration in the brain.

However, the analysis of complementary data obtained with these and other neuroimaging techniques, described in Chapters 4, 5, and 8, may yield more comprehensive information than data acquired with a single imaging modality. Studies using multimodal neuroimaging techniques have in fact started to be used in the investigation of the complexity of the neurophysiological processes associated with

VPT birth, which will be discussed later in this chapter [19–21].

Experimental design and analysis in functional neuroimaging studies

A variety of experimental designs may be employed in functional neuroimaging studies, and their choice mainly depends on the experimental question and characteristics of sample(s) investigated.

The main designs are "block" and "event-related." In blocked-task paradigms several stimuli of the same type are presented in sequence and signal change is then averaged across the entire block. In event-related-task paradigms, stimuli (or trial events) are presented individually and sometimes even broken down in subcomponents.

Likewise, several methods are available for the analysis of functional neuroimaging data and their choice is dependent upon the type of assumption about the data collected (i.e., linearity). Petersson and colleagues [22] argued that no functional neuroimaging analysis method currently available is optimal for all purposes, and in order to use the available methods in an optimal way it is important to be aware of the limits of applicability. Statistical model selection is essential for the validity of data interpretation [22].

Typical functional neuroimaging studies identify aspects of functional anatomy, as measured by regionally specific differences in hemodynamic responses, that differ between conditions and/or that are "typical" of a group.

Cognitive subtraction can be used, which assumes that the difference between two conditions can be regarded as a separable cognitive or sensorimotor component. However, differences in BOLD signal can be also the result of an interaction between a cognitive component and preexisting components, rather than the evocation of the cognitive component of interest (e.g., a button press response to an infrequently occurring visual cue may differ from a button press response to a semantic judgment) [23].

Another issue about subtraction concerns the fact that although different brain regions may show different engagement between conditions/groups, these may not be either necessary or sufficient for task completion or exclusively pertinent for only one of the groups investigated. In addition, brain areas which display BOLD signal during a cognitive task may not be necessary for the completion of the specific task. Adding to these considerations, Ment and Constable recently pointed out in a review of fMRI studies of prematurely born children that only brain areas that are involved in separate conditions would show signal change in activation maps, whereas areas that are equally engaged in different conditions or that are not involved in any of the conditions would not appear in results [24].

In order to address these potential problems, cognitive conjunction approaches have been proposed [25], which can be regarded as an extension of subtraction techniques. Subtraction analyses test a *single* hypothesis concerning the activation in one task relative to another. Conjunction analyses test *several* hypotheses, investigating whether all activations, in a series of tasks, are jointly significant. The idea is that if there is only one cognitive component (e.g., response inhibition), which is common to differences in a series of conditions, and it emerges as an underlying brain region in difference maps, then the region which activates in all the corresponding subtractions can be related to the common cognitive component. Conjunction analyses can be used to exclude the possibility of a given fMRI signal being the result of an interaction between the cognitive component of interest and preexisting components. A conjunction design is also particularly useful in multi-subject neuroimaging studies in which contrasts, testing for activation, are specified separately for each subject. A conjunction analysis has been described as being "the joint refutation of multiple null hypotheses, in this instance, of no activation in any subject" [26].

Neonatal studies

The use of invasive functional neuroimaging techniques in VPT and VLBW neonatal samples presents several logistic problems as the amount of radiation allowed is approximately one tenth of that allowed in older samples. Nevertheless, PET and SPECT studies have been performed on VPT infants.

Early developmental changes in cerebral (blood-to-brain) glucose transport (CTXglc) and regional cerebral metabolic rate for glucose consumption (CMRglc) have been studied with PET in VPT infants during the first week of life. Data with regard to energy metabolism were comparable to those observed in normal human adults, but reduced CTXglc values were observed in VPT neonates [27]. Another PET study investigating babies with known neonatal complications, such as periventricular leukomalacia (PVL), described poorly developed metabolic activity in the primary sensorimotor cortex [18].

Distortions in rCBF in VPT infants with normal cerebral ultrasound studied with SPECT in the first 5 weeks of life showed a flow distribution similar to flow in other newborn mammals, with respect to the basal ganglia, cerebellum, and fronto-temporal cortex. However, the gray–white matter contrast was greater in infants who were born VPT, suggesting that blood flow to the white matter was extremely low [28].

The use of non-invasive fMRI techniques in VPT and VLBW neonatal samples also presents complex and challenging problems. Erberich and colleagues [29] suggested that neonates need a controlled microenvironment and close monitoring during the MRI study in order to preserve respiratory and cardiovascular functions, body temperature, and fluid and electrolyte homeostasis. To minimize motion artifacts, dedicated coils have been used, as well as sedation with chloral hydrate. However, sedation increases the risk of respiratory depression affecting the infant's capacity to maintain satisfactory ventilation and oxygenation during scanning [29]. Furthermore, a constant temperature of 22 °C is normally maintained in MRI suites, while incubators used in neonatal units maintain a temperature similar to the infant's bodily temperature, around 36–7 °C. It has in fact been suggested that the somewhat hostile MRI room environment may result in infants developing hypothermia and consequent changes in cardiac output associated with alterations in cerebral blood flow [30]. These limitations may explain the paucity of fMRI studies in newborn infants.

Resting-state networks, or spontaneous brain activity, during sleeping were studied with fMRI in VPT infants at term and consistent activation patterns were identified in the primary visual cortex, somatosensory and motor cortices bilaterally, bilateral temporal/inferior parietal cortex encompassing the primary auditory cortex, parts of the parietal cortex, cerebellum, and medial and lateral sections of the anterior prefrontal cortex [31]. Activation was in fewer networks than those observed in adults, and was predominantly non-lateralized.

Findings of other studies indicate that the refinement of hemispheric lateralization may occur only in the postnatal period. The development of lateralization systems in preterm and term neonates was recently studied in the somatosensory system located in the regions of the pre- and postcentral gyri using a passive task involving the opening of the infant's hand [32]. Results for term, 3- to 9-month-old term, and preterm neonates revealed responses that were unilateral and contralateral to the stimulated hand. Results for the neonatal cohort reported unilateral, contralateral as well as bilateral responses to the stimulated hand, suggesting only a non-significant trend for contralateral lateralization of the somatosensory system at around term, in line with the results of Fransson and colleagues [31] of brain activity during resting states.

Sensory development in infants has been investigated with fMRI using passive visual, tactile, and auditory tasks. In control samples, during photic stimulation, a BOLD signal increase in the visual cortex has been described in children under 8 weeks of age, and a signal decrease in older children, possibly underlying changes in oxygen consumption associated with rapid synapse formation starting at 48 weeks and accompanying increased metabolism [33]. Response to changes in luminance through closed eyelids was studied in a sample of VPT infants and controls [34]. Children < 60 weeks' postmenstrual age (PMA) exhibited either BOLD signal increases or decreases in visual cortex, while in the older participants a BOLD signal decrease was observed, irrespective of chronological age at assessment. The BOLD signal decrease during activation has been interpreted as reflecting a fall in rCBF, an increase in oxygen extraction or an increase in cerebral blood volume [35]. The observation of BOLD signal increase only in those infants < 60 weeks' PMA therefore suggests developmental immaturity.

The study of passive sensorimotor and visual function in VPT infants revealed activated regions above a statistical threshold in most participants [29]. During sensorimotor tasks decreased as well as increased BOLD signal was detected ipsilaterally, contralaterally, and bilaterally in motor and sensory areas of the precentral gyrus, being consistent with the early myelination of the posterior limb of the internal capsule and the corona radiata [36], and in the frontal cortex. Increased signal in the brainstem was observed for the least mature infants born at 32 weeks. The authors interpreted their results as evidence that neonatal brain function may fundamentally differ from childhood and adult function, possibly due to differences in synaptic density characterizing various stages of brain maturation. During the visual experiment, BOLD signal was detected in the occipital lobe, where the primary visual cortex is located [29]. However, both location and size of the activation was different from results observed in adults, in line with previous studies on term neonates and infants (0–2 years) [33,34].

Auditory cortical activation in non-sedated neonates was studied in a group of VPT and term infants and adult controls. Participants were presented with a frequency-modulated pure tone and increased BOLD signal was demonstrated in adult controls in the superior temporal areas compared to both groups of infants. Detected in BOLD signal decreases were instead during auditory stimulation in most infants [37]. Auditory system development could be particularly disrupted by preterm birth, as the onset of hearing in healthy samples has been estimated to occur at around 29 weeks of gestation [38]. A relation between fetal auditory system development and later language functions has been described [39], possibly accounting at least in part for language deficits reported in VPT and VLBW samples later in life [11,40] (see Chapter 13 for further details).

To summarize, these studies suggest that increased BOLD signal characterizes sensory stimulation in the human newborn cortex [29,34,37] and that the association between neural activity and vascular responses may be dependent on subjects' gestational as well as postmenstrual age. It has been suggested that the neonate's vascular system may be unable to meet increased oxygen demands by increasing local cerebral blood flow, resulting in a negative BOLD signal brought about by a decrease in the ratio of oxy- to deoxyhemoglobin [41]. Furthermore, the above studies, summarized in Table 7.1, suggest that different sensory modalities may become lateralized and start to respond to stimulation at different stages of development, namely the auditory system may develop earlier than the visual system.

Childhood studies

One of the most consistently reported areas of impaired cognitive function in VPT and VLBW individuals compared to controls is language. At school age, developmental language delays have been described [42], as well as deficits in reading skills [43], and receptive/listening vocabulary scores [44]. It is therefore not surprising that the majority of fMRI studies with VPT children published to date have investigated the neural correlates of language processing [44–46]. These are summarized in Table 7.2. Participants for these studies were recruited from a multisite randomized trial of indomethacin use to prevent intraventricular hemorrhage [47].

Peterson *et al.* [46] investigated the neural correlates of phonological (encoding and processing of

Table 7.1 Functional neuroimaging studies in VPT and VLBW neonatal samples

Study	Cases	Controls	Imaging method	Analysis software	Variables of interest	Findings
Powers et al. [27]	6 VPT, F = 1 (estimated GA range 25–34, range BW 770–2280 g) during the first week of life	None reported	ECAT 961 EXACT HR PET	PROMIS algorithm	CTXglc and CMRglc	CMRglc comparable to values in normal human adults, CTXglc reduced in VPT
Higuchi et al. [18]	2 VPT, F = 1, with periventricular leukomalacia (GA 28 and 30, BW 1308 and 1476 g), corrected ages 18 and 34 days	None reported	PCT3000W, PET	ROI for brainstem and sensorimotor area	CMRglc	Low CMRglc in SMC
Borch & Greisen [28]	12 VPT, F = 3 (mean GA = 27.7, range 25–32; mean BW = 915 g, range 550–2680 g) during the first 5 weeks of life	None reported	SPECT	ROI for basal ganglia, lateral cortex, subcortical white matter, cerebellum	rCBF	rCBF distribution similar to other newborn mammals in BG, CER and fronto-temporal cortex. Gray–white matter contrast greater in VPT
Fransson et al. [31]	12 VPT, F = 5 (GA range 24–27; BW range 499–1325 g) at term; 5 VPT IVH grade 1 or 2	1 CTRL adult	1.5 Tesla fMRI	SPM2	Resting-state during sleeping, 10 minutes	Activation in 5 areas: primary VC; SMC bilaterally; bilateral temporal/IPL including PAC and parts of PC; CER; and anterior PFC compared to 10 areas identified in adults
Erberich et al. [32]	42 term and VPT neonates (mean PMA = 42, range 38–49), some had mild US abnormalities	6 CTRL (PMA range 3–9 months)	1.5 Tesla, neonatal volume head coil fMRI	SPM99	Passive motor stimulation	CTRL: BOLD responses unilateral and contralateral to the stimulated hand. All neonates: BOLD signal in SMC from unilateral, stimulation was contralateral, unilateral, and bilateral in TH and PFC (in 42%) CTRL: no activation in these areas
Born et al. [34]	15 VPT (mean GA = 30.9, range 25–37) PMA 29–61	12 children with visual deficit (PMA 41–338); 12 CTRL (PMA 39–179)	1.5 Tesla fMRI	STIMULATE	Stroboscopic light stimulation, 1 or 8 Hz alternated with 30 seconds darkness	Children < 60 weeks' PMA exhibited either BOLD signal increases or decreases in VC, older participants showed signal decrease, irrespective of age

Table 7.1 Continued

Study	Cases	Controls	Imaging method	Analysis software	Variables of interest	Findings
Erberich et al. [29]	7 VPT, F = 2 (mean GA = 28.6, range 24–39; range BW 1200–4600 g); PMA range 34–58	None reported	1.5 Tesla, neonatal volume head coil fMRI	SPM99	2 passive sensorimotor tasks and one visual task (gantry light flickering 2 Hz)	Sensorimotor tasks: unilateral hand stimulation resulted in decreased (5 out of 6 infants) as well as increased (3/6) BOLD signal in contralateral SMC. Increased signal in brainstem in VPT (GA 32) for both hands Visual task: BOLD signal in OL (6/7)
Anderson et al. [37]	20 healthy neonates (13 term, F = 6, PMA range 39.5–47.5; 7 VPT, F = 3, mean GA = 29, range 25–32; PMA range 33.5–36), normal US, at term	4 CTRL, all M (mean age 34 years, range 23–49)	1.5 Tesla, fMRI	SPM99b	60–80 dB tone centered at 1.3 kHz and modulated over range ±1 kHz at a rate of 8 Hz	Neonates: BOLD signal decrease in 64% and increases in the remaining subjects in STG bilaterally CTRL: positive BOLD signal in similar areas

BG = basal ganglia; BW = birth weight; CER = cerebellum; CMRglc = regional cerebral metabolic rate for glucose consumption; CTRL = healthy controls; CTXglc = cerebral (blood-to-brain) glucose transport; GA = gestational age in weeks; F = female; IPL = inferior parietal lobule; IVH = intraventricular hemorrhage; M = male; OL = occipital lobe; PAC = primary auditory cortex; PC = parietal cortex; PFC = prefrontal cortex; PMA = postmenstrual age in weeks; rCBF = regional cerebral blood flow; ROI = region of interest; SMC = sensorimotor cortex; SPM2 = Statistical Parametric Mapping 2002; SPM99 = Statistical Parametric Mapping 1999; STG = superior temporal gyrus; TH = thalamus; US = ultrasound in the neonatal period; VC = visual cortex.

Table 7.2 Functional neuroimaging studies in VPT and VLBW childhood samples

Study	Cases	Controls	Imaging method	Analysis software	Variables of interest	Findings
Peterson et al. [46]	23 VPT, F = 9; mean age 8.6 years (mean GA = 28.8, range 26–33; range BW 700–1240 g)	11 CTRL, F = 6, age matched, 4 adults, F = 3 (mean age 36.5 years)	1.5 Tesla, fMRI	SPM99	Passive auditory listening task, 3 stimuli: semantic processing, phonological processing, and phonemic randomization (no semantic processing)	Semantic processing: VPT < CTRL lateral PFC, ventral CG; similar areas activated in CTRL during phonological processing. VIQ correlated with activations VPT in Wernicke's area, AG, and DLPC
Ment et al. [44]	47 VPT, F = 22 (mean GA = 28; BW range 600–1250 g); mean age 8 years, normal US; 22/47 VPT saline; 25/47 VPT indomethacin	23 CTRL, matched for age, sex, maternal education, and ethnicity	1.5 Tesla, fMRI	SPM99	Passive auditory listening task, 3 stimuli: semantic processing, phonological processing, and phonemic randomization (no semantic processing)	Treatment-by-gender effect in phonological but not semantic contrast in left IPL, IFG (Broca's area), and right DLPC. "VPT indomethacin" boys showed BOLD signal similar to controls rather than "VPT saline"; girls showed no indomethacin effect
Ment et al. [45]	14 VPT, mean age 12 years old, normal US (range BW 600–1250 g)	10 CTRL matched for age, sex, and ethnicity	1.5 Tesla, fMRI	SPM99	Passive auditory listening task, 3 stimuli: semantic processing, phonological processing, and phonemic randomization (no semantic processing)	Semantic processing: VPT and CTRL positive and negative BOLD signal in similar brain areas including left IFG and posterior CG; % signal change VPT < CTRL. Phonological processing: VPT positive signal in left PHG, right anterior MTG, posterior CG, and left middle/STG. CTRL negative signal in same regions

AG = angular gyrus; BW = birth weight; CG = cingulate gyrus; CTRL = healthy controls; DLPC = dorsolateral prefrontal cortex; GA = gestational age in weeks; F = female; IFG = inferior frontal gyrus; IPL = inferior parietal lobule; MTG = middle temporal gyrus; PHG = parahippocampal gyrus; PFC = prefrontal cortex; SPM99 = Statistical Parametric Mapping 1999; STG = superior temporal gyrus; US = ulltrasound; VIQ = verbal intelligence quotient.

phonemes, the basic sounds of speech) and semantic (understanding the meaning conveyed by speech) language processing in VPT children aged 8 years and controls. Results suggested that the preterm children with the poorest language comprehension scores did not engage the same brain regions during the semantic tasks as controls. Instead, this subgroup of VPT children engaged the neural pathways which controls used when processing meaningless phonological sounds. Specifically, during the semantic processing task, VPT children showed decreased BOLD signal in lateral prefrontal and ventral cingulate regions; similar brain areas were activated in controls during phonological processing tasks. Verbal comprehension IQ scores correlated with fMRI activations in the VPT group only in regions including Wernicke's area, angular gyrus, and dorsal prefrontal cortex bilaterally. These findings suggest that, in at least a subset of VPT children, language impairments may be due to differences in neural organization.

The same passive listening language task used by Peterson was studied in a larger group of preterm-born school-age children (n = 47) with no evidence of intraventricular hemorrhage on neonatal cranial echoencephalography [44]. One of the aims of the study was to assess the possible benefits of neonatal indomethacin treatment on subsequent functional brain activation across genders. In terms of neurodevelopmental outcome in childhood, the VPT group showed lower scores than controls in full-scale, verbal, and performance IQ, as well as receptive/listening vocabulary scores. In the randomized indomethacin study some neonates received saline and some were assigned to indomethacin. Preterm boys in the saline group tended to have lower neurodevelopmental scores than preterm boys in the indomethacin group and all preterm girls.

Investigation of BOLD signal indicated a significant treatment-by-gender effect in the phonological but not in the semantic contrast in areas known to be implicated in the phonological processing of language, namely the left inferior parietal lobule, left inferior frontal gyrus (Broca's area), and right dorsolateral prefrontal cortex. Preterm boys in the indomethacin group showed patterns of neural activations which were similar to those observed in controls rather than to those of preterm boys in the saline group, whilst girls did not show a significant effect of early indomethacin at the neuronal level during verbal processing.

Another study by Ment et al. [45] included slightly older VPT participants, aged 12 years, with no evidence

of neonatal brain injury and controls using the passive listening task of language, evaluating both phonologic and semantic processing, described above. Offline language function testing revealed differences in estimated IQ between VPT children and controls, as well as differences on language scales, measuring the understanding of language and sight word recognition, but no differences in phonology scores.

Functional MRI data analyses were performed adjusting for IQ and results demonstrated that the groups differentially engaged the neural systems underlying auditory language processing. During semantic processing, VPT participants and controls exhibited positive and negative BOLD signals in similar brain areas, including the left inferior frontal gyrus and posterior cingulate gyrus, but the percent of signal change was greater in controls than VPT children, i.e., controls were significantly more likely to activate systems for the semantic processing of language. When investigating the neural correlates of phonologic processing, children born VPT showed a positive BOLD signal in left parahippocampal gyrus, right anterior middle temporal gyrus, posterior cingulate gyrus, and left middle/superior temporal gyrus. In controls, a negative BOLD signal was found in the same regions, even after adjusting for verbal IQ and subjects' age at assessment.

These results suggest that, in the absence of overt differences in phonological processing, VPT children engage different and broader neural networks for phonologic processing than controls. In line with Peterson's results, some of the areas which were found to be activated in VPT children during phonological processing have been associated with semantic processing [48] and further behavioral evidence indicates that children with suboptimal phonological processing skills have the tendency to rely on lexico-semantic information to process phonological material [49].

Altered neuronal activation during phonological processing in preterm populations may contribute to the development of other neurodevelopmental impairments often described in VPT samples. For instance, phonological processing is required for the acquisition of reading and spelling skills, which have been found to continue to be poorer in early adulthood in VPT individuals compared to controls [8]. Poor phonological skills may in addition contribute to the need for special services in school received by large proportions of VPT children [44,50] (see also Chapter 16).

Adolescent and adult studies

A number of functional neuroimaging studies during the adolescent, and recently, the early adult period, have investigated VPT and VLBW samples (see Table 7.3). Our group recruited VPT adolescents from the University College Hospital London (UCHL) cohort [50] and studied visual and auditory, language, response inhibition, and memory processing.

A first study used visual and auditory tasks requiring callosal transfer in a cohort of VPT individuals and controls aged 18–20 years [21]. A subgroup of the VPT individuals had damaged corpus callosum (CC) visualized on structural MRI (referred to as "callosal group"), whilst another subgroup had no CC damage. The visual task consisted of stimuli presented bilaterally in the right and in the left visual field, and unilaterally in one hemifield. The auditory task involved timbre discrimination presented monaurally to the left or the right ear.

Results showed that the VPT individuals with damaged CC had significantly different activation patterns compared with controls, and with a group of VPT adolescents without any evidence of brain damage. In the visual modality, increased BOLD signal was seen in the right dorsolateral prefrontal cortex of the callosal group, which the authors interpreted as possibly reflecting an alternative strategy used to perform the task, involving the storage of information in working memory. On the auditory task, increased BOLD signal was seen in the right temporal lobe and precentral gyrus bilaterally of the callosal group. These findings suggested a plasticity of function compensating for early CC damage. However, differences in performance were observed between the groups: in the visual modality the callosal group was significantly slower at completing the task although accuracy was comparable to VPT individuals with no CC damage and controls; in the auditory task the callosal group showed poorer performance and was significantly slower at completing the task compared to the other two groups.

One interpretation of the fMRI auditory results could be that the callosal group had difficulties accessing the timbre discrimination area, i.e., the right temporal lobe [51], which resulted in both slower reaction time and increased activation in this area. Differences in task performance and reaction times, in addition to VPT status and callosal damage, may have thus contributed to the interpretation of neural activation maps, as the authors acknowledged.

Another study tested the hypothesis that adolescents who were born VPT and who exhibited radiological evidence of CC thinning would display incomplete lateralization of language function [20]. The CC has been found to be reduced in size in VPT adolescents compared to controls, and to be related to language function [7]. Some authors (e.g., [52]) have suggested that this may be due to the role of the CC in the development of hemispheric lateralization (for example left hemisphere dominance for language function).

Rushe and colleagues [20] compared the patterns of activation for VPT individuals and controls matched for age, handedness (all right-handed) and gender (all males) for a non-word rhyming task, testing phonological skills, and a letter case judgment task, assessing orthographic skills. The two groups did not show differences in task performance, but different patterns of neural activation for the groups were detected.

During the phonological processing trials, relative to controls, VPT adolescents showed reduced BOLD signal in the left hemisphere, including the peristriate cortex and cerebellum; they also showed a reduction in activation in right parietal association areas. The VPT group showed increased BOLD signal in the right precentral gyrus and the right supplementary motor area (SMA). During the orthographic processing trials, VPT individuals displayed reduced activation compared to controls in left peristriate cortex and left precuneus. Thus, peristriate cortex seemed to show decreased neural activity during both the orthographic and phonological tasks. There is evidence from imaging studies in normal subjects that this region is active in early orthographic processing of linguistic stimuli [53].

Rushe and colleagues suggested that reduced activation in peristriate cortex might have been the result of an inefficient or developmentally delayed network implicated in orthographic processing, and that the VPT participants reached comparable task performance by employing a more effortful phonological approach than the controls.

We recently investigated verbal fluency processing with differential cognitive loading ("easy" and "hard" letter trials) in VPT-born 20-year-old individuals [54]. We found that group membership, level of task difficulty, and gestational age all had significant effects on brain activation.

In the absence of significant between-group differences in task performance, during "easy" letter trials, VPT-born individuals showed attenuated activation in anterior cingulate gyrus, right caudate nucleus and left inferior frontal gyrus compared to controls. During "hard" letter trials, the VPT-born group showed both

Table 7.3 Functional neuroimaging studies in VPT and VLBW adolescent and adult samples

Study	Cases	Controls	Imaging method	Analysis software	Variables of interest	Findings
Santhouse et al. [21]	9 VPT, all M (GA > 33), age range 18–20 years; VPT with damaged CC (DCC) and VPT with normal CC (NCC)	7 CTRL, age, sex matched	1.5 Tesla, fMRI	SPM99	Visual task: stimuli presented bilaterally and unilaterally Auditory task: timbre discrimination presented monaurally	Visual task: DCC > NCC > CTRL in right DLPC. Auditory task: DCC > NCC > CTRL in right TL, PRG bilaterally
Rushe [20]	6 VPT, all M (mean GA = 28.8; mean BW 1360 g), mean age at study 18.1 years	6 CTRL, age, sex matched	1.5 Tesla, fMRI	XBAM (non-parametric)	Non-word rhyming task (phonological) and letter case judgment task (orthographic)	Phonological processing: CTRL > VPT in left PSC, CER, right PC. VPT > CTRL in right PRG and right SMA Orthographic processing: VPT < CTRL in left PSC and left precuneus
Gimenez et al. [19]	14 VPT (mean GA = 29.4) mean age 16 years, all had anoxia, PVH, or fetal suffering; mean age 14.7 years, range 12–18	14 CTRL, age matched	1.5 Tesla, fMRI	SPM2 ROI for HI	Encoding: novel face–name pairs (target task); recognition of two repeated face–name pairs (control task)	Encoding: VPT > CTRL right HI
Nosarti et al. [55]	8 VPT, all M (mean GA = 27.8; mean BW = 1105.9 g), mean age 16 years	14 CTRL, age matched	1.5 Tesla, fMRI	XBAM (non-parametric)	Go/No-go (response inhibition) and Oddball tasks (attention allocation)	Oddball: VPT < CTRL in ACG, left vPMC, VPT > CTRL in IFG/ orbital/mesial PFC, posterior CER Response inhibition: VPT < CTRL in CER, right CN, TH, left IFG, left ACG. VPT > CTRL in TL
Curtis et al. [61]	9 VPT (mean GA = 30.2, range 27–35; mean BW = 1519.2 g) 5 IVH; mean age of both samples 13.8 years, range 12.5–16.2 years	9 CTRL, age matched	4.0 Tesla, fMRI	STIMULATE ROI for HI and CN	5 tasks: delayed match to sample (DMS), delayed non-match to sample (DNMS), spatial memory span, 2 perceptuo-motor tasks	Spatial memory span encoding: VPT > CTRL in right CN. Spatial memory span recognition: VPT < CTRL in right CN Perceptuo-motor tasks: similar patterns

Study	VPT sample	Controls	Scanner	Software	Task	Results
Carmody et al. [64]	10 VPT, F = 7 (mean GA = 32.1, range 28–35), with no evidence of IVH on neonatal US, aged 15–16 years	None	1.5 Tesla, fMRI	AFNI	fMRI attentional task: response to target letter and response inhibition when any letter other than the target. Scores of cumulative medical and environmental risk	Lower medical complications scores: increased activation in left PC. Lower environmental complications scores: increased activation in TL bilaterally Improved task performance: increased activation in left IPL, SMG, and STG
Lawrence et al. [56]	26 VPT, F = 10 (mean GA = 28.7; mean BW = 1336.8 g), mean age 20 years	21 CTRL, age matched	1.5 Tesla, fMRI	XBAM (non-parametric)	Go/No-go (response inhibition) and Oddball tasks (attention allocation)	Oddball: VPT < CTRL in IFG, PRG, CER, SMG Response inhibition: VPT > CTRL in MTG, PCG, precuneus
Narberhaus et al. [60]	21 VPT, F = 9 (mean GA = 26.6), mean age 20 years	22 CTRL, age and sex matched	1.5 Tesla, fMRI	XBAM (non-parametric)	Visual paired associates encoding and recognition	Encoding: VPT < CTRL in IFG VPT > CTRL in CN, cuneus, SPL Recognition: VPT > CTRL in CER, IFG
Nosarti et al. [54]	28 VPT, F = 11 (mean GA = 28.8), mean age 20 years	26 CTRL, age and sex matched	1.5 Tesla, fMRI	XBAM (non-parametric)	Verbal fluency, "easy" and "hard" letters	Easy: VPT < CTRL in IFG, CN, ACG Hard: VPT < CTRL in MFG VPT > CTRL in ACG, GA correlated with activation in ACG and CN

ACG = anterior cingulate gyrus; AFNI = Analysis of Functional Neuroimages Package; BW = birth weight; CC = corpus callosum; CER = cerebellum; CN = caudate nucleus; CTRL = healthy controls; DLPC = dorsolateral prefrontal cortex; GA = gestational age in weeks; F = female; HI = hippocampus; IFG = inferior frontal gyrus; IPL = inferior parietal lobule; IVH = intraventricular hemorrhage; M = males; MFG = middle frontal gyrus; MTG = middle temporal gyrus; PC = parietal cortex; PCG = posterior cingulate gyrus; PFC = prefrontal cortex; PRG = precentral gyrus; PSC = peristriate cortex; SPL = superior parietal lobule; PVH = periventricular hemorrhage; ROI = region of interest; SMA = supplementary motor area; SMG = supramarginal gyrus; SPM2 = Statistical Parametric Mapping 2002; SPM99 = Statistical Parametric Mapping 1999; STG = superior temporal gyrus; TH = thalamus; TL = temporal lobe; US = ultrasound; VC = visual cortex; vPMC; = ventrolateral premotor cortex; XBAM = Brain Activation Map.

decreased and increased BOLD signal compared to controls, in left middle frontal and anterior cingulate gyrus, respectively (Fig. 7.3). The BOLD signal in caudate nucleus and anterior cingulate gyrus, in regions with peaks close to areas where between-group differences were observed, was linearly associated with gestational age. Analysis of structural MRI data showed altered gray matter distribution in the preterm-born group compared to controls. However, fMRI results were only partly explained by structural changes, and were interpreted as possibly reflecting processes of functional plasticity for the successful completion of executive-type operations.

Another study from our group studying adolescents from the UCHL cohort employed event-related fMRI to investigate the hypothesis that individuals who were born VPT may use alternative neuronal pathways during performance of a task involving selective attention and response inhibition compared to controls [55].

We used Oddball trials to measure perceptive selective attention allocation and Go/No-go trials to assess response selection and motor response inhibition in response to a visual stimulus.

Although task performance was similar in VPT adolescents and controls, between-group differences in functional neuroanatomy were observed. During the Oddball condition, adolescents who were born VPT showed decreased BOLD signal response bilaterally (with cluster local maxima on left side) in the anterior cingulate cortex and in a left ventrolateral premotor area, compared to controls. They also displayed increased activation in the right hemisphere in a large area of the prefrontal gyrus and posterior cerebellum. During successful response inhibition trials the VPT subjects showed decreased neuronal activation in cerebellum, right caudate nucleus and thalamus, left lateral globus pallidus and inferior frontal/anterior

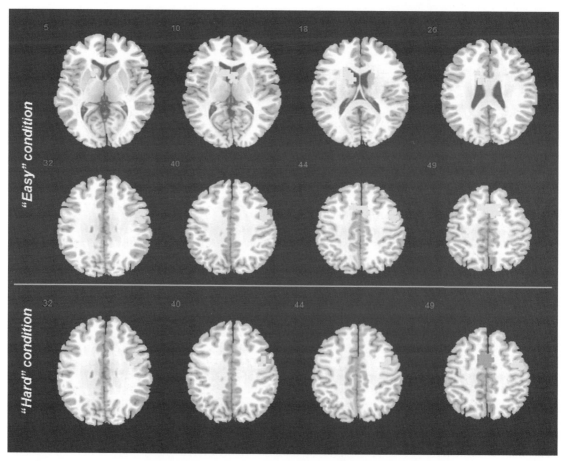

Fig. 7.3. Two-dimensional representative slices are presented for group data with activations displayed on a template image. Numbers indicate z coordinate in standard Talairach space. Brain regions with decreased (yellow) and increased (blue) activation in VPT participants compared with controls during "easy" and "hard" letter trials (adapted from [54]). See plate section for color version.

cingulate areas bilaterally compared to controls. They also showed increased response mainly in prefrontal and temporal regions.

This suggests that despite good task performance, VPT individuals may activate different neural networks and use alternative strategies when challenged with attention allocation and motor response inhibition processing. We hypothesized that the hyperactivation observed in the above brain areas in both conditions may have compensated for a possible dysfunction of cingulo-frontal and frontal-striatal-cerebellar connectivity, by recruiting secondary response pathways, resulting in a modified, yet effective attentional circuitry.

We recently used the same Go/No-go task in another group of VPT-born individuals aged 20 and controls. Very preterm young adults showed reduced activation in a fronto-parietal-cerebellar network during attention allocation, and increased activation in posterior brain regions during inhibitory control, which the authors interpreted as possibly reflecting developmental delay [56].

Another brain area which has been consistently found to be altered in VPT and VLBW samples is the hippocampus [6,57], possibly due to its vulnerability to hypoxic-ischemic damage [58]. Hippocampal damage may thus contribute to the explanation of at least some of the memory deficits observed in preterm populations [59].

Gimenez and colleagues used fMRI to investigate hippocampal activation during a declarative memory (e.g., conscious explicit memory) task in VPT adolescents and controls [19]. Participants were requested to learn novel face–name pairs (target task), and then to recognize two repeated face–name pairs (control task). Group comparison revealed that BOLD signal in the encoding phase of the experiment was increased in the right hippocampus in VPT adolescents compared to controls. Furthermore, the volume of the left hippocampus was smaller in VPT adolescents than in the control group and right hippocampal volume was positively associated in the VPT group with right hippocampal BOLD signal during the recognition phase of the experiment.

In order to explain these results, the authors mentioned the possibility that left hippocampal tissue loss may be associated with an increase in contralateral brain activity, which may reflect compensatory processes, but are however not sufficient for the achievement of normal performance in the VPT group, which scored significantly lower than controls in the recognition phase of the experiment.

A study from our group also investigated the neural correlates of visual paired-associate learning [60]. Participants were requested to memorize pairs of pictures and then recognize previously associated pairs from novel pairs. Analysis of fMRI data revealed that during encoding VPT young adults (mean age 20 years) showed reduced BOLD signal response compared to controls in right inferior frontal gyrus and increased response in left caudate nucleus, right cuneus and left superior parietal lobule. In the absence of differences in the number of correctly recognized items and response times, during recognition, VPT-born participants again showed increased BOLD signal response in right cerebellum and in anterior cingulate gyrus bilaterally.

The fMRI data were additionally analyzed controlling for structural differences in the hippocampi bilaterally, where the VPT group showed decreased probability of the absolute amount of gray matter compared to controls. Results remained unaltered except from the loss of statistical significance in a cluster with local maxima in the cerebellum, observed during the recognition phase of the experiment.

Once more, these results suggest that VPT individuals may use alternative cortical activations during learning and memory processing. Decreased activation in prefrontal cortex, possibly due to structural alterations [8], may be compensated for by increased recruitment of brain areas known to be involved in mnemonic and attentional processes.

The neural correlates of another type of memory, object working memory, was studied with fMRI by Curtis and colleagues [61]; working memory refers to the ability to maintain and manipulate information that is no longer available in the environment. Object working memory deficits have been described in preterm preschool children, and were predicted by measures of early brain injury [62].

This study used delayed match to sample (DMS) and delayed non-match to sample (DNMS) tasks, classically divided into encoding, mnemonic maintenance and recognition phases, during which subjects were asked to choose either a familiar (DMS) or unfamiliar (DNMS) stimulus. In this type of task, cognitive load can be manipulated by increasing the duration of the maintenance delay, with a corresponding increase in response latency and reduction in response accuracy. In addition, a spatial memory span task was used on the basis of deficits observed in an earlier assessment of a larger cohort of VPT children [63], and baseline tasks consisting of two analogous perceptuo-motor paradigms. The main aim of the study was to investigate whether preterm early adolescents would show differential activation of the hippocampus (tested with the DMS and DMNS tasks) and caudate nucleus (tested with spatial memory span task) compared to controls.

Task performance and hippocampal activation did not differ between the two groups. Functional MRI results revealed that, during the spatial memory span task, VPT adolescents displayed *increased* BOLD signal during encoding and *decreased* signal during recognition in the right caudate nucleus. Similar patterns of activation were detected during the DMS perceptuo-motor and spatial span perceptuo-motor tasks, which were baseline tasks placing no cognitive demands on memory.

The authors interpreted their results as possibly reflecting group differences in the planning and execution of a motor response, with reduced BOLD signal in the VPT group underlying functional impairments in the execution of a complex motor response and increased activation in the encoding phase reflecting greater cognitive effort needed by VPT individuals to maintain unimpaired on-line performance.

A different approach to the study of functional neuroanatomy in VPT adolescents was adopted by Carmody *et al.* [64], who investigated neonatal medical complications (i.e., early cumulative medical risk) and the pre- and postnatal environment in which infants are reared (i.e., cumulative environmental risk) in relation to BOLD signal. Cumulative neonatal medical risk has been associated with motor development in the first few years of life and a cumulative environmental risk has been found to predict cognitive and language outcome [65]. Furthermore, interventions aimed at reducing environmental risk have been found to result not only in improved neurodevelopmental function, but to have an impact on brain development, specifically on white matter maturation in frontal and occipital cortices [66].

Using an attentional task similar to a Go/No-go task, where participants were asked to squeeze a bulb when a target letter appeared on the screen and not to squeeze the bulb when any letter other than the target was presented, Carmody and colleagues found that BOLD signal was associated with differential risk type scores [64].

Lower medical complications scores were associated with increased activation in the left parietal cortex and lower environmental complications scores were related to increased activation in temporal lobes bilaterally. In addition, improved task performance was associated with increased activation in the left hemisphere in inferior parietal lobule, and supramarginal and superior temporal gyri.

These results could be interpreted in the context of functional maturation of fronto-parietal networks. Age and increased efficiency in the completion of a variety of cognitive tasks has in fact been associated with increased BOLD signal in parietal brain regions during tasks involving cognitive control [67]. These findings therefore indicate that early risk is associated with more immature patterns of brain activation, including reduced efficiency of attentional processing.

Methodological considerations

The study of neuronal activity using functional neuroimaging techniques provides the opportunity to improve the understanding of the neurodevelopmental processes associated with the sequelae of VPT birth and ascertain differences in the degree, profile, and specificity of possible impairments in this group, as well as possible mechanisms underlying recovery from brain injury and processes of neural plasticity.

The studies described above have used different designs which could be grouped as follows: (1) metabolic and functional brain correlates, as affected by developmental changes associated with gestational and postmenstrual age; (2) the study of the effect of structural brain alterations on functional neural activity [19–21]; (3) the study of the neural correlates of specific cognitive functions in VPT samples with normal neonatal ultrasound results, some of whom did and some of whom did not show differences in performance during fMRI scanning [45,55,68]; (4) studies which examined the effect of environmental factors, including medical interventions, on subsequent brain function [44,64].

All these designs, as the majority of functional neuroimaging studies, are prone to be affected by potential methodological problems. The remaining part of this chapter will attempt to address methodological considerations and issues related to data interpretation.

Neonatal studies have described low blood flow and poorly developed metabolic activity in VPT infants [18,27,69]. As far as we are aware, no similar studies have been conducted so far in older groups of VPT individuals, therefore a methodological concern refers to the possibility that the observed modality- and task-specific between-group differences observed in most studies with VPT groups reviewed in this chapter may be affected by differences between VPT individuals and controls in functional activation in resting-state neural networks, which can be regarded as representing a physiological baseline.

Another important point to consider when interpreting neurodevelopmental processes in VPT samples is the age of subjects being studied. During normal brain development, neural systems responsible for specific cognitive processes progress from diffuse, undifferentiated systems to specialized systems. The bulk of this "fine tuning" process occurs during the last trimester of gestation and a few years postnatally [70]. However, developmental dynamic processes of brain maturation have been observed in normative samples at least up to the second decade of life.

Typically, gray matter volume in the frontal lobes increases during preadolescence, followed by a decline in teenage years with the prefrontal cortex not being fully mature until late adolescence. In temporal lobes, gray matter development is also non-linear; the peak being reached at about 16–17 years [71] (see also Chapter 6). Consequently, the existence of critical periods during which marked changes in functional organization occur with increasing age and skill have been postulated [67,72].

In a comprehensive review of the literature on injury and recovery in the developing brain, which focused on fMRI studies in VPT individuals, Ment and Constable [24] suggested a "hyperfrontality" of response in VPT individuals during tasks involving language, which may underlie functional developmental delays, as there is evidence of a shift from diffuse to focal cortical activity during childhood development [73], although this may be dependent on the task, modality and developmental stage being studied, as age and increased skills have also been associated with increased BOLD signal in selective brain regions [67].

A few of the functional neuroimaging studies we have described selected VPT participants on the basis of structural brain alterations, and found that the "structurally different" VPT group, e.g., with thinning of the CC, exhibited different neural activation from VPT individuals with no CC damage and controls [20,21]; significant associations between the size of a chosen brain structure (e.g., the hippocampus) and BOLD signal were also observed [19]. Furthermore, some VPT samples have included individuals with evidence of periventricular hemorrhage and other neonatal ultrasound abnormalities [18,19,31,61], who are likely to show a greater extent of cortical and subcortical alterations in adolescence than VPT individuals with normal ultrasound results [8].

Given the extent of structural brain alterations reported in VPT samples and described in detail in Chapters 4, 5, and 6, Ment and Constable [24] discussed methodological limitations with respect to the employment of fMRI neuroimaging analysis techniques which

use registration to a common (often standard) reference space, especially for VPT individuals with enlarged lateral ventricles, and stressed the importance of developing statistical atlases for neonates and children of various ages.

Brett and colleagues [74] gave an example of how different anatomy between two groups may confound interpretability of BOLD signal differences using intersubject averaging analysis: if functional areas are not well aligned amongst individuals, then fMRI analysis may fail to identify a location in which there is an average increase/decrease in activation even if all subjects have activated/deactivated an homologous region. On this basis, it could be concluded that there are no differences between the two groups, when in fact the difference would be in terms of brain anatomy.

A customized brain template has been used to address difficulties in normalizing images with substantial distortion in their anatomy in a structural MRI study of VPT adolescents [8]. Another option would be to localize activation relative to an individual's own microstructural anatomy, rather than to rely on estimates derived from group averaging [74]. The analysis of fMRI data could be, for instance, informed by diffusion tension imaging (DTI) techniques, which are comprehensively summarized in relation to VPT research in Chapter 8.

Differences in task performance are other potential confounders in the interpretation of fMRI data, and these have been reported in fMRI studies with VPT groups [19,21]. There is evidence that neural activation is affected as a function of duty cycle (the time spent in completing a task) or the pace of completion [75] and differences in response times have been reported in online fMRI performance in VPT adolescents [21].

The observed greater activation of selective brain areas during a variety of cognitive tasks may have underlined increased difficulty in completing the task, although this did not necessarily result in poorer task performance. Increased activity, especially of prefrontal cortices, may have other interpretations, including greater monitoring of cognitive operations in VPT groups [76], a partial failure to avoid superfluous processing of information non-specific to the task being completed [77], and high arousal and stress during task completion [78]. In addition, it would be important to measure and account for intra-individual performance variability within the VPT individuals, as this has been shown to correlate with brain activation in attentional networks [79].

Developmental effects on brain function, as well as structure, may be affected by sexual dimorphism, therefore the effects of gender should be taken into account when interpreting functional neuroimaging results. Ment and colleagues described a significant effect of early indomethacin at the neuronal level during verbal processing in boys but not in girls [44]. Gender effects in structural MRI in VPT children have been reported [80] (see also Chapter 5), as well as in the relationship between the size of selective brain areas and cognitive and behavioral function [7,81]. Furthermore, there is evidence that differences in cortical thickness affect fMRI signal and are gender specific [82].

Studies investigating the neural correlates of specific cognitive functions in VPT samples with normal neonatal ultrasound results in the absence of differences in on-line performance have nevertheless identified significant differences when compared to age- and sex-matched control samples [45,55]. One explanation could be that morphological brain alterations may be present, yet not have been detected by neonatal cranial ultrasound, which is much less sensitive to diffuse white matter abnormalities than MRI [83] and is therefore likely to under-represent children with earlier cerebral abnormalities. We have previously shown that the posterior part of the CC was 10.5% smaller in the preterm compared to the control group, even in the absence of any brain injury detected on neonatal ultrasound [7].

Another interpretation involves processes of neural plasticity (i.e., whereby compensatory neural events facilitate the reorganization of existing brain tissue). Possible mechanisms of brain reorganization and sparing of function may occur at different levels in VPT individuals (see [84] for further discussion).

At the neuronal level, ultrastructural changes in neurons and their connections have been reported in autopsy studies [85]. In response to injury, the mammalian brain shows healing responses, including the establishment of new limiting membranes that function as boundaries, and creation of conditions conducive to rapid sprouting of neurites that underlie circuit reorganization [86].

At the level of cortical and subcortical circuits, other brain areas may become alternative substrates for the particular functions subserved by the brain region that is damaged. Altered patterns of structure–function relationships may be observed following early brain injury because functions are remapped onto other undamaged areas of the brain [87].

Alternatively, changes at the level of cognitive strategies may occur: for example, the fMRI experiments cited above in which working memory appears to be

recruited to compensate for the lack of efficient transfer across a damaged CC [21].

These three potential mechanisms are not, of course, mutually exclusive and it is likely that all three occur following VPT birth [84]. Some authors have gone as far as arguing that developmental disorders are associated with altered development of the entire brain, and that the end-state functional architecture of developmentally altered systems may possess modules that are not to be found in the normally developing brain, or in other words are characterized by "different functional structures" [88]. Very preterm birth with subsequent neurodevelopmental alterations could be studied within this theoretical framework.

However, there may be adverse consequences of such processes of reorganization. An early brain lesion can have different functional consequences as the individual advances in age. For instance, animal studies have shown that a lesion may remain relatively silent until the neuronal system affected reaches a degree of maturity, at which point abnormal behavior results [89]. Likewise, studies with humans have suggested that certain early lesions may produce little impairment in childhood, but profound behavioral disturbance in adult life [90,91].

Chapter 18 of this book elegantly describes the ways in which development is malleable and can be enhanced at every stage of early maturation in VPT infants. We have recently reported that gray and white matter volume in selective brain regions mediate the relationship between VPT birth and adolescent cognitive impairment, and could be clinically used as a marker for the identification of those individuals at increased risk for cognitive impairment, at whom targeted interventions could be directed [8]. Furthermore, structural and functional brain changes in "late developing" cortices could potentially allow for interventions aimed at minimizing the impact of anatomical and neural alterations to be devised, as it has been demonstrated with respect to white matter in frontal and occipital cortices [66], so as to preserve the functional attributes of these brain regions.

References

1. Freud S. *On Aphasia: A Critical Study (E. Stengel Transl.)*. London: Imago; 1953.

2. Hack M, Fanaroff AA. Outcomes of children of extremely low birthweight and gestational age in the 1990's. *Early Hum Dev* 1999; **53**(3): 193–218.

3. United Nations Children's Fund,and World Health Organization. *Low Birthweight: Country, Regional and Global Estimates*. New York: UNICEF; 2004.

4. Abernethy LJ, Palaniappan M, Cooke RW. Quantitative magnetic resonance imaging of the brain in survivors of very low birth weight. *Arch Dis Child* 2002; **87**(4): 279–83.

5. Inder TE, Warfield SK, Wang H, Huppi PS, Volpe JJ. Abnormal cerebral structure is present at term in premature infants. *Pediatrics* 2005; **115**(2): 286–94.

6. Nosarti C, Al Asady MH, Frangou S, *et al.* Adolescents who were born very preterm have decreased brain volumes. *Brain* 2002; **125**(Pt 7): 1616–23.

7. Nosarti C, Rushe TM, Woodruff PW, *et al.* Corpus callosum size and very preterm birth: relationship to neuropsychological outcome. *Brain* 2004; **127**(Pt 9): 2080–9.

8. Nosarti C, Giouroukou E, Healy E, *et al.* Grey and white matter distribution in very preterm adolescents mediates neurodevelopmental outcome. *Brain* 2008; **131**(Pt 1): 207–15.

9. Peterson BS, Anderson AW, Ehrenkranz R, *et al.* Regional brain volumes and their later neurodevelopmental correlates in term and preterm infants. *Pediatrics* 2003; **111**(5 Pt 1): 939–48.

10. Hack M, Taylor HG. Perinatal brain injury in preterm infants and later neurobehavioral function. *JAMA* 2000; **284**(15): 1973–4.

11. Nosarti C, Giouroukou E, Micali N, *et al.*Impaired executive functioning in young adults born very preterm. *J Int Neuropsychol Soc* 2007; **13**(4): 571–81.

12. Woodward LJ, Anderson PJ, Austin NC, Howard K, Inder TE. Neonatal MRI to predict neurodevelopmental outcomes in preterm infants. *N Engl J Med* 2006; **355**(7): 685–94.

13. Taylor HG, Minich NM, Klein N, Hack M. Longitudinal outcomes of very low birth weight: neuropsychological findings. *J Int Neuropsychol Soc* 2004; **10**(2): 149–63.

14. Ogawa S, Lee TM, Kay AR, Tank DW. Brain magnetic resonance imaging with contrast dependent on blood oxygenation. *Proc Natl Acad Sci U S A* 1990; **87**(24): 9868–72.

15. Thulborn KR, Waterton JC, Matthews PM, Radda GK. Oxygenation dependence of the transverse relaxation time of water protons in whole blood at high field. *Biochim Biophys Acta* 1982; **714**(2): 265–70.

16. Ogawa S, Lee TM. Magnetic resonance imaging of blood vessels at high fields: in vivo and in vitro measurements and image simulation. *Magn Reson Med* 1990; **16**(1): 9–18.

17. Logothetis NK, Pauls J, Augath M, Trinath T, Oeltermann A. Neurophysiological investigation of the basis of the fMRI signal. *Nature* 2001; **412**(6843): 150–7.

18. Higuchi Y, Maihara T, Hattori H, *et al.* [18F]-fluorodeoxyglucose-positron emission tomography findings in protein infants with severe periventricular leukomalacia and hypsarrhythmia. *Eur J Pediatr* 1997; **156**(3): 236–8.

19. Gimenez M, Junque C, Vendrell P, *et al.* Hippocampal functional magnetic resonance imaging during a face-name learning task in adolescents with antecedents of prematurity. *Neuroimage* 2005; **25**(2): 561–9.

20. Rushe TM, Temple CM, Rifkin L, *et al.* Lateralisation of language function in young adults born very preterm. *Arch Dis Child Fetal Neonatal Ed* 2004; **89**(2): F112–18.

21. Santhouse AM, Ffytche DH, Howard RJ, *et al.* The functional significance of perinatal corpus callosum damage: an fMRI study in young adults. *Brain* 2002; **125**(Pt 8): 1782–92.

22. Petersson KM, Nichols TE, Poline JB, Holmes AP. Statistical limitations in functional neuroimaging. I. Non-inferential methods and statistical models. *Philos Trans R Soc Lond B Biol Sci* 1999; **354**(1387): 1239–60.

23. Aguirre GK, D'Esposito M. Experimental design for brain fMRI. In: Mooneen CTW, Bandettini PA, eds. *Functional MRI*. Berlin: Springer. 2000; 369–80.

24. Ment LR, Constable RT. Injury and recovery in the developing brain: evidence from functional MRI studies of prematurely born children. *Nat Clin Pract Neurol* 2007; **3**(10): 558–71.

25. Price CJ, Friston KJ. Cognitive conjunction: a new approach to brain activation experiments. *Neuroimage* 1997; **5**(4 Pt 1): 261–70.

26. Friston KJ, Holmes AP, Price CJ, Buchel C, Worsley KJ. Multisubject fMRI studies and conjunction analyses. *Neuroimage* 1999; **10**(4): 385–96.

27. Powers WJ, Rosenbaum JL, Dence CS, Markham J, Videen TO. Cerebral glucose transport and metabolism in preterm human infants. *J Cereb Blood Flow Metab* 1998; **18**(6): 632–8.

28. Borch K, Greisen G. Blood flow distribution in the normal human preterm brain. *Pediatr Res* 1998; **43**(1): 28–33.

29. Erberich SG, Friedlich P, Seri I, Nelson MD, Jr., Bluml S. Functional MRI in neonates using neonatal head coil and MR compatible incubator. *Neuroimage* 2003; **20**(2): 683–92.

30. O'Hare B, Bissonnette B, Bohn D, Cox P, Williams W. Persistent low cerebral blood flow velocity following profound hypothermic circulatory arrest in infants. *Can J Anaesth* 1995; **42**(11): 964–71.

31. Fransson P, Skiold B, Horsch S, *et al.* Resting-state networks in the infant brain. *Proc Natl Acad Sci U S A* 2007; **104**(39): 15531–6.

32. Erberich SG, Panigrahy A, Friedlich P, *et al*. Somatosensory lateralization in the newborn brain. *Neuroimage* 2006; **29**(1): 155–61.

33. Yamada H, Sadato N, Konishi Y, *et al*. A rapid brain metabolic change in infants detected by fMRI. *Neuroreport* 1997; **8**(17): 3775–8.

34. Born AP, Miranda MJ, Rostrup E, *et al*. Functional magnetic resonance imaging of the normal and abnormal visual system in early life. *Neuropediatrics* 2000; **31**(1): 24–32.

35. Ogawa S, Lee TM, Barrere B. The sensitivity of magnetic resonance image signals of a rat brain to changes in the cerebral venous blood oxygenation. *Magn Reson Med* 1993; **29**(2): 205–10.

36. Gilles FH, Leviton A, Dooling EC. *The Developing Human Brain – Growth and Epidemiologic Neuropathology*. Boston, MA: PSG Inc.; 1983.

37. Anderson AW, Marois R, Colson ER, *et al*. Neonatal auditory activation detected by functional magnetic resonance imaging. *Magn Reson Imaging* 2001; **19**(1): 1–5.

38. Kisilevsky BS, Pang L, Hains SM. Maturation of human fetal responses to airborne sound in low- and high-risk fetuses. *Early Hum Dev* 2000; **58**(3): 179–95.

39. Kisilevsky BS, Davies GA. Auditory processing deficits in growth restricted fetuses affect later language development. *Med Hypotheses* 2007; **68**(3): 620–8.

40. Rushe TM, Rifkin L, Stewart AL, *et al*. Neuropsychological outcome at adolescence of very preterm birth and its relation to brain structure. *Dev Med Child Neurol* 2001; **43**(4): 226–33.

41. Meek JH, Firbank M, Elwell CE, *et al*. Regional hemodynamic responses to visual stimulation in awake infants. *Pediatr Res* 1998; **43**(6): 840–3.

42. Magill-Evans J, Harrison MJ, Van der Zalm J, Holdgrafer G. Cognitive and language development of healthy preterm infants at 10 years of age. *Phys Occup Ther Pediatr* 2002; **22**(1): 41–56.

43. Hall A, McLeod A, Counsell C, Thomson L, Mutch L. School attainment, cognitive ability and motor function in a total Scottish very-low-birthweight population at eight years: a controlled study. *Dev Med Child Neurol* 1995; **37**(12): 1037–50.

44. Ment LR, Peterson BS, Meltzer JA, *et al*. A functional magnetic resonance imaging study of the long-term influences of early indomethacin exposure on language processing in the brains of prematurely born children. *Pediatrics* 2006; **118**(3): 961–70.

45. Ment LR, Peterson BS, Vohr B, *et al*. Cortical recruitment patterns in children born prematurely compared with control subjects during a passive listening functional magnetic resonance imaging task. *J Pediatr* 2006; **149**(4): 490–8.

46. Peterson BS, Vohr B, Kane MJ, *et al*. A functional magnetic resonance imaging study of language processing and its cognitive correlates in prematurely born children. *Pediatrics* 2002; **110**(6): 1153–62.

47. Ment LR, Oh W, Ehrenkranz RA, *et al*. Low-dose indomethacin and prevention of intraventricular hemorrhage: a multicenter randomized trial. *Pediatrics* 1994; **93**(4): 543–50.

48. Hoenig K, Scheef L. Mediotemporal contributions to semantic processing: fMRI evidence from ambiguity processing during semantic context verification. *Hippocampus* 2005; **15**(5): 597–609.

49. Shaywitz SE, Shaywitz BA, Fulbright RK, *et al*. Neural systems for compensation and persistence: young adult outcome of childhood reading disability. *Biol Psychiatry* 2003; **54**(1): 25–33.

50. Stewart AL, Rifkin L, Amess PN, *et al*. Brain structure and neurocognitive and behavioural function in adolescents who were born very preterm. *Lancet* 1999; **353**(9165): 1653–7.

51. Mazziotta JC, Phelps ME, Carson RE, Kuhl DE. Tomographic mapping of human cerebral metabolism: auditory stimulation. *Neurology* 1982; **32**(9): 921–37.

52. Temple CM, Ilsley J. Phonemic discrimination in callosal agenesis. *Cortex* 1993; **29**(2): 341–8.

53. Price CJ, Wise RJ, Warburton EA, *et al*. Hearing and saying. The functional neuro-anatomy of auditory word processing. *Brain* 1996; **119**(Pt 3): 919–31.

54. Nosarti C, Shergill SS, Allin MP, *et al*. Neural substrates of letter fluency processing in young adults who were born very preterm: alterations in frontal and striatal regions. *Neuroimage* 2009; **47**(4): 1904–13.

55. Nosarti C, Rubia K, Smith A, *et al*. Altered functional neuroanatomy of response inhibition in adolescent males who were born very preterm. *Dev Med Child Neurol* 2006; **48**(4): 265–71.

56. Lawrence EJ, Rubia K, Murray RM, *et al*. The neural basis of response inhibition and attention allocation as mediated by gestational age. *Hum Brain Mapp* 2009; **30**(3): 1038–50.

57. Peterson BS, Vohr B, Staib LH, *et al*. Regional brain volume abnormalities and long-term cognitive outcome in preterm infants. *JAMA* 2000; **284**(15): 1939–47.

58. Nakamura Y, Nakashima T, Fukuda S, Nakashima H, Hashimoto T. Hypoxic-ischemic brain lesions found in asphyxiating neonates. *Acta Pathol Jpn* 1986; **36**(4): 551–63.

59. Isaacs EB, Lucas A, Chong WK, *et al*. Hippocampal volume and everyday memory in children of very low birth weight. *Pediatr Res* 2000; **47**(6): 713–20.

60. Narberhaus A, Lawrence EJ, Allin MP, *et al*. Neural substrates of visual paired associates in young adults with a history of very preterm birth: alterations

in fronto-parieto-occipital networks and caudate. *Neuroimage* 2009; **47**(4): 1884–93.

61. Curtis WJ, Zhuang J, Townsend EL, Hu X, Nelson CA. Memory in early adolescents born prematurely: a functional magnetic resonance imaging investigation. *Dev Neuropsychol* 2006; **29**(2): 341–77.

62. Woodward LJ, Edgin JO, Thompson D, Inder TE. Object working memory deficits predicted by early brain injury and development in the preterm infant. *Brain* 2005; **128**(Pt 11): 2578–87.

63. Curtis WJ, Lindeke LL, Georgieff MK, Nelson CA. Neurobehavioural functioning in neonatal intensive care unit graduates in late childhood and early adolescence. *Brain* 2002; **125**(Pt 7): 1646–59.

64. Carmody DP, Bendersky M, Dunn SM, *et al*. Early risk, attention, and brain activation in adolescents born preterm. *Child Dev* 2006; **77**(2): 384–94.

65. Bendersky M, Lewis M. Effects of intraventricular hemorrhage and other medical and environmental risks on multiple outcomes at age three years. *J Dev Behav Pediatr* 1995; **16**(2): 89–96.

66. Als H, Duffy FH, McAnulty GB, *et al*. Early experience alters brain function and structure. *Pediatrics* 2004; **113**(4): 846–57.

67. Rubia K, Smith AB, Woolley J, *et al*. Progressive increase of frontostriatal brain activation from childhood to adulthood during event-related tasks of cognitive control. *Hum Brain Mapp* 2006; **27**(12): 973–93.

68. O'Carroll CM, Nosarti C, McGuire PK, Rifkin L, Murray RM. Altered neuronal activation during processing of verbal episodic memory in preterm adolescents. *Schizophr Bull* 2005; **31**(2): 429.

69. Borch K, Greisen G. Blood flow distribution in the normal human preterm brain. *Pediatr Res* 1998; **43**(1): 28–33.

70. Aram DM, Eisele JA. Plasticity and recovery of higher cognitive function following early brain damage. In: Boller F, Grafman J, eds. *Handbook of Neuropsychology*. Amsterdam: Elsevier. 1992; 73–91.

71. Sowell ER, Trauner DA, Gamst A, Jernigan TL. Development of cortical and subcortical brain structures in childhood and adolescence: a structural MRI study. *Dev Med Child Neurol* 2002; **44**(1): 4–16.

72. Casey BJ, Tottenham N, Liston C, Durston S. Imaging the developing brain: what have we learned about cognitive development? *Trends Cogn Sci* 2005; **9**(3): 104–10.

73. Durston S, Davidson MC, Tottenham N, *et al*. A shift from diffuse to focal cortical activity with development. *Dev Sci* 2006; **9**(1): 1–8.

74. Brett M, Johnsrude IS, Owen AM. The problem of functional localization in the human brain. *Nat Rev Neurosci* 2002; **3**(3): 243–9.

75. D'Esposito M, Zarahn E, Aguirre GK, *et al*. The effect of pacing of experimental stimuli on observed functional MRI activity. *Neuroimage* 1997; **6**(2): 113–21.

76. van Veen V, Holroyd CB, Cohen JD, Stenger VA, Carter CS. Errors without conflict: implications for performance monitoring theories of anterior cingulate cortex. *Brain Cogn* 2004; **56**(2): 267–76.

77. Boksman K, Theberge J, Williamson P, *et al*. A 4.0-T fMRI study of brain connectivity during word fluency in first-episode schizophrenia. *Schizophr Res* 2005; **75**(2–3): 247–63.

78. Critchley HD, Mathias CJ, Josephs O, *et al*. Human cingulate cortex and autonomic control: converging neuroimaging and clinical evidence. *Brain* 2003; **126**(Pt 10): 2139–52.

79. Rubia K, Smith AB, Brammer MJ, Taylor E. Temporal lobe dysfunction in medication-naive boys with attention-deficit/hyperactivity disorder during attention allocation and its relation to response variability. *Biol Psychiatry* 2007; **62**(9): 999–1006.

80. Reiss AL, Kesler SR, Vohr B, *et al*. Sex differences in cerebral volumes of 8-year-olds born preterm. *J Pediatr* 2004; **145**(2): 242–9.

81. Nosarti C, Allin M, Frangou S, Rifkin L, Murray R. Decreased caudate volume is associated with hyperactivity in adolescents born very preterm. *Biol Psychiatry* 2005; **13**(6): 339.

82. Sowell ER, Peterson BS, Kan E, *et al*. Sex differences in cortical thickness mapped in 176 healthy individuals between 7 and 87 years of age. *Cereb Cortex* 2007; **17**(7): 1550–60.

83. Volpe JJ. Cerebral white matter injury of the premature infant-more common than you think. *Pediatrics* 2003; **112**(1 Pt 1): 176–80.

84. Allin M, Nosarti C, Rifkin L, Murray RM. Brain plasticity and long term function after early cerebral insult: the example of very preterm birth. In: Keshavan MS, Kennedy JL, Murray RM, eds. *Neurodevelopment and Schizophrenia*, 1st edn. Cambridge: Cambridge University Press. 2004; 89–110.

85. Marin-Padilla M. Developmental neuropathology and impact of perinatal brain damage. III: gray matter lesions of the neocortex. *J Neuropathol Exp Neurol* 1999; **58**(5): 407–29.

86. Ide CF, Scripter JL, Coltman BW, *et al*. Cellular and molecular correlates to plasticity during recovery from injury in the developing mammalian brain. *Prog Brain Res* 1996; **108**: 365–77.

87. Stiles J, Reilly J, Paul B, Moses P. Cognitive development following early brain injury: evidence for neural adaptation. *Trends Cogn Sci* 2005; **9**(3): 136–43.

88. Thomas M, Karmiloff-Smith A. Are developmental disorders like cases of adult brain damage? Implications from connectionist modelling. *Behav Brain Sci* 2002; **25**(6): 727–50.

89. Sams-Dodd F, Lipska BK, Weinberger DR. Neonatal lesions of the rat ventral hippocampus result in hyperlocomotion and deficits in social behaviour in adulthood. *Psychopharmacology (Berl)* 1997; **132**(3): 303–10.

90. Murray RM, Lewis SW. Is schizophrenia a neurodevelopmental disorder? *Br Med J (Clin Res Ed)* 1987; **295**(6600): 681–2.

91. Weinberger DR. Implications of normal brain development for the pathogenesis of schizophrenia. *Arch Gen Psychiatry* 1987; **44**(7): 660–9.

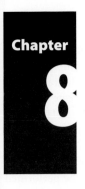

Diffusion tensor imaging findings in preterm and low birth weight populations

Matthew P. G. Allin

Introduction

Premature birth represents a significant cause of peri-natal morbidity and mortality. In Europe and North America, driven by improvements in neonatal inten-sive care, more preterm and low birth weight babies are surviving, even with extreme degrees of prema-turity. The sequelae of premature birth may be ser-ious, and include cerebral palsy and learning disability, but many individuals are free of these complications. Nevertheless, developmental problems are becoming apparent even in individuals who come through the neonatal period relatively unscathed. If we are to opti-mize the health of these individuals as they grow and mature into adults we will require a better understand-ing of the pathological and developmental processes involved in recovery from this early adversity.

This chapter will focus on the white matter of the brain, in part because it is especially vulnerable to injury in the premature infant [1,2], but also because development and maturation of white matter may be crucial in enabling individuals to overcome the effects of early adversity [3]. Relatively recent developments in MRI technology have made it possible for us to look at white matter in startling detail in the living brain, and are providing new information about its structure and function. This chapter will introduce one such technique, diffusion tensor imaging (DTI), and dis-cuss how it can be used to study preterm and low birth weight populations.

A non-physicist's guide to DTI

Diffusion tensor imaging (DTI; DT-MRI) exploits a physical property of water molecules – their Brownian motion. That is, on the microscopic scale, molecules of H_2O in liquid water are always on the move. Diffusion tensor imaging is an MRI sequence that is sensitive to the Brownian motion of water molecules [4]. Vertebrates such as Homo sapiens have a high water content – but not all of this water is as free to diffuse as it would be in, for example, a cup of tea, and this is exploited by DTI to differentiate between different types of tissue. For example, in a volume of cerebrospinal fluid, water molecules are able to diffuse in any direction – diffu-sion is *isotropic*. However, in white matter, where tissue is arranged in bundles, diffusion of water is greater in the direction of axon fascicles than it is perpendicular to them – that is, diffusion is *anisotropic* [4,5] . In gray matter, the diffusion of water molecules is hindered by cellular and extracellular structures, but this effect is the same in all directions, so that the diffusion in gray matter is also largely *isotropic*.

During a typical 50 ms diffusion time in an MRI scanner, water molecules move on average by around 10 μm. To get as complete a picture as possible of dif-fusion in three dimensions, at least six MRI sequences are applied, each in a different direction. Three eigen-values are calculated (designated λ1, λ2, and λ3), rep-resenting diffusion in three dimensions. The property known as "diffusivity" (also called D, D_{av}) is the mean of these three eigenvalues. Mean diffusivity (MD) and apparent diffusion coefficient (ADC), often reported in the literature, are roughly equivalent parameters, being indices of water diffusion independent of its directionality. Diffusion may also be represented by a tensor, which is a mathematical description of a sys-tem of multidimensional vectors. The diffusion tensor has a preferred orientation in each voxel, and can be used to calculate *fractional anisotropy* (FA), the most commonly reported DTI parameter. Other similar measures which are reported in the literature include lattice anisotropy index (LAI) and relative anisotropy (RA). These measures reflect the degree to which diffu-sion in a voxel is constrained in a particular direction. Fractional anisotropy values lie between 0 and 1, with higher values indicating tissue that is more coherent

Neurodevelopmental Outcomes of Preterm Birth, ed. Chiara Nosarti, Robin M. Murray, and Maureen Hack. Published by Cambridge University Press. © Cambridge University Press 2010.

and directionally organized. Fractional anisotropy is therefore high in white matter, lower in gray matter and very low in cerebrospinal fluid [6].

The tissue and cellular correlates of DTI

Diffusion tensor imaging began to be developed as a research and diagnostic tool in the mid 1980s [5], with an early clinical application in identifying the neural correlates of stroke [7], where diffusion changes are evident before lesions become visible on structural MRI. Diffusion tensor imaging is thus still relatively new, and it is not yet entirely clear what cellular and extracellular factors it may be measuring. In the case of white matter, one obvious possibility is myelination. Certainly, developmental changes in FA would at least partially support this interpretation, such as the study of Klingberg *et al.* [8], showing that maturational changes in temporoparietal white matter FA are related to reading ability in teenagers.

However, anisotropy is detectable in the brains of preterm neonates before myelination commences [9], so white matter constituents other than the myelin sheath must contribute to FA. Basser [6] suggests that FA is affected by many cellular and extracellular characteristics – such as large, oriented macromolecules, organelles, and cell membranes. He says "determining tissue microstructural and architectural features from the NMR (nuclear magnetic resonance) signal remains a challenging ill-posed inverse problem." Budde *et al.* [10], in a mouse model, co-registered histological sections with DTI images to attempt to examine this directly. They measured radial diffusivity (diffusivity perpendicular to axon tracts) and axial diffusivity (parallel to them). They reported that the parameter of axial diffusivity is associated with axonal injury and dysfunction, whereas radial diffusivity is associated with deficits in myelination. They also suggested that DTI is actually more sensitive than histopathology, in that diffusion changes were present in tissue that was microsopically normal. It is probable that DTI can detect some very early tissue changes which occur before histological changes become evident.

In spite of the remaining uncertainties there is general consensus that reduced FA and elevated MD are indicators of poorer white matter "integrity" [11].

Is DTI just pretty pictures?

Figure 8.1 shows a false-color FA map of an 18-year-old very preterm (VPT) individual. Some structures

are labeled on this picture, to give an idea of the information that DTI can provide that is complementary to structural MRI. Combined with tractography (see below) similar maps have been used to create atlases of white matter tracts based on the living brain [12]. Such atlases are highly consistent with post-mortem dissections of white matter of the century-before-last (e.g., [13]). Of course, DTI has the substantial advantage over anatomical methods in that it can be performed in vivo, and can also be applied to selected patient or healthy groups. The individual shown in Fig. 8.1 was born at 26 gestational weeks, and abnormalities of brain structure, especially enlargement of the lateral ventricles, are prominent. One of the problems with using "standard" white matter atlases to assess individuals born preterm is that they may have "non-standard" white matter anatomy.

There are broadly three ways in which DTI information can be analyzed, and I will briefly introduce them:

Region of interest

Region-of-interest approaches usually take the FA maps of individual subjects (such as that shown in Fig. 8.1) and manually place anatomically or geometrically defined regions onto a particular slice. The diffusion parameters within that region are then sampled, and can be used to perform group comparisons using a standard statistics program. An example of this approach is the study of Miller *et al.* [14], which measured the diffusion parameters in different white matter regions in preterm neonates. The main limitation of such methods is that the placement of regions is operator dependent and may be prone to error. For example, when the outline of an anatomical structure is traced manually, its mean FA may be substantially reduced if any non-white matter tissue is accidentally included. Geometric shapes (e.g., squares or ellipses) must also be placed in exactly the same position within a tract in each individual's map. This is perhaps feasible in large structures like the corpus callosum, but is difficult for smaller tracts. Additionally, altering the position of the region of interest within a tract can alter the results that are obtained, since white matter composing a tract is not necessarily homogeneous in its properties throughout that tract.

Tractography

Since the diffusion tensor has a dominant direction in each voxel, algorithms have been developed that

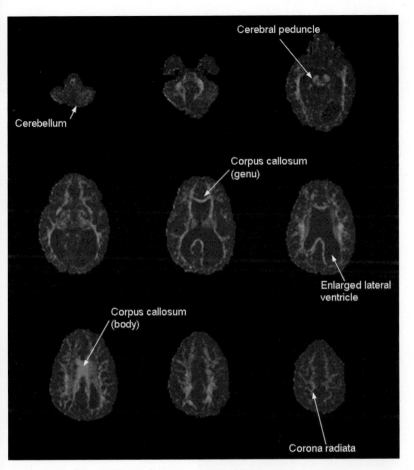

Fig. 8.1 Selected axial cross-sections through the brain of a VPT individual, with color-coding indicating the main orientation of fibers. Red fibers (e.g., corpus callosum) traverse left–right in the plane of the image. Green fibers run antero-posteriorly in the plane of the image. Blue fibers run perpendicular to the plane of the image. This scan is of an 18-year-old female, born at 26 gestational weeks. Enlargement of the lateral ventricles is prominent (University College Hospital London and Institute of Psychiatry Preterm Birth Follow-Up Study). See plate section for color version.

can "join up" vectors in adjacent voxels, and so track the path of a white matter bundle through the brain. This method can be used to reconstruct and visualize white matter tract anatomy in vivo (e.g., [15]), and is known as *tractography*. Such methods can trace the pathway of greatest FA through the brain in three dimensions [15–21].

The starting point for the tracking algorithm is usually defined manually on each subject's FA map, and provides "seed points" from which the tractography procedure can commence. The tracking algorithm then follows the direction of maximum FA from each seed point, until FA falls below a set threshold, or a maximum length is attained. A refinement of this technique [15] uses a two-region approach, where only paths that pass through both regions are reconstructed. This reduces the potential for operator error in placement of the regions to affect the result. Using such techniques, tractography can allow reconstruction of all the major white matter tracts of the brain [12]. Its disadvantages are that it can be time-consuming and

is still potentially subject to some operator bias. More importantly, tractographic methods may underestimate white matter complexity because deterministic tractography algorithms do not cope well with crossing fibers. In voxels where fibers cross, there will be two directions of maximum FA, but this is not resolvable by the algorithm, which instead sees that the FA of that voxel has reduced (with two preferred vectors, pulling in different directions). More recent developments in probabilistic tractography may help to reduce these discrepancies (for a review, see [22]). Tractographic images may be examined radiologically for anatomical differences, and DTI parameters such as FA and MD can be extracted from reconstructed tract. These can then be used to make group comparisons, or to seek associations between DTI and neurological, cognitive, or behavioral outcome (as for region-of-interest studies). Figure 8.2 is an example of tractographic reconstruction of the genu of the corpus callosum, illustrating the region used to derive the seed points and the reconstructed tracts.

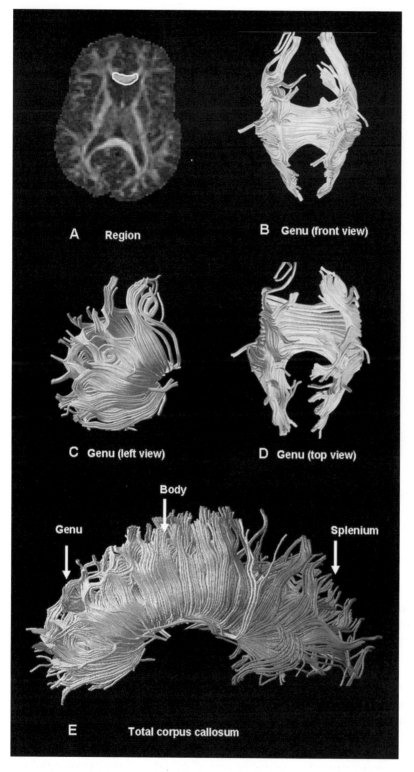

A   Region

B   Genu (front view)

C   Genu (left view)

D   Genu (top view)

E   Total corpus callosum

Body

Genu

Splenium

Fig. 8.2 Tractographic reconstruction of the genu of the corpus callosum. (A) A sample region of interest for tracking the genu is shown in yellow on this single axial slice from the FA map of a single (healthy control) subject. Only one slice is shown, for clarity, but typically the region of interest might extend over several axial slices. Tracts passing through this region are shown in three-dimensional views: (B) from the front; (C) from the left side; (D) from the top. (E) Reconstruction of tracts passing through the whole corpus callosum: genu (yellow); body (green); splenium (red). See plate section for color version.

Tractographic methods may be able to cope better with "non-standard" brain anatomy than voxel-based methods (see below). The study of Berube *et al.* [23] used DTI tractography to define the white matter anatomy in a group of individuals with an arteriovenous malformation (AVM) in one hemisphere. They found that tracts were altered in their morphology in the presence of an AVM, and that this was also related to their function. Thus, fronto-occipital and inferior longitudinal fasciculus alterations were associated with impaired vision, while abnormalities of the arcuate fasciculus were associated with speech disorder. Berube *et al.* [23] were able to use these DTI indices to predict the outcome of neurosurgery – perhaps in the future we may be able to use tract anatomy and integrity in an analogous way to predict cognitive and behavioral outcomes in preterm and low birth weight individuals.

Voxel-based morphometry (VBM)

Voxel-based methods use automated image processing software that was originally developed for use with functional and structural MRI (e.g. Statistical Parametric Mapping; Wellcome Department of Imaging Neurosciences, University College London, UK). These methods are useful for comparing large numbers of scans between two or more groups, and are not subject to bias in the same way as the two methods outlined above. They also do not require a starting hypothesis, and their results could be used to generate hypotheses that may be tested further by other methods.

Voxel-based morphometry methods make intensive use of computer processing resources, and rely on a number of common processing steps [24]. Firstly, non-brain tissues are removed ("stripped"); then tissue is "segmented" – that is assigned a probability of belonging to a particular tissue class (e.g. gray matter vs. white matter). Scans must also be "smoothed" – that is blurred using a Gaussian filter, which allows individual differences in gross brain structure to be softened. The next processing step subjects the data to a series of mathematical transformations ("warping"), so that the scans for each subject will fit into a common template. This template may be a preexisting one (e.g., [25]), or may be constructed from the scans in the study [26]. The use of study-specific gray matter and white matter templates may at least partially deal with some of the registration problems that are encountered when applying VBM to preterm and low birth weight populations. Diffusion tensor imaging data – which have low spatial resolution – are often registered to

high-resolution structural MRI images [27]. The final step is to compare the groups of scans at each voxel, for differences DTI parameters (usually FA). Packages such as SPM (Statistical Parametric Mapping) or XBAM (Brain Activation Map) (Institute of Psychiatry, London, UK: www.brainmap.co.uk/) implement basic statistics (such as general linear models, correlations, and *t*-tests) to examine group differences and control for confounding variables. These approaches can also be used to look for relationships between FA and other parameters, such as cognitive performance [27]. The results are usually displayed as color-coded "blobs" on a template image, demonstrating the areas where differences or correlations are found. An example of such an image is given in Fig. 8.3.

A potential limitation of VBM is the potential to generate mis-registration artifacts [28,29]. This is particularly evident in preterm and low birth weight populations, where the high prevalence of structural brain abnormalities such as ventriculomegaly can interfere with registration [30]. Such problems can be mitigated by excluding scans with extremely large ventricles, although this results in loss of power.

Another approach is to use the "optimized VBM" methodology of Good *et al.* [26], in which scans are registered to study-specific gray/white matter templates, thus minimizing the transformations required to warp data to the template. As with tractography, complexity of white matter anatomy (such as crossing fibers) may cause problems for voxel-based methods. Snook *et al.* [29] performed a head-to-head comparison of region-of-interest and VBM analyses in healthy subjects at different ages. Luckily, both methods produced consistent results in this instance, but perhaps inevitably the differences in methodology mean that there may be some discrepancies. Thus group differences may be evident on region-of-interest studies, but not found using VBM. Snook *et al.* [29] believe that this is likely to be due to anatomical variation between participants that is lost in the processing required for VBM analysis. Variability of structures such as the splenium of the corpus callosum may mean that VBM analyses are limited in their ability to detect differences in this area, for example. Conversely, VBM methods, because they are not confined to a particular region, can examine parts of the brain that are difficult to include in region-of-interest analyses. For example, areas of the brain that lack obvious anatomical boundaries, such as functional subdivisions of the prefrontal cortex, would not be so amenable to region-of-interest studies.

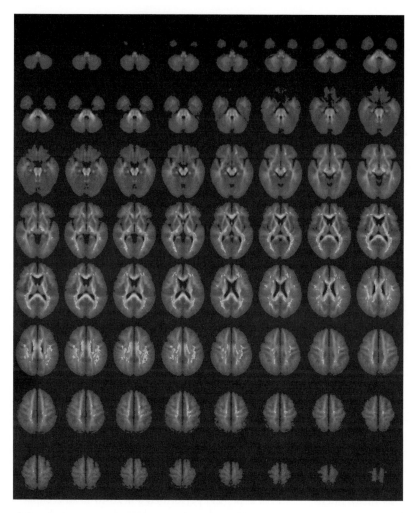

Fig. 8.3 Results of an "optimized VBM" group analysis of FA comparing preterm and term-born adults, using SPM2 (Wellcome Department of Imaging Neurosciences, University College London, UK) and XBAM (Institute of Psychiatry, London, UK: www.brainmap. co.uk/). Serial axial sections are shown, displayed on an FA template. This is the result of a comparison between a group of VPT individuals (born before 33 weeks' gestation) (n = 87) and a group born at term (n = 49), at mean age 19.13 years (range 17–22 years) and 18.54 years (range 17–22 years), respectively. Blue areas indicate significantly lower FA in the preterm group (p = 0.0075); red areas indicate higher FA in the preterm group. See plate section for color version.

Early brain development and DTI

Using DTI to look at the development of white matter after preterm birth still poses some challenges, not the least of which is that the DTI characteristics of normally developing white matter across the lifespan are still being worked out. Diffusion tensor imaging sequences and analysis procedures are usually developed in adults, and may not be immediately applicable to neonates and infants, where brain tissue may have a different composition [31]. In general, diffusivity is high and anisotropy relatively low in the immature brain compared to the adult, and normal development is accompanied by an increase in anisotropy together with a decrease in diffusivity. White matter development is of course a protracted process, and may well not peak until early adulthood [32]. The early postnatal developmental changes in DTI parameters may be a reflection of several underlying changes in brain structure. Firstly, water content decreases in the brain in the neonatal period. Secondly, membranes and other structures that hinder diffusion, become more tightly packed. Thirdly, myelin begins to be formed. In the developing infant's brain, FA change takes place in two steps [33,34]. The first wave of FA increase occurs before the start of myelination, and may reflect changes in axonal membranes and axonal diameter, which are required to allow increased axonal conduction speed. Numbers of oligodendrocytes may also be increasing at the same time. The second wave of increasing FA, which lasts at least until early adulthood, is associated with the appearance and subsequent consolidation of myelin.

There are indications that white matter development may be heterogeneous from an early stage. Provenzale *et al.* [35] performed DTI, analyzed by a region-of-interest method, in 53 healthy infants, ranging in age from 38.5 to 51.5 gestational weeks (GW) equivalents. They found that at term peripheral white matter was less "mature" than deep white matter (the corpus callosum and internal capsule). Apparent diffusion coefficient decreased and FA increased, as expected, but they did so at different rates in different white matter compartments. Thus the early rate of fall of ADC was twice as great in peripheral white matter than in central white matter. Over the same time, the FA rise was half as great in central white matter compared to peripheral. From this, it seems likely that ADC and FA measure different aspects of white matter microstructure, and also that white matter development is regionally heterogeneous. It should be noted that this was a cross-sectional study, and not truly longitudinal, however. That white matter is heterogeneous is also indicated by the study of Qiu et al. [36], who looked at DTI in children who had received cranial radiotherapy (for medulloblastoma). They found that the frontal lobe white matter appeared to be more sensitive to radiation damage than that of the parietal lobe. This may be a reflection of different stages of maturation of white matter.

Using DTI to study white matter development after premature birth

White matter damage is common in premature infants – perhaps even commoner than has been generally recognized [1]. Several characteristic patterns of brain injury can be detected by ultrasound (US) in very preterm (VPT; less than 33 weeks' gestation) neonates, and all of them are likely to have a direct or indirect effect on white matter structure. Bleeding may occur from immature vessels in the germinal matrix (germinal matrix hemorrhage; GMH) and may also involve the ventricles (intraventricular hemorrhage; IVH). Periventricular hemorrhagic infarction (PHI) of white matter may occur, usually causing localized rather than diffuse injury [37]. Necrosis of developing axons and oligodendrocytes may occur in the destructive lesions of periventricular leukomalacia (PVL) [38]. Periventricular leukomalacia is usually localized to the white matter in the centrum semiovale [39], and is associated with more severe adverse outcomes, including cerebral palsy. It may also have effects on later myelination [37]. The autopsy studies of Marin-Padilla [40–42] demonstrated that localized lesions in the preterm brain can also cause distant alterations of cell structure and connectivity, as static lesions interact with the dynamic processes of brain development and plasticity.

In addition to discrete lesions, certain types of cell may be vulnerable to damage in premature birth. One such population of cells is important in white matter development – precursors of oligodendrocytes. These oligodendrocyte precursor cells are in an immature state of differentiation prior to 32 gestational weeks, and it has been suggested that they may be killed or damaged by hypoxia in the neonatal period, thus causing diffuse white matter injury [2,43]. Again, this would also have the effect of impairing or delaying later waves of myelination. Neonatal US underestimates the prevalence of white matter pathology in premature neonates, and MRI, with its superior spatial resolution, shows that "diffuse excessive high-signal intensities" (DEHSI) are present in up to 79% of VPT infants at term-equivalent age [1]. Dyet et al. [44] carefully examined T2-weighted scans of preterm infants, looking for low intensities (which would be hyperintense on T1) and found white matter pathology in 80% (see also Chapters 2, 3 and 4).

After white matter injury, diffusivity decreases rapidly, and this is the first change to be detectable on DTI [45]. Diffusivity subsequently rises, and remains high through the chronic phase of the injury. In contrast, anisotropy changes occur several days or even weeks after the injury. An early case-report using diffusion-weighted imaging in a preterm infant [46] found diffusion abnormalities in white matter areas which appeared "normal" on conventional MRI scanning. Followed up at 10 weeks, this infant had the MRI features of cystic PVL in the regions where diffusion had been abnormal. Fan et al. [47] assessed children with PVL and controls aged 4–12 years in a region-of-interest study. They found that the PVL group had reduced FA in numerous long association tracts, including the posterior limb of the internal capsule, the arcuate fasciculus, the cingulum, the superior longitudinal fasciculus, and the corpus callosum. This group did not also assess cognitive and behavioral outcome, so the clinical effects of these FA changes are not clear. The diffusion-weighted imaging study of Counsell et al. [48] sheds further light on these lesions. This group found diffusivity changes in infants with DEHSI, which included elevated radial diffusivity in the splenium of the corpus callosum and the posterior limb of the internal capsule, and elevation of both radial and axial diffusivity in the centrum semiovale and frontal, periventricular, and occipital white matter. They suggest that DEHSI represent a widespread abnormality of oligodendrocytes or axons (or both).

Miller *et al.* [14] measured ADC rates serially in a group of VPT infants up to term-equivalent age. In normally developing infants, ADC decreases between 28 and 40 weeks, and FA increases, perhaps as a result of the beginning of central nervous system myelination. Very preterm infants with DEHSI did not show this fall in ADC, suggesting that their white matter development is already being disrupted. Fractional anisotropy has been found to be correlated with gestational age in preterm neonates [49], and different regions display different patterns of maturation (FA is greater in the motor system than the sensory system, for example) [50]. Partridge *et al.* [51], again studying preterm neonates, found that early-maturing tracts such as the corpus callosum, cerebral peduncles, and internal capsules had higher FA and lower MD than later maturing tracts (such as subcortical projection and intrahemispheric association pathways). For a summary of DTI studies in VPT/very low birth weight (VLBW) populations see Table 8.1.

Normally developing white matter is characterized by rising FA and falling MD, although it is likely that regional heterogeneity exists in the trajectory of these changes. At any rate, DTI may provide more sensitive imaging of early white matter injury than conventional MRI. It has even been used to image transient cortical laminae in vivo in extremely preterm infants [54]. These are structural features of the developing cerebral cortex which were hitherto only seen on histopathological examination. Additionally, it has recently become possible to apply DTI to fetuses in utero [60], which will allow a more complete picture of human brain development to be built up.

Diffusion tensor imaging in the early neonatal period may turn out to be useful as a predictor of outcome. Arzoumanian *et al.* [52] found that infants with reduced FA in the posterior limb of the internal capsule had worse neurological outcomes at 18–24 weeks. Drobyshevsky *et al.* [57] performed serial DTI from 30 to 36 GW in premature infants, and analyzed their data using regions of interest placed in all the major fiber systems. Infants with severe brain injury had higher ADC in the central and occipital white matter, and in the corona radiata, along with lower FA in the optic radiations. Infants with the lowest FA at 30 GW had the poorest psychomotor functioning at 2 years, assessed with Bayley developmental scales. This group was also able to look at the effect of maturation of white matter on outcome. They found that those babies in whom FA increased the most between 30 and 36 GW were more

likely to have poor outcome at 2 years. Since increasing FA is a normal developmental finding, this appears contradictory at first sight. Possibly it means that those with the lowest initial FA are the worst affected, and that early white matter maturation cannot "catch up" enough to mitigate these effects. Despite the "catch-up" growth, FA values attained by 36 GW in the severe injury group were still low.

Tractographic methods have also been applied in preterm neonates. Van Pul *et al.* [61] were able to use DTI tractography successfully in term-born neonates with hypoxia-ischemia, and Yoo *et al.* [9] have also demonstrated that fiber-tracking algorithms can be applied to DTI of neonates ranging in gestational age from 28 to 40 weeks. Nagae *et al.* [58] used fiber-tracking techniques in preterm children and adolescents with a history of PVL and cerebral palsy. They did not extract DTI parameters for statistical analysis, but evaluated the resultant images with a rating scale, and found that white matter anatomy was highly variable in this group, with alterations in the anatomy of several tracts. These included the internal capsule, posterior thalamic radiation, superior corona radiata, and commissural fibers.

White matter abnormalities persist beyond childhood and into adolescence in preterm and low birth weight individuals [30,62]. Specific white matter tracts may be affected, such as the corpus callosum, which is smaller, particularly in the splenium, in preterm adolescents compared to controls [63]. Diffusion tensor imaging shows abnormalities in consistent regions – thus in preterm 11-year-olds with attention deficits, Nagy *et al.* [53] demonstrated reduced FA in the posterior corpus callosum and the internal capsules. They also produced a measure of organization of axons within fasciculi, which they termed "coherence." This is a measure of how well the main direction of diffusion in a voxel is aligned with the directions of diffusion in the surrounding voxels [4]. This measure did not differ between preterm children and term-born controls, so Nagy *et al.* [53] concluded that the differences in FA that they found were more likely to be related to restriction of axon diameter, reduced numbers of axons, or deficits of myelination (or a combination of the three) in preterm children, rather than to disorganization of fibers.

A study by our group [59] also demonstrated white matter abnormalities in the corpus callosum, persisting into adulthood. This study showed altered diffusivity in the genu of the corpus callosum in young adult

Table 8.1 Table of studies of DTI in preterm birth and low birth weight, listed by year of publication

Paper	Sample characteristics	Control group?	Measure	Mode of analysis	Outcome measure	Brief summary of findings
Inder et al. [46]	Case study, single preterm infant	No	DWI	ROI	Conventional MRI at 10 postnatal weeks	Diffusion abnormalities in "normal" appearing white matter. These areas later took on the appearance of cystic PVL
Miller et al. [14]	23 preterm neonates (less than 36 GW)	No	DTI	ROI	Serial measures of anisotropy and ADC	Developmental changes in FA and ADC did not occur in preterm infants with white matter damage
Arzoumanian et al. [52]	63 LBW (< 1800 g) infants	No	DTI	ROI	Neurodevelopmental assessment at 18–24 months	Infants with low FA in the posterior limb of the internal capsule had worse neurological outcome
Nagy et al. [53]	9 preterm children (11 years) with attention-deficit (mean 26.8 GW)	Yes	DTI	VBM	FA	Lower FA in posterior corpus callosum and bilateral internal capsules
Partridge et al. [51]	Neonates 25–34 GW; severe brain injuries excluded	No	DTI	ROI	Second DTI at interval of 5 weeks	Maturational changes of FA and diffusivity. Early-maturing tracts (including corpus callosum) had higher FA and lower MD than late-maturing ones
Maas et al. [54]	2 extremely preterm neonates, 25 and 27 GW	No	DTI	Automated segmentation	None	Transient, developmental cortical laminae could be seen
Yoo et al. [9]	6 preterm neonates, 28–40 weeks	One 28-year-old man	DTI	Tractography	None	Tracts could be traced despite low anisotropy. Anisotropy was detectable before onset of myelination
Deipolyi et al. [49]	37 infants, 28–35 GW	No	DTI	ROI	None	FA was correlated with gestational age, with regional heterogeneity
Fan et al. [47]	Children with PVL. Age 4–12 years	Yes, 12 age-matched	DTI	ROI	None	Reduced FA in association tracts in the PVL group
Counsell et al. [48]	38 preterm individuals at term-equivalent age	Yes, 8 term-born infants	DTI	ROI	None	Widespread alterations of diffusivity in infants with DEHSI, interpreted as oligodendrocyte or axonal pathology
Vangberg et al. [55]	34 VLBW individuals at 15 years	Yes, 47 NBW; 42 SGA	DTI	VBM	None	Reduced FA in corpus callosum, internal capsule, and superior fasciculus in VLBW group

Table 8.1 Continued

Paper	Sample characteristics	Control group?	Measure	Mode of analysis	Outcome measure	Brief summary of findings
Skranes et al. [56]	34 VLBW individuals at 15 years	Yes. 47 term-born, NBW	DTI	VBM	Neuropsychometry, psychosocial	Reduced FA in multiple tracts. Correlations between FA and psychiatric, cognitive, and social outcomes
Drobyshevsky et al. [57]	24 preterm infants, less than 32 GW	Stratified by degree of US abnormality	Serial DTI	ROI	Bayley scales of infant development	Infants with severe brain injury had lower FA and higher ADC. Those with highest rate of increase of FA had the worst outcomes
Nagae et al. [58]	24 children with PVL and cerebral palsy	Yes	DTI	Tractography	None	High variability of tract anatomy in the PVL group, including internal capsule, posterior thalamic radiation, superior corona radiata, and commissures
Kontis et al. [59]	Young adults (19 years) born before 33 GW	Yes	DTI	Tractography	Neuropsychometry	Abnormalities of corpus callosum white matter persisted until adulthood

ADC = apparent diffusion coefficient; DEHSI = diffuse excessive high-signal intensity; DTI = diffusion tensor imaging; DWI = diffusion-weighted imaging; FA = fractional anisotropy; GW = gestational weeks; LBW = low birth weight; MD = mean diffusivity; NBW = normal birth weight; PVL = periventricular leukomalacia; ROI = region of interest; SGA = small for gestational age; US = ultrasound; VBM = voxel-based morphometry; VLBW = very low birth weight.

females who were born before 33 weeks' gestation (see Fig. 8.3) .

Two related and recently published studies report DTI findings in preterm adolescents. Firstly, Vangberg et al. [55] compared VLBW, small-for-gestational-age (SGA), and normal birth weight individuals at age 15. They found reduced FA in the VLBW group compared to controls in corpus callosum, internal capsule, and superior fasciculus. This was a VBM study, and the authors acknowledge problems with spatial normalization, but express the view that artifacts could only account for one third of their positive findings. They used a study-specific template, to try to minimize this. There were no significant differences between SGA and control groups. Interestingly, there were also areas in which the VLBW group had higher FA than the control group. Such apparently discrepant results (higher FA) could be a result of decreased white matter complexity in the preterm group, as discussed above. Thus, if there were fewer branching or crossing fibers in a certain region in the preterm group, this would result in those areas having apparently higher FA than the control group. Another possibility is that part of the plastic response to injury in the preterm brain is to increase the FA of certain fiber systems. The related study of Skranes et al. [56] looked at VLBW 15-year-olds, and also examined their neurological, cognitive, and behavioral outcomes. They found reduced FA in the internal and external capsules, corpus callosum, and superior, middle superior and inferior fasciculi.

These studies tell us that white matter "microstructure" or "integrity" is abnormal in prematurely born individuals, and that this is detectable from birth. Although white matter continues to mature into early adulthood, with increases in white matter density and organization [11,64], differences in white matter are still detectable in adolescents born prematurely. Thus, white matter development does not attenuate these microstructural abnormalities. Questions that remain to be answered include how parameters such as ADC, MD, and FA change over development. This is beginning to be done in normal populations, despite the technical and statistical challenges [6]. For instance, McLaughlin et al. [32], in a cross-sectional study across the lifespan, found that the corpus callosum increases in size until it reaches a peak in young adulthood, with subsequent slight decline into old age. The FA characteristics of the corpus callosum followed a similar pattern, with FA increase until early adulthood, followed by stability and non-significant decline in old age.

Our research group followed VPT individuals at 15 and 19 years, and found disproportionate growth of the corpus callosum in VPT compared to term-born individuals over this time [65]. It is not known whether this growth in callosal size is also reflected in a change of DTI parameters over this time, because unfortunately we were unable to conduct a longitudinal DTI evaluation. Ashtari et al. [66] performed another cross-sectional study in adolescent males, and found age-related changes in the arcuate fasciculus, with increasing FA and no change in radial diffusivity, which they interpret as fiber bundles becoming straighter and better organized during adolescence. Zhang et al. [67] found evidence that the fiber orientation of the superior longitudinal fasciculus is changing during childhood, not just its state of myelination.

White matter and plasticity

Perinatal destructive brain lesions can be compensated for remarkably by the plastic brain. For example, Heller et al. [68] report a case of a 44-year-old man who had suffered a left hemisphere stroke. Functional MRI indicated that speech had been transferred to the right hemisphere, and DTI tractography indicated a paucity of left hemisphere connections, with a richer pattern of right hemispheric connectivity. Thomas et al. [69], in a region-of-interest study, compared individuals with hemiparetic cerebral palsy to controls and found reduced FA and increased MD in the corticospinal and corticobulbar tracts and the superior thalamic radiation of the lesioned hemisphere, along with evidence of reorganization of connections in the unaffected hemisphere. Tovar-Moll et al. [70] studied individuals with dysgenesis of the corpus callosum with DTI tractography, and were able to define their connectional anatomy. They found an extra white matter tract (the Probst bundle) connecting frontal and occipital cortices within each hemisphere. This connection was already known from gross anatomical studies. They also found a previously undefined tract which they called the "sigmoid bundle," connecting the frontal cortex to the contralateral occipital cortex. This is another example of how plastic reorganization of white matter may produce "non-standard" connectional anatomy.

There is accumulating evidence that experience can also affect white matter connectivity. For example, Bengtsson et al. [71], using DTI, found that FA was increased in the corpus callosum and internal capsule of individuals who practiced the piano in childhood. They also found that white matter can be reconfigured over shorter timescales – piano practice in adulthood was correlated with increased FA in the arcuate fasciculus. Electrical activity by axons can stimulate myelination (this process can also be inhibited by blocking axonal action potentials) [72], and this provides one plausible mechanism to link practice and FA.

Unfortunately, being deprived of appropriate environmental stimulation early in life can also affect white matter. Children who survived upbringing in Romanian orphanages, with extreme social and emotional neglect, have cognitive and behavioral deficits and also show reduced FA in the uncinate fasciculus [73]. In preterm babies, attempts to mitigate the potentially harsh early experiences of neonatal intensive care may be beneficial. A program of supportive developmental interventions for preterm babies known as NIDCAP (Newborn Individualized Developmental Care and Assessment Program) was associated with increased FA in the left corticospinal tract, as well as increased fronto-occipital electroencephalography (EEG) coherence and improved behavioral outcome [74].

Thus it seems clear that white matter is a dynamic, plastic system, capable of changing its properties on a timescale ranging from weeks to years. The genetic, constitutional, and experiential influences on this are yet to be fully determined, but we are starting to see how such plasticity allows premature brains to functionally recover from significant early injury. However, does large-scale reconfiguration of white matter come at a cost?

White matter development and cognitive function

Compared to other primates, Homo sapiens has a disproportionately large prefrontal cortex. Interestingly, the gray matter volume of the human frontal lobes is roughly what would be predicted for a primate brain of human size. The disproportionate size of the frontal lobes in our species is actually accounted for by an increased amount of white matter [75]. This expanded connectivity is expensive for the brain to maintain, and is highly likely to serve an adaptive function [76]. Cognitive function and complex adaptive behavior are properties of spatially distributed neural assemblies, and require rich white matter connectivity [7]. As we saw earlier, changes in connectivity may underlie cognitive development – for example, Klingberg et al. [8] showed that reading ability correlated with DTI measures in temporoparietal white matter. Schmithorst

et al. [11] used VBM to correlate DTI with cognitive function in term-born children and adolescents (up to 18 years old). They found positive correlations between FA and IQ in what they described as "association areas." Because FA and cognitive function may both be correlated with age, this confounder must be considered carefully in such analyses. The tractographic study of Catani et al. [77] showed relationships between FA of the arcuate fasciculus (a structure involved in language comprehension and expression) and verbal learning and memory in young adults.

Fewer studies have examined such structure–function relationships in people born prematurely. The impressive VBM study of Skranes et al. [56] did report associations between FA and various outcome measures in VLBW 15-year-olds. Areas where the VLBW group had lower FA were associated with perceptual, motor, cognitive, and mental health outcomes. Complex cognitive functions such as visuomotor integration, arithmetic, and attention were associated with more widespread abnormalities – including areas that did not have lower FA on the group comparison maps. Very low birth weight individuals with relatively low IQ had associations between IQ and FA which were localized to long association tracts. These authors also found that attention-deficit symptoms were correlated with FA in the internal capsule and superior and middle fasciculi, and suggested that deficits in social skills in VLBW adolescents were related to dysfunctional connectivity in association fiber bundles.

White matter and resilience

What are the factors that govern the degree of recovery from perinatal brain injuries? How come some individuals escape without major deficits while others are severely disabled, despite having similar perinatal brain injuries? Some tantalizing possibilities are starting to appear at the interface between genetics and neuroimaging. White matter volume appears to be under some degree of genetic control, as demonstrated by the review of imaging studies of twins reported by Peper et al. [78]. This report concluded that brain volumes, including white matter volume, are highly heritable. Pfefferbaum et al. [79] estimated the proportion of structural variance attributable to genetic or environmental effects in the corpus callosum in twins. They found that there is regional heterogeneity in the heritability of corpus callosum structure, with DTI parameters in the splenium being more under genetic control than the genu. One of the candidate genes which may be involved in this is oligodendrocyte lineage transcription factor 2 (OLIG2) [80]. Interestingly, single nucleotide polymorphisms (SNPs) of the OLIG2 gene are associated with obsessive compulsive disorder in adults [81]. Obsessive compulsive disorder has been shown to be associated with reduced FA in the anterior cingulate [82]. It is worth mentioning that young adults born before 33 weeks' gestation have an increased rate of psychiatric morbidity [83], including obsessive symptoms.

Williams syndrome is a genetic disorder caused by a hemideletion on chromosome 7. Marenco *et al.* [84] performed a tractographic study in individuals with this syndrome and found altered white matter structure – an effect which they considered to be genetically mediated. Of course, genetic and environmental factors are likely to interact, and the relationship between them may not be straightforward. A recent example of such a "gene–environment interaction" comes from the study of Caspi *et al.* [85], who found that children who were breast-fed tend to have higher IQs, but only if they also have a particular variant of the fatty acid desaturase 2 (FADS2) gene. This gene is involved in controlling fatty acid metabolism – it is worth pointing out that one of the high consumers of fatty acids during development is myelinating white matter [86]. The study of genetic and environmental influences on brain, and white matter, development is still in its infancy, but in the future, it may be instructive to examine the interactions between perinatal brain injury, genetics, and white matter structure in premature individuals.

Other possible future developments

One of the obvious gaps in the state of knowledge about white matter development is the lack of genuinely longitudinal studies of brain development in premature birth populations, using DTI and other imaging modalities. Longitudinal studies may even help to disentangle the question of what FA and MD and ADC changes mean on a cellular or tissue level [6]. These studies are not straightforward to conduct, and are time-consuming and require a somewhat long-term strategy on the part of funding bodies. Other developments currently taking place include the integration of DTI with data from other imaging modalities, such as functional MRI [87], and the introduction of higher field-strength magnets in MRI scanners, which may make it possible to produce DTI images with enhanced spatial resolution, improving the accuracy of anatomical localization of microstructural changes.

Conclusion

Diffusion tensor imaging is a relatively new technique that provides information about white matter structure that is complementary to conventional structural MRI. Diffusion tensor imaging is starting to be used to look at white matter development, but many questions remain to be answered. It has been applied to preterm individuals, from the neonatal period to adolescence, and has produced useful insights into white matter development and plasticity, and how the brain reorganizes itself in response to perinatal injury. Diffusion tensor imaging is more than just a way of producing "pretty pictures" or wiring diagrams – it provides information about the white matter of the living brain that is not available by any other means.

Acknowledgments

Diffusion tensor images are from the University College Hospital London and Institute of Psychiatry Preterm Birth Follow-Up Study, funded by the Wellcome Trust. Analysis software for DTI images was written by Professor Derek Jones, Cardiff University. Dr. Marco Catani advised on tractography methods, and Dr. Dimitris Kontis performed the tractographic analysis illustrated in Fig. 8.2, and the VBM analysis in Fig. 8.3.

References

1. Volpe JJ. Cerebral white matter injury of the premature infant-more common than you think. *Pediatrics* 2003; **112**: 176–80.

2. Back SA. Perinatal white matter injury: the changing spectrum of pathology and emerging insights into pathogenetic mechanisms. *Ment Retard Dev Disabil Res Rev* 2006; **12**: 129–40.

3. Allin M, Nosarti C, Rifkin R, Murray RM. Brain plasticity and long term function after early cerebral insult: the example of very preterm birth. In: Keshavan M, Kennedy J, Murray R, eds. *Neurodevelopment and Schizophrenia*. Cambridge: Cambridge University Press. 2005; 89–110.

4. Basser PJ, Pierpaoli C. Microstructural and physiological features of tissues elucidated by quantitative-diffusion-tensor MRI. *J Magn Reson* B 1996; **111**: 209–19.

5. Le Bihan D, Mangin JF, Poupon C. Diffusion tensor imaging: concepts and applications. *J Magn Reson Imaging* 2001; **13**: 534–46.

6. Basser PJ. Diffusion-tensor MR imaging fundamentals. In: Edelman RR, Hesselink JR, Zlatkin MB, Crues III, JV, eds. *Clinical Magnetic Resonance Imaging*, 3rd edn. China: Saunders Elsevier. 2006; 320–32.

7. Catani M, Ffytche DH. The rises and falls of disconnection syndromes. *Brain* 2005; **128**: 2224–39.

8. Klingberg T, Hedehus M, Temple E, *et al.* Microstructure of temporo-parietal white matter as a basis for reading ability: evidence from diffusion tensor magnetic resonance imaging. *Neuron* 2000; **25**: 493–500.

9. Yoo SS, Park HJ, Soul JS, *et al.* In vivo visualization of white matter fiber tracts of preterm- and term-infant brains with diffusion tensor magnetic resonance imaging. *Invest Radiol* 2005; **40**: 110–15.

10. Budde MD, Kim JH, Liang HF, *et al.* Toward accurate diagnosis of white matter pathology using diffusion tensor imaging. *Magn Reson Med* 2007; **57**: 688–95.

11. Schmithorst V, Wilke M, Dardzinski BJ, Holland SK. Cognitive functions correlate with white matter architecture in a normal pediatric population: a diffusion tensor MRI study. *Hum Brain Mapp* 2005; **26**: 139–47.

12. Mori S, Oishi K, Faina AV. White matter atlases based on diffusion tensor imaging. *Curr Opin Neurol* 2009; **22**: 362–9.

13. Dejerine J. *Anatomie des Centres Nerveux*, vol. 1. Paris: Rueff et Cie; 1895.

14. Miller SP, Vigneron DB, Henry RG, *et al.* Serial quantitative diffusion tensor MRI of the premature brain: development in newborns with and without injury. *J Magn Reson Imaging* 2002; **16**: 621–32.

15. Catani M, Howard RJ, Pajevic S, Jones DK. Virtual in vivo interactive dissection of white matter fasciculi in the human brain. *Neuroimage* 2002; **17**: 77–94.

16. Mori S, Crain BJ, Chacko VP. Three-dimensional tracking of axonal projections in the brain by magnetic resonance imaging. *Ann Neurol* 1999; **45**: 265–9.

17. Mori S, Kaufmann WE, Davatzikos C, *et al.* Imaging cortical association tracts in the human brain using diffusion-tensor-based axonal tracking. *Magn Reson Med* 2002; **47**: 215–23.

18. Conturo TE, Lori NF, Cull TS, *et al.* Tracking neuronal fiber pathways in the living human brain. *Proc Natl Acad Sci U S A* 1999; **96**: 10422–7.

19. Hagmann P, Thiran JP, Jonasson L, *et al.* DTI mapping of human brain connectivity: statistical fibre tracking and virtual dissection. *Neuroimage* 2003; **19**: 545–54.

20. Jones DK, Simmons A, Williams SC, Horsfield MA. Non-invasive assessment of axonal fiber connectivity in the human brain via diffusion tensor MRI. *Magn Reson Med* 1999; **42**: 37–41.

21. Basser PJ, Pajevic S, Pierpaoli C, Duda J, Aldroubi A. In vivo fiber tractography using DT-MRI data. *Magn Reson Med* 2000; **44**: 625–32.

22. Nucifora PGP, Verma R, Lee S-K, Melhem ER. Diffusion-tensor MR imaging and tractography: exploring brain microstructure and connectivity. *Radiology* 2007; **245**: 367–84.

23. Berube J, McLaughlin N, Bourgouin P, Beaudoin G. Bojanowski MW. Diffusion tensor imaging analysis of long association bundles in the presence of an arteriovenous malformation. *J Neurosurg* 2007; **107**: 509–14.

24. Jones DK, Griffin LD, Alexander DC, *et al.* Spatial normalization and averaging of diffusion tensor MRI data sets. *Neuroimage* 2002; **17**: 592–617.

25. Talairach J, Tournoux P. *Co-planar Stereotaxic Atlas of the Human Brain.* New York: Thieme Medical Publishers; 1988.

26. Good CD, Johnsrude IS, Ashburner J, *et al.* A voxel-based morphometric study of ageing in 465 normal adult human brains. *Neuroimage* 2001; **14**: 21–36.

27. Moseley M, Bammer R, Illes J. Diffusion-tensor imaging of cognitive performance. *Brain Cogn* 2002; **50**: 396–413.

28. Kanaan RA, Shergill SS, Barker GJ, *et al.* Tract-specific anisotropy measurements in diffusion tensor imaging. *Psychiatry Res* 2006; **146**: 73–82.

29. Snook L, Plewes C, Beaulieu C. Voxel based versus region of interest analysis in diffusion tensor imaging of neurodevelopment. *Neuroimage* 2007; **34**: 243–52.

30. Allin M, Henderson M, Suckling J, *et al.* The effects of very low birth weight on brain structure in adulthood. *Dev Med Child Neurol* 2004; **46**: 46–53.

31. Hüppi PS, Dubois J. Diffusion tensor imaging of brain development. *Semin Fetal Neonatal Med* 2006; **11**: 489–97.

32. McLaughlin NC, Paul RH, Grieve SM, *et al.* Diffusion tensor imaging of the corpus callosum: a cross-sectional study across the lifespan. *Int J Dev Neurosci* 2007; **25**: 215–21.

33. Wimberger DM, Roberts TP, Barkovich AJ, *et al.* Identification of 'premyelination' by diffusion-weighted MRI. *J Comput Assist Tomogr* 1995; **19**: 28–33.

34. Hüppi PS, Maier SE, Peled S, *et al.* Microstructural development of human newborns cerebral white matter assessed in vivo by diffusion tensor MRI. *Pediatr Res* 1998; **44**: 584–90.

35. Provenzale JM, Liang L, DeLong D, White LE. Diffusion tensor imaging assessment of brain white matter maturation during the first postnatal year. *AJR Am J Roentgenol* 2007; **189**: 476–86.

36. Qiu D, Kwong DLW, Chan GCF, Leung LHT, Khong P-L. Diffusion tensor magnetic resonance imaging finding of discrepant fractional anisotropy between the frontal and parietal lobes after whole-brain irradiation in childhood medulloblastoma survivors: reflection of regional white matter radiosensitivity? *Int J Radiat Oncol Biol Phys* 2007; **69**: 846–51.

37. Volpe J. Neurologic outcome of prematurity. *Arch Neurol* 1998; **55**: 297–300.

38. Paneth N, Rudelli R, Kazam E, Monte W. *Brain Damage in the Preterm Infant*. Cambridge: Mac Keith Press/ Cambridge University Press; 1994.

39. Dammann O, Kuban KC, Leviton A. Perinatal infection, fetal inflammatory response, white matter damage, and cognitive limitations in children born preterm. *Ment Retard Dev Disabil Res Rev* 2002; **8**: 46–50.

40. Marin-Padilla, M. Developmental neuropathology and impact of perinatal brain damage. I: Hemorrhagic lesions of neocortex. *J Neuropathol Exp Neurol* 1996; **55**: 758–73.

41. Marin-Padilla, M. Developmental neuropathology and impact of perinatal brain damage. II: White matter lesions of neocortex. *J Neuropathol Exp Neurol* 1997; **56**: 219–35.

42. Marin-Padilla, M. Developmental neuropathology and impact of perinatal brain damage. III: Gray matter lesions of neocortex. *J Neuropathol Exp Neurol* 1999; **58**: 407–29.

43. Johnston MV. Selective vulnerability in the neonatal brain. *Ann Neurol* 1998; **44**: 155–6.

44. Dyet LE, Kennea N, Counsell SJ, et al. Natural history of brain lesions in extremely preterm infants studied with serial magnetic resonance imaging from birth and neurodevelopmental assessment. *Pediatrics* 2006; **118**: 536–48.

45. Rutherford M, Counsell S, Allsop J, et al. Diffusion-weighted magnetic resonance imaging in term perinatal brain injury: a comparison with site of lesion and time from birth. *Pediatrics* 2004; **114**: 1004–14.

46. Inder T, Huppi PS, Zientara PG, et al. Early detection of periventricular leukomalacia by diffusion-weighted magnetic resonance imaging techniques, *J Pediatr* 1999; **134**: 631–4.

47. Fan GG, Yu B, Quan SM, Sun BH, Guo QY. Potential of diffusion tensor MRI in the assessment of periventricular leukomalacia. *Clin Radiol* 2006; **61**: 358–64.

48. Counsell SJ, Shen Y, Boardman JP, et al. Axial and radial diffusivity in preterm infants who have diffuse white matter changes on magnetic resonance imaging at term-equivalent age. *Pediatrics* 2006; **117**: 376–86.

49. Deipolyi AR, Mukherjee P, Gill K, et al. Comparing microstructural and macrostructural development of the cerebral cortex in premature newborns: diffusion tensor imaging versus cortical gyration. *Neuroimage* 2005; **27**: 579–86.

50. Berman JI, Mukherjee P, Partridge SC, et al. Quantitative diffusion tensor MRI fiber tractography of sensorimotor white matter development in premature infants. *Neuroimage* 2005; **27**: 862–71.

51. Partridge SC, Mukherjee P, Henry RG, et al. Diffusion tensor imaging: serial quantitation of white matter tract maturity in premature newborns. *Neuroimage* 2004; **22**: 1302–14.

52. Arzoumanian Y, Mirmiran M, Barnes PD, et al. Diffusion tensor brain imaging findings at term-equivalent age may predict neurologic abnormalities in low birth weight preterm infants. *AJNR Am J Neuroradiol* 2003; **24**: 1646–53.

53. Nagy Z, Westerberg H, Skare S, et al. Preterm children have disturbances of white matter at 11 years of age as shown by diffusion tensor imaging. *Pediatr Res* 2003; **54**: 672–9.

54. Maas LC, Mukherjee P, Carballido-Gamioa J, et al. Early laminar organization of the human cerebrum demonstrated with diffusion tensor imaging in extremely premature infants. *Neuroimage* 2004; **22**: 1134–40.

55. Vangberg TR, Skranes J, Dale AM, et al. Changes in white matter diffusion anisotropy in adolescents born prematurely. *Neuroimage* 2006; **32**: 1538–48.

56. Skranes J, Vangberg TR, Kulseng S, et al. Clinical findings and white matter abnormalities seen on diffusion tensor imaging in adolescents with very low birth weight. *Brain* 2007; **130**: 654–66.

57. Drobyshevsky A, Bregman J, Storey P, et al. Serial diffusion tensor imaging detects white matter changes that correlate with motor outcome in premature infants. *Dev Neurosci* 2007; **29**: 289–301.

58. Nagae LM, Hoon AH, Jr., Stashinko E, et al. Diffusion tensor imaging in children with periventricular leukomalacia: variability of injuries to white matter tracts. *Am J Neuroradiol* 2007; **28**: 1213–22.

59. Kontis D, Catani M, Cuddy M, et al. Diffusion tensor MRI of the corpus callosum and cognitive function in adults born preterm. *Neuroreport* 2009; **20**: 424–8.

60. Bui T, Daire J-L, Chalard F, et al. Microstructural development of human brain assessed in utero by diffusion tensor imaging. *Pediatr Radiol* 2006; **36**: 1133–40.

61. van Pul C, Buijs J, Vilanova A, Roos FG, Wijn Pff. Infants with perinatal hypoxic ischemia: feasibility of fiber tracking at birth and 3 months. *Radiology* 2006; **240**: 203–14.

62. Stewart AL, Rifkin L, Amess PN, et al. Brain structure and neurocognitive and behavioural function in adolescents who were born very preterm. *Lancet* 1999; **353**: 1653–7.

63. Nosarti C, Rush TM, Woodruff PWR, et al. Corpus callosum size and very preterm birth: relationship to neuropsychological outcome. *Brain* 2004; **127**: 2080–9.

64. Snook L, Paulson LA, Roy D, Phillips L, Beaulieu C. Diffusion tensor imaging of neurodevelopment

in children and young adults. *Neuroimage* 2005; **26**: 1164–73.

65. Allin M, Nosarti C, Narberhaus A, *et al.* Growth of the corpus callosum in adolescents born preterm. *Arch Pediatr Adolesc Med* 2007; **161**: 1183–9.

66. Ashtari M, Cervellione KL, Hasan KM, *et al.* White matter development during late adolescence in healthy males: a cross-sectional diffusion tensor imaging study. *Neuroimage* 2007; **35**: 501–10.

67. Zhang Z, Evans A, Hermoye AL, *et al.* Evidence of slow maturation of the superior longitudinal fasciculus in early childhood by diffusion tensor imaging. *Neuroimage* 2007; **38**: 239–47.

68. Heller SL, Heier LA, Watts R, *et al.* Evidence of cerebral reorganisation following perinatal stroke demonstrated with fMRI and DTI tractography. *J Clin Imaging* 2005, **29**: 283–7.

69. Thomas B, Eyssen M, Peeters R, *et al.* Quantitative diffusion tensor imaging in cerebral palsy due to periventricular white matter injury. *Brain* 2005; **128**: 2562–77.

70. Tovar-Moll F, Moll J, de Oliveira-Souza R, *et al.* Neuroplasticity in human callosal dysgenesis: a diffusion tensor imaging study. *Cereb Cortex* 2007; **17**: 531–41.

71. Bengtsson SL, Nagy Z, Skare S, *et al.* Extensive piano practicing has regionally specific effects on white matter development. *Nat Neurosci* 2005; **8**; 1148–50.

72. Demerens C, Stankoff B, Logak M, *et al.* Induction of myelination in the central nervous system by electrical activity. *Proc Natl Acad Sci USA* 1996; **93**: 9887–92.

73. Eluvathingal TJ, Chugani HT, Behen ME, *et al.* Abnormal brain connectivity in children after early severe socioemotional deprivation: a diffusion tensor imaging study. *Pediatrics* 2006; **117**: 2093–100.

74. Als H, Duffy FH, McAnulty GB, *et al.* Early experience alters brain function and structure. *Pediatrics* 2004; **113**: 846–57.

75. Schoenemann PT, Sheehan MJ, Glotzer LD. Prefrontal white matter volume is disproportionately larger in humans than in other primates. *Nat Neurosci* 2005; **8**: 242–52.

76. Laughlin SB, Sejnowski TJ. Communication in neuronal networks. *Science* 2003; **301**: 1870–4.

77. Catani M, Allin M, Husain M, *et al.* Symmetries in human brain language pathways correlate with verbal recall. *PNAS* 2007; **104**: 17163–8.

78. Peper JS, Brouwer RM, Boomsma DI, Kahn RS, Hulshoff Pol HE. Genetic influences on human brain structure: a review of brain imaging studies in twins. *Hum Brain Mapp* 2007; **28**: 464–73.

79. Pfefferbaum ACA, Sullivan EV, Carmelli D. Genetic regulation of regional microstructure of the corpus callosum in late life. *Neuroreport* 2001; **12**: 1677–81.

80. Zhou Q, Choi G, Anderson DJ. The bHLH transcription factor Olig2 promotes oligodendrocyte differentiation in collaboration with Nkx2.2. *Neuron* 2002; **31**: 791–807.

81. Stewart SE, Platko J, Fagerness J, *et al.* A genetic family-based association study of OLIG2 in obsessive-compulsive disorder. *Arch Gen Psychiatry* 2007; **64**: 209–14.

82. Szeszko PR, Ardekani BA, Ashtari M, *et al.* White matter abnormalities in obsessive-compulsive disorder: a diffusion tensor imaging study. *Arch Gen Psychiatry* 2005; **62**: 782–90.

83. Walshe M, Rifkin L, Rooney M, *et al.* Psychiatric disorder in young adults born very preterm: role of family history. *Eur J Psychiatry* 2008; **23**: 527–31.

84. Marenco S, Siuta MA, Kippenhan JS, *et al.* Genetic contributions to white matter architecture revealed by diffusion tensor imaging in Williams syndrome. *PNAS* 2007; **104**: 15117–22.

85. Caspi A, Williams B, Kim-Cohen J, *et al.* Moderation of breastfeeding effects on the IQ by genetic variation in fatty acid metabolism. *Proc Natl Acad Sci U S A* 2007; **104**: 18860–5.

86. Madhavarao CN, Arun P, Moffett JR, *et al.* Defective N-acetylaspartate catabolism reduces brain acetate levels and myelin lipid synthesis in Canavan's disease. *PNAS* 2005; **102**: 5221–6.

87. Casanova R, Srikanth R, Baer A, *et al.* Biological parametric mapping: a statistical toolbox for multimodality brain image analysis. *Neuroimage* 2007; **34**: 137–43.

Behavioral outcome of preterm birth in childhood and adolescence

Elaine Healy

Introduction

Although the numbers of live births registered in most industrialized nations have remained relatively stable in recent years, the incidence of preterm birth (birth at less than 37 completed weeks of gestation) and of low birth weight (LBW; birth weight less than 2500 g) has increased. The shorter the gestation, the smaller the baby and the higher the risk of death, morbidity, and disability. Survival rate among these vulnerable infants has improved considerably throughout the 1990s. As survival rates have improved, concern about the long-term outcome of the survivors of very preterm (VPT) birth (birth at less than 32 completed weeks of gestation) has risen. Poor outcomes in early childhood include global cognitive delay, cerebral palsy, blindness, and deafness. Given these neurosensory and cognitive disadvantages, which are described in detail in Chapter 3 and Chapters 11–15, preterm-born children and adolescents are at increased risk of adverse mental health outcomes. Clear characterization of the emotional and behavioral outcomes of preterm birth and of mediating and/or moderating biological and experiential variables may offer the opportunity for interventions that improve prognosis, both in the neonatal intensive care unit and after discharge.

This chapter reviews the literature on mental health outcomes of preterm birth in childhood and adolescence, with a particular emphasis on attention and hyperactivity problems, emotional difficulties, and socialization problems. It concludes with a discussion on the pathways to psychopathology in these neonatally compromised young people.

Behavioral outcome of preterm birth in childhood

A meta-analysis of behavioral outcomes in school-age children who were born preterm conducted by Bhutta

et al. [1] showed a higher prevalence of attention problems and of internalizing and externalizing behaviors compared with term-born controls, although these differences were not present in all studies. The following sections will describe outcomes with regard to the three most commonly reported behavioral outcomes in childhood: attention and hyperactivity problems, emotional difficulties, and socialization problems.

Attention and hyperactivity problems

Several groups have reported an excess of attention problems (i.e., lack of persistence in tasks that require cognitive involvement) and hyperactivity problems (i.e., tendency to move from one activity to another without completing any one, together with disorganized, ill-regulated, and excessive activity) in children born preterm or with LBW [1–5]. For example, using data from the American 1981 National Health Interview Survey, McCormick et al. [3] found that children born with a birth weight of less than 1500 g (very low birth weight; VLBW) were significantly more likely than peers to have higher scores on the hyperactivity subscale of the Behavior Problem Index; furthermore, hyperactivity score was an independent risk factor for school difficulties.

Using standard diagnostic criteria, such as Diagnostic and Statistical Manual IV (DSM-IV) [6] or International Classification of Diseases 10 (ICD-10) [7], facilitates interstudy comparison. The DSM-IV diagnosis of attention deficit hyperactivity disorder (ADHD) is made when functionally impairing and persistent symptoms of inattention and/or hyperactivity-impulsivity are present to a developmentally inappropriate extent, with the impairment being evident in two or more situations. The ICD-10 defines the narrower syndrome of hyperkinetic disorder and requires the full syndrome of inattention, hyperactivity, and impulsivity symptoms to be present in

Neurodevelopmental Outcomes of Preterm Birth, ed. Chiara Nosarti, Robin M. Murray, and Maureen Hack. Published by Cambridge University Press. © Cambridge University Press 2010.

two independent situations. A number of studies of preterm survivors have measured the prevalence of disorders, as defined by such classification systems, as distinct from behavioral problems [8–12]. Preterm-born children from the six studies in the meta-analysis by Bhutta et al., which used formal diagnostic criteria (DSM-III, DSM-III-R, DSM-IV) had a pooled relative risk of ADHD of 2.64 (95% confidence interval [CI] = 1.85–3.78) [1]. Botting et al. [8], who used the Child and Adolescent Psychiatric Assessment interview (CAPA), a standardized investigator-based interview, to study the frequency of psychiatric disorders in 136 VPT/VLBW survivors aged 12 years, reported an elevated prevalence of DSM-IV ADHD/attention deficit disorder (ADD) (23% vs. 6% full-term-born [FTB; born between 38 and 42 completed weeks of gestation]). Elgen et al. determined DSM III-R diagnoses, based on Child Assessment Schedule (CAS) interview, of an 11-year-old Norwegian LBW sample (defined as less than 2000 g in this study) and normal birth weight (NBW) controls [9]. They found that 27% of these Norwegian LBW children compared with 9% of controls met the clinical criteria for a child psychiatric disorder. One LBW child in four was inattentive, but only 10% of the LBW sample was diagnosed as having ADHD, supporting the concept of attention problems without hyperactivity being more common than "classical" ADHD in LBW children.

Linnet and colleagues conducted a nested case-control study based on data from four Danish longitudinal registers that confirmed this association; compared with children born at term, those with a gestational age below 34 completed weeks had a three-fold increased risk of ICD-10 hyperkinetic disorder [13]. Adjusting for possible confounders, such as socioeconomic status and parental age, did not substantially reduce the risk. The median age for these children with hyperkinetic disorder was 8.8 (interquartile range 3). In a population-based sample of 1480 twin pairs born in the period 1985–6 ascertained from the Swedish twin registry, LBW was a risk factor for symptoms of ADHD and the association did not diminish when controlled for genetic influence [14]. The lighter twin in birth weight-discordant pairs had on average 12–13% higher ADHD symptom scores in middle childhood and early adolescence than the heavier twin. The twin design eliminated to a large extent possible confounding variables including parents' socioeconomic status, maternal lifestyle factors, and psychosocial stressors during the pregnancy. Mick

and colleagues [15] examined the relative effect of LBW in a large case-control study of clinically referred ADHD and control subjects. ADHD cases were three times as likely to have been born LBW than were their peers, after controlling for potential confounders such as prenatal exposure to drugs and alcohol, parental ADHD and/or antisocial behavior disorders, and socioeconomic class.

Breslau et al. used a cohort study that oversampled LBW children in order to study the association of LBW and the later development of inattention/hyperactivity in a large-scale sample of children followed longitudinally [16]. At age 6, children with LBW had increased incidence of ADHD but not of anxiety or oppositional-defiant disorder. This relationship was stronger in an urban than suburban subsample. This effect was more pronounced at 11-year-old follow-up with LBW urban children, but not suburban children, having an excess of inattention/hyperactivity, suggesting that social disadvantage (in this case regarded as urban living) may increase the vulnerability of LBW to the development of these difficulties [17]. Breslau's group have shown that LBW has independent effects on ADHD, in contrast to the association between prenatal smoking exposure and ADHD, where the association is confounded by maternal education and maternal history of substance use disorder [18].

Given that deficits in attention and motor control only contribute towards a diagnosis of ADHD if they are excessive for a child's IQ as well as age, and that children born with VLBW show lower IQ scores than peers, some researchers consider it is important to factor out the effect of IQ when studying behavioral outcome [19]. The EPICure study was designed to describe survival and health problems for infants born before 26 completed weeks of gestational age in the United Kingdom and Ireland, and to date has followed survivors up until 10 years of age. In the 6-year-old EPICure population, Wolke reported that the difference in the prevalence of pervasive ADHD between preterm-born children and FTB controls was no longer evident when IQ was adjusted for, suggestive of age-inappropriate but cognitive-appropriate development of attention and motor control [20]. In an 8-year-old sample, the increased risk for ADHD associated with LBW was also completely attenuated by IQ [5]. Elgen and colleagues reported slower mean reaction time on tests of alternating attention and demonstrated more errors of omission on neuropsychological assessment of 130 LBW subjects compared with 130 controls, which regression analysis showed could be attributed to confounding group differences in parental factors and/or the child's intellectual abilities [21]. An increased risk of vigilance problems (i.e., having more difficulty maintaining the alert state required for information processing), which was evident in LBW boys compared to peers, persisted when IQ and parental factors were controlled for. Botting et al. noted a significantly lower IQ in children with ADHD than in non-ADHD children in both VLBW and NBW groups in their 12-year-old sample [8]. A 3.7-fold increased risk of ADHD was attenuated to a 1.8-fold increased risk, after adjusting for IQ, attainment measures (including maths score which was the only variable other than birth status to enter the model), and motor impairment. Others suggest that controlling for IQ in ADHD research is methodologically tenuous, because decrements in overall ability are a feature of the disorder, making statistical "control" impossible. The association between ADHD symptoms and lower IQ is largely due to a shared genetic etiology suggestive of below average IQ and ADHD being indicators of the same disease process, in which case, attempting to control for IQ would signify over-adjusting the analysis.

The gender distribution of ADHD in preterm-born populations is more balanced than in the general population [8]. Martel and colleagues explored sex differences in the pathways from LBW to inattention/hyperactivity [22]. They used a continuous measure of inattention/hyperactivity symptoms, and reported a stronger relationship between birth weight and inattention/hyperactivity in boys than in girls, although the difference was not significant (boys: $r = -0.24$, $p < 0.01$; girls: $r = -0.18$, $p < 0.01$). There was a modest difference by sex for motor control, suggesting that the higher incidence of neurological motor symptoms in boys may contribute to their tendency to show a higher incidence of ADHD. Jeyaseelan and colleagues have demonstrated that neurosensory motor and developmental difficulties identified at 2 years in extremely low birth weight (ELBW; < 1000 g) survivors are associated with an increased likelihood of clinically significant school-age attentional difficulties [23].

The studies reviewed above suggests that LBW and preterm children are more likely to experience a "pure," non-comorbid form of attention deficit hyperactivity, strongly suggesting a more biologically determined ADHD in those born preterm compared with FTB peers [5,8,9]. This view is supported by a cross-cultural comparison study of 408 children aged 8–10

years, weighing 1000 g or less at birth [24], which used the Child Behavior Checklist (CBCL) completed by parents. All four cohorts (from the USA, Canada, Germany, and the Netherlands) showed increased problems in the dimensions of social, thought, and attention difficulty; the mean scores of these subscales were 0.5–1.2 standard deviation (SD) higher than their country-specific norms or NBW control scores.

Emotional outcomes

In Bhutta's meta-analysis, most of the ten studies that explored internalizing problems reported significant emotional difficulties relative to peers [8,10,25–29], though other groups using equally robust measures such as CBCL or DSM criteria failed to find differences between groups [11,30,31]. The Victorian Infant Collaborative Study Group recently reported on 8-year-old outcomes of ELBW or extremely preterm birth (EPT; < 28 completed weeks of gestation) survivors; both parent and teacher reports suggested an excess of mild internalizing symptoms (parents reported an excess of somatic complaints; teachers an excess of depressive symptoms) and fewer adaptive skills compared to peers [2].

Two groups have reported on diagnostic outcomes of VLBW survivors in late childhood. At 12 years, 8% of Botting's sample of 136 VLBW children met criteria for CAPA-generated DSM-IV diagnosis of generalized anxiety disorder compared with 1% of peers [8]. Very low birth weight young people were more likely than controls to score on two out of seven of the CAPA depression screening questions, these being "feeling unloved" and "suicidal behavior." Very low birth weight children showed a trend towards increased depression with 34% having experienced at least one depressive symptom compared with 22% classroom controls; however, the number of children meeting clinical criteria for major depression was very small (2/136 VLBW; 2/148 control group). Similar results were reported by Rice and colleagues using the CASTANET (Cardiff Study of All Wales and North West England Twins) database: being small for gestational age increased the risk of depression in childhood [32]. Low birth weight for gestation and genetic/familial factors coacted and interacted in influencing early parent-rated depressive symptoms. Elgen et al. [9] reported mental health findings in 130 prospectively followed-up LBW young people and noted elevated anxiety/depression scales on the CBCL compared to peers. Although psychiatric disorder was three times more common in these LBW

11-year-olds than in controls, there was no increased diagnosis of depression, separation anxiety, or phobia; moreover, bipolar mood disorders and psychotic disorders were not evident in either group [9]. However, possible precursors of major mental illness such as thought problems, anxiety, and social withdrawal were 2- to 4-fold higher in LBW subjects. A clearer picture of any increased risk of psychotic illness in VPT/VLBW groups will only emerge when these vulnerable subjects are followed up beyond the period of maximum risk for psychosis. Please refer to Chapter 10 for further discussion of adult psychiatric outcome.

Socialization difficulties

Some researchers suggest that major mental health disorder is not a problem for preterm-born children, but that they experience difficulties in socialization and peer relationships. Preterm-born toddlers, especially those with severe neonatal problems or a very low gestational age or birth weight, risk developmental problems in the sociocommunicative domain [33]. In the first three, years of life, LBW children are as responsive as NBW children to parental social overtures. However, regardless of medical risk, they show greater difficulty in initiating social interactions and slower rates of increase in initiating such behaviors across the first 36 months [34].

Hoy and colleagues noted higher social withdrawal scores and lower scores for both social skills and peer acceptance at school age in 183 VLBW children compared with peers matched for age, gender, social class, parity, and maternal age [35]. Whitfield et al reported similar findings of higher parent-reported problem scores with regard to social skills and social withdrawal in 8- to 9-year-old ELBW children compared to peers [29]. The Stanford Binet Behavior Scale, which was rated by the examiner during psychoeducational assessment, suggested more dependent behavior, a greater need for examiner praise and encouragement, and poorer establishment of rapport in the ELBW subjects. In Hille's comparison of middle childhood outcomes of ELBW survivors across the USA, Canada, Germany, and the Netherlands, in each country CBCL social problems scores were higher in cases than in controls [24]. Elgen and coauthors (2002) also noted more social problems in 11-year-old LBW survivors than peers as reported by parents and teachers [9]. Finally, Schothorst and van Engeland reported stability of this trait between middle childhood and 11 years of age in a heterogeneous group of 145 non-handicapped preterm-born children

who had been in a neonatal intensive care unit (NICU); scores were also very stable between early childhood and preadolescence in the VPT subgroup [36].

Recent reports, based on screening assessments, have suggested that autism may be prevalent among preterm children [37,38]. Johnson et al. reported in an abstract that a British cohort of 11-year-old children born at < 26 weeks' gestation had higher levels of the autism spectrum disorder on the Social Communication Questionnaire compared to controls [39]. Two studies in the USA found that 26% and 22% of children who were born < 1500 g birth weight and < 28 weeks' gestation respectively screened positive on the Modified Checklist for Autism in Toddlers (M-CHAT) at age 2 [38,40].

There may be many routes to preterm-born children displaying socialization difficulties. For example, functionally limiting deficits in neuromotor development could account for behavioral problems. A study comparing M-CHAT rates (measuring autistic spectrum disorder) in VPT-born children with cerebral palsy, cognitive impairment, and vision and hearing impairments with those in preterm children without such deficits revealed that major motor, cognitive, visual, and hearing impairments accounted for more than half of the positive M-CHAT screens in 2-year-olds with an extremely low gestational age. However, even when the authors excluded those children with impairments from their analyses, 10% of their sample, which is nearly double the expected rate, screened positive [41]. Another study demonstrated that functionally limiting delays in neuromotor development may lead to sensitive isolated behavior in 7-year-old preterm-born children [42]. Playground activities such as skipping, hopping, and toe-walking are compromised by these developmental delays. Sometimes parents and teachers are not aware of what may be subtle deficits, but school peers are acutely aware, and peer rejection and peer victimization may ensue.

It is likely that the lower cognitive level of some preterm-born children and specific difficulties, such as deficits in simultaneous information processing and/or processing speed, increase the risk of peer relationship problems. In Elgen's preadolescent LBW group, there was a high correlation between the CBCL attention and social problems scale leading the authors to suggest that poor self-regulatory function manifesting as difficulties with adaptability, impulsivity, and sustaining attention could contribute to reported problems in peer relationships and subsequently to the lower self-esteem and reduced social activity reported by teenagers with LBW [9]. Attention deficit hyperactivity disorder/social impairment comorbidity has also been described in FTB children. Further exploration of the possibly common etiology for attention deficit and social relational problems in VLBW/VPT-born survivors may not only suggest interventions appropriate for preterm-born children but may also improve the understanding of the development of this comorbidity in all children.

Another factor which may contribute to social difficulties in preterm subjects is parental behavior. The immature behavioral organization of the preterm infant is a challenge to parents and to the development of parent–child interactions [43]. Life-threatening events in the perinatal period may induce overprotective parental behavior, which leads to differences in parental perception of the child's behavior, and may result in inadequate socioemotional adjustment in the child [44,45]. Pathways to psychopathology in VPT/VLBW children and adolescents will be further discussed later in this chapter.

Behavioral outcome of preterm birth in adolescence

Adolescence is a time of considerable development at the level of behavior, cognition, and the brain. It is characterized by dramatic changes in identity, self-consciousness, and cognitive flexibility, and by the development of cognitive abilities, such as executive function and social cognition. It is a time of transition from dependency on parents to autonomy and independence. The academic, behavioral, and general developmental difficulties experienced by preterm children raise concern as to how they will function as they approach adulthood. It has been proposed that preterm-born subjects "catch up" developmentally with their FTB peers by adolescence, secondary to the highly canalized, genetically mediated mechanisms of normal brain maturation; in addition, the plasticity of the developing brain may facilitate functional compensation. Others have speculated that preterm survivors are more impaired in adolescence than earlier in childhood as a result of peripubertal refinement of neural connections and/or the increasingly complex environment in which the young person lives. Recent reports have suggested that preterm-born adolescents experience ongoing neurosensory and cognitive problems and poorer educational attainments than peers [31,46–54]. Very low birth weight and/or VPT-born

adolescents appear to be at greater risk of parent-reported attention, emotional and socialization difficulties and seem more behaviorally cautious than peers [55–57].

Attention and hyperactivity problems

Only three adolescent outcome studies met inclusion criteria for Bhutta's meta-analysis on cognitive and/or behavioral outcomes in young people who were born preterm [28,31,58] and of these, two reports indicated there was no difference between VLBW teenagers and NBW peers in hyperactivity measures [28,31]. Stevenson et al administered the Rutter Questionnaire to parents and teachers of a regional cohort of non-disabled VLBW children and school-matched controls at age 8 and age 14 [28]. In both Stevenson's group and Saroj Saigal's Ontario ELBW cohort [59], there was a reduction in hyperactivity symptoms/ADHD between childhood and adolescence, reflecting changes observed in FTB subjects. Levy-Shiff and colleagues reported more behavioral disturbance at home and at school in 83 VLBW Israeli adolescents born between 25 and 35 weeks' gestation than in controls [58].

More recent reports suggest that difficulties with attention occur in VLBW/preterm-born adolescent subjects, but not excessive activity levels [56,57,60]. The report from the population-based study by Indredavik suggested that 56 Norwegian VLBW adolescents had higher teacher-rated inattention scores than peers without significant differences in hyperactivity scores on a teacher-completed ADHD rating scale [61]. Twenty-five percent of the VLBW subjects had "attention problems" (defined as ADHD symptoms greater than or equal to 75% of diagnostic criteria on child and parent Kiddie-Schedule for Affective Disorder and Schizophrenia for School-Age Children [K-SADS]), but only 7% were diagnosed as having ADHD [61]. In a follow-up of the University College Hospital London (UCHL) birth cohort, VPT-born adolescents (mean age 15 years) scored significantly higher than controls on the Rutter Hyperactivity score. In addition, in VPT-born boys only, left caudate volume was negatively correlated with Hyperactivity score [62]. Extremely preterm-born teenagers had higher CBCL attention problems scores than either FTB or VPT-born adolescents and were substantially more likely than peers to have difficulty concentrating according to parents (16% EPT-born, 6% VPT-born, 3% FTB) [56]. Eleven percent of EPT adolescents were described by a parent as having difficulty following through on instructions or jumping from one uncompleted activity to another compared with 5% of other adolescents, and they were significantly more likely than peers to act before thinking and to interrupt others. However, only 5% of EPT-born adolescents compared with 3% FTB peers met DSM criteria for ADHD.

The low prevalence of ADHD diagnoses reported in VLBW/preterm-born adolescents is consistent with syndrome remission in adolescence, a phenomenon that may reflect the natural history of ADHD or the developmental insensitivity of operationally defined diagnoses [63,64]. The DSM-IV diagnostic criteria for ADHD were developed and field-tested with children and adolescents aged 6–14 years and may be less appropriate for older adolescents. Although on the face of it, ADHD appears to attenuate over time, the diagnostic status of non-persistence in preterm-born and FTB adolescents could be attributed to a large number of subthreshold cases with persisting clinical symptoms and ongoing functional impairment [64].

When Levy-Shiff's group included full-scale IQ and visuomotor score as covariates, differences between preterm-born and FTB children were substantially diminished, with the school behavior difference no longer meeting statistical significance [58]. In contrast, Kulseng and colleagues suggest that attention problems persist even when IQ is controlled for. Attention and executive function problems were particularly frequent in the subgroup of VLBW adolescents who had a low estimated IQ (defined as 2SD below the mean value of the control group), but persisted even when these adolescents were excluded from analysis [65]. Further studies are needed to explore the prevalence and nature of attention difficulties in preterm-born/VLBW adolescents.

Emotional outcomes

Most but not all case-control studies and birth cohort studies suggest that VLBW/VPT-born adolescents are emotionally vulnerable [8,9,31,46,58,61,66,67]. More than a decade ago, Levy-Shiff reported that 13- to 14-year-old VLBW Israeli children manifested a wide array of self-reported emotional problems, such as anxiety and depression [58]. Both parents and teachers reported a higher prevalence of emotional and behavioral problems in VLBW teenagers in Stevenson's Merseyside sample [28]. Saigal's population-based comparison of 143 Canadian ELBW children (mean gestational age 27 weeks) with peers at age 12–16 years demonstrated significantly higher depression

subscale scores on the parent-reported Ontario Child Health Study-Revised (OCHS-R) questionnaire; there was no difference between groups on self-report [59]. In another Canadian ELBW group, clinically significant levels of internalizing problems were reported by parents in 30% of 53 ELBW teenagers compared with 7% peers; boys were disproportionately affected [55]. Botting et al. reported that parents and their VLBW children reported significantly higher scores on the Moods and Feelings Questionnaire (MFQ) and on the Revised Children's Manifest Anxiety Scale (RCMAS) [8].

In contrast, Rickards et al reported no emotional differences by parent- or self-report between 130 Australian VLBW young people prospectively followed up at 14 years old and NBW peers though VLBW adolescents scored significantly lower on self-esteem [31]. Dahl et al used mailed questionnaire to explore mental health outcomes in Norwegian VLBW adolescents [68]. They and their parents reported no excess of emotional difficulties. Similar findings were reported by Cooke in a UK young adult VLBW group; there were no differences between groups on the Hospital Anxiety and Depression Scale [69]. Healy studying the adolescent outcomes of the UCHL cohort reported no excess of internalizing symptoms or disorders in preterm-born subjects [56]. Generalized anxiety disorder was present in 5/110 (5%) preterm-born subjects compared with 2/68 (3%) peers. Indredavik and colleagues reported that 14% of their 14-year-old VLBW group had a diagnosis of anxiety disorder compared with 4% of peers, but they were no more likely to suffer from clinical depression [61].

Recent birth cohort studies support the view of LBW/preterm-born survivors being emotionally vulnerable, but differing in the age of symptom emergence and in gender-specific risk [66,67]. The 16-year-old follow-up of the 1970 British Birth Cohort did not show any association between birth weight and risk of psychological distress in girls; LBW boys were more likely than peers to be psychologically distressed (odds ratio [OR] = 1.6, 95% CI = 1.1–2.5) [66]. At 26-year follow-up, LBW women had an increased risk of depression (OR = 1.3, 95% CI = 0.9–1.8) and LBW men were more likely than peers to report a history of depression (OR = 1.6, 95% CI = 1.1–2.3). Patton et al. explored the association between prematurity/LBW and adolescent depressive disorder using a case-control design within a prospective cohort study of 2032 Australian adolescents [67]. Odds for self-reported depressive disorder were 11-fold higher in preterm-born/LBW adolescents after regression adjusting for major confounding factors (parental education, parental separation, maternal age at birth, maternal smoking in pregnancy, and serious illness in the first year of life and parental depressive disorder). This was particularly evident in preterm/LBW adolescent girls who had a 30-month cumulative prevalence of 15% for depressive disorder in contrast to 1.8% of FTB, NBW girls. This increased risk to depressive disorder secondary to LBW or gestational age seems to hold true even with the NBW and/or gestational age ranges [70,71]. Wals *et al.* described mental health outcomes in adolescent and young adult offspring of a parent with bipolar mood disorder [71]. In these young people with a genetic liability to depression, LBW within the normal range (just 4 of the sample of 140 young people having birth weights less than 2500 g) appeared to be an independent factor in increasing risk of mood disorder.

Clearly, the vast majority of children born VPT do not experience clinical levels of emotional disturbance, and some groups report no excess of internalizing symptomatology relative to FTB peers. Such resilient functioning is among the most intriguing and adaptive phenomena of human development. The mechanisms that underlie the association between low gestational age and LBW and a greater probability of affective psychopathology are unclear, but are likely to include genetic mechanisms and early physiological adaptation of the hypothalamic–pituitary–adrenal axis to adverse intra- and extrauterine events [32,72]. Early nurturing parent–child relations may buffer the developing child from stress [73]; in rat models in the first 6 days of life, a high level of tactile maternal care reduces methylation of part of the promoter region of glucocorticoid receptors which increases gene expression and results in more glucocorticoid receptors in the hippocampus and decreased reaction to stress [74].

Further exploration is warranted of the evolution of internalizing symptomatology in VPT/VLBW survivors, including clarification of risk and resilience factors. Finding ways to enhance resiliency is a major task for child mental health professionals. Understanding the phenomenon of resilience will inform efforts to translate research on positive adaptation in the face of adversity into the development of interventions to promote resilient functioning.

Eating disorders

Anorexia and bulimia nervosa are multiply determined. Risk factors include insecure attachment and unresolved loss in mothers of cases contributing to emotional processing difficulties in the daughters, both of which are more likely to occur in preterm survivors than in FTB controls. A population-based, case-control study, using the Swedish Inpatient Register, explored pregnancy and perinatal factors that increased the risk of anorexia nervosa in girls who were born between 1973 and 1984. An increased risk (OR = 3.2) was found in VPT girls, with those who were also small for gestational age being most at risk (OR = 5.7) [75]. However, Feingold and coworkers failed to find statistically significant differences between a low and high composite variable of pregnancy/perinatal complications and eating disorder symptomatology or distortion of body shape in VPT-born adolescents [76]. The possible association between perinatal factors and maladaptive eating patterns across infancy, childhood, and adolescence merits further investigation in longitudinal studies.

Risk-taking

Adolescents who were born preterm are less likely to demonstrate risk-taking than FTB peers. Most studies have reported less alcohol and substance use [59,77]. In a UK geographically defined cohort of EPT adolescents, Johnson *et al* found that fewer EPT teenagers who were attending mainstream school used alcohol and soft drugs than FTB peers (never drank 41% vs. 20%; never used cannabis 92% vs. 76%) [77]; Saigal *et al* also reported less alcohol use than in a control population: 8% of the ELBW teenage group had consumed 3 or more drinks of alcohol at a time compared with 25% of peers [59]. An older study of Danish teenagers noted similar rates of alcohol and drug use for VLBW young adults and controls [78]. The consensus that VLBW adolescents are more likely to be behaviorally cautious or risk-averse contradicts predictions from older studies of sociopathic outcomes in adulthood (see Chapter 10).

Socialization difficulties

An important development task during adolescence is increasingly independent socialization and the formation of close mutual friendships. Given the physical and psychosocial changes that occur during puberty, any preexisting vulnerability in socialization is likely to become more evident [79]. Previous socialization difficulties are likely to be further compounded by the more complex social networks in which the adolescent finds him/herself. Most groups agree that birth weight- or gestational age-compromised adolescents are at increased risk of socialization difficulties [31,55,56,61,68]. In epidemiological samples, birth weight is a significant predictor of scores on peer relationship problems scales [80,81]. Rickards and colleagues described more teacher-reported social rejection (being isolated from and not being accepted by the peer group) compared to peers in 130 14-year-old Australian VLBW, preterm-born survivors [31]. Increased CBCL social problems scores have been reported in Norwegian VLBW adolescents, in Canadian ELBW survivors, and in British VPT-born adolescents [55,56,68]; in the UCHL group, EPT adolescents themselves reported lower social competence than controls [56]. Indredavik and colleagues noted that VLBW subjects had higher mean scores on the Autism Spectrum Screening Questionnaire (ASSQ), with higher scores on the following items: lives somewhat in a world of his own with restricted idiosyncratic intellectual interests, has literal understanding of ambiguous and metaphorical language, uses language freely but fails to make adjustment to fit social contexts or the needs of different listeners, lacks empathy, wishes to be sociable but fails to make relationships with peers [61]. They hypothesized that VLBW adolescents might struggle with encoding and interpreting subtle cues of social relations.

As previously described in this chapter, there are many routes to preterm-born survivors displaying socialization difficulties. Echoing Elgen's report of a high correlation between the CBCL attention and social problems scale in 11-year-olds, Indredavik noted a significant correlation between ADHD total score and ASSQ score [9,82]. Teenager survivors may be additionally vulnerable because of their disadvantage in growth attainment [49,83], with males being more affected than females [84]. The fact that preterm-born males are likely to be smaller and lighter than their peers in adolescence may have social implications though only anecdotal evidence supports short stature being associated with a psychological burden. In their follow-up of Canadian ELBW adolescents, Saigal and colleagues found that weight-by-age z scores but not height-by-age z scores contributed to a positive self-rating of close friendships [85].

Time trends

De Kleine and colleagues reporting from Leiden in the Netherlands compared 5-year-old outcomes of VPT survivors in 1983 and in 1993 [86]. The incidence of disabling cerebral palsy increased over time and that of visual difficulties decreased; there were no changes in incidence of hearing problems, the need for special education, and the incidence of behavioral problems (17.5% vs. 22%). The exploration of behavioral problems was limited to 15 problem items of the CBCL that discriminated best between children referred and not referred to mental health services. A more comprehensive exploration of time trends in mental health outcomes of VPT survivors is warranted.

Pathways to psychopathology in VPT/VLBW children and adolescents

Many preterm-born children and adolescents show none of the deficits described in this chapter and therefore, to understand outcomes, it is necessary to consider other mental health risk factors associated with prematurity, including brain development, neonatal medical complications, and the social environment in which these at-risk children are raised [87,88].

Preterm birth affects the complex temporally and spatially ordered sequence of brain development that starts soon after conception and continues into the second decade of life [89,90]. Whitaker showed an association between brain lesions identified by ultrasound and behavioral problems at 6 years [91]. Stewart and colleagues reported that more than half of the VPT adolescents they followed up had abnormal MRI scans (enlarged ventricles, thinning of corpus callosum, white matter signal change) at adolescence [54]. Very preterm adolescents with abnormal scans had higher Rutter scores than FTB controls; those with normal or equivocal scans had similar scores to controls.

Voxel-based morphometry studies of the brains of VPT adolescents suggest that developmental changes following VPT birth and early brain insult do not simply result in gray and white matter tissue loss, but in complicated patterns of cortical and subcortical alterations [56,92,93]. Increased gray matter probability has been described in frontal and limbic lobes bilaterally and in the cerebellum in preterm-born children and adolescents [56,93]. A consistent finding is less temporal lobe gray matter [56,93–97]. These structural findings are consistent with a delay in cortical maturation [56,93,94,97–100].

When VPT children engage in cognitive processing, they may be limited in the brain resources they can recruit, given their smaller brains and multiple foci of brain injury. It can be therefore speculated that the capacity of the brain for specialization may be diminished and immature processing strategies in preterm/LBW individuals may be more likely to persist. Activation patterns studied with functional magnetic resonance imaging (fMRI) for children with immature processing strategies generally show a more distributed pattern of activation than adults. The findings of Nosarti and colleagues of differential neuronal activation between VPT and FTB male adolescents during performance of a simple response inhibition task is consistent with a delay in fronto-striatal cortical organization and with a more diffuse, immature, though perhaps no less effective, pattern of activation in VPT-born adolescents [101]. Preterm-born adolescents with higher medical and environmental risk scores show less mature patterns of brain activation during attention tasks than those with low risk scores [102]. For additional information on these and other fMRI studies in preterm/LBW samples see also Chapter 7.

There is ample evidence to show that cumulative neonatal medical complication scores are negatively related to cognitive and motor outcomes and to attainments and behavior. Minor motor dysfunction at aged 2 years is associated with clinical measures of attention at school age. For instance, Davis and colleagues involved in the Victorian Infant Collaborative Study Group noted that ELBW/VPT children with developmental coordination disorder (DCD) exhibited more problems in adaptive and externalizing behaviors than ELBW/VPT children without DCD [103].

The social and psychological environment in which the prematurely born child grows and is nurtured also has a significant influence on his/her development [104–108]. Sociodemographic variables, such as socioeconomic status, ethnicity, and parental education account for some of the variance associated with outcome (see Chapter 17). Proximal environmental stresses may include parental stress and/or insecure attachments. Parents of children with shorter gestation experience more stress and in particular feel more socially isolated and show more partner-relationship difficulties 18 months after the preterm birth [109].

In addition, preterm birth impacts upon early infant–mother relationships and may be associated with compromised attachment relationships and/or an atypical style of parenting [110–114]. Very preterm babies are not as ready to receive or respond to social stimuli as are FTB babies [115–119]; they are less able to organize responses in the gaze, affective, and motor

modalities into coherent affective configurations [120], which decreases the parent's capacity to read and respond to the infant's social cues. Interactions between premature infants and their mothers have been described as suboptimally coordinated, with less maternal behavior in the gaze, affect, and touch modalities, and poorer coordination of these behaviors with moments of infant alertness [121–124]. The extent of mother–child a synchrony correlates with the level of infant medical risk at birth, suggesting that the degree of central nervous system insult plays an important role in the development of mother–infant reciprocity [125]. Some researchers have proposed that maternal "overwhelming" influences on VPT infants in the context of high maternal stress is associated with an excessively responsive hypothalamic–pituitary axis and poor quality of focused attention in the first year of life [126]. Emotional, social, and attention difficulties in VPT adolescents could be manifestations of insecure attachment in some preterm-born teenagers [127–131].

Parents of preterm-born children may be overprotective in their parenting. After controlling for socioeconomic status, ethnicity, sex, and age of child, parents of 8-year-old ELBW children reported higher Parental Protection Scale scores [45]. These Parent Protection Scale findings were not significant when the 36 children with neurosensory impairments were excluded from analysis, although parental overprotection remained a significant difference between groups.

Complex interactional effects are likely to exist between neurobiological vulnerability and environmental variables [87]. One of the models proposed is an additive interactional model, in which intrinsic developmental disorders in vulnerable children increase the susceptibility to disorganization by lowering the child's resilience to suboptimal parenting factors [132]. The subsequent insecure attachments are more predictive of behavior problems in children growing up in higher-risk environments than in children growing up in low-risk environments [127].

In order to optimize developmental outcomes in preterm-born survivors, both biomedical risk reduction strategies and biopsychosocial interventions are needed. Interventions such as the enrichment of the neonatal and early childhood environment, as reviewed in Chapter 18, and early diagnosis and treatment of maternal postnatal mental health difficulties should be particularly targeted at preterm-born neonates and their families.

References

1. Bhutta AT, Cleves MA, Casey PH, Cradock MM, Anand KJ. Cognitive and behavioral outcomes of school-aged children who were born preterm – a meta-analysis. *JAMA* 2002; **288**(6): 728–37.

2. Anderson P, Doyle L W. Neurobehavioral outcomes of school-age children born extremely low birth weight or very preterm in the 1990s. *JAMA* 2003; **289**(24): 3264–72.

3. McCormick MC, Gortmaker SL, Sobol AM. Very-low-birth-weight children – behavior problems and school difficulty in a national sample. *J Pediatr* 1990; **117**(5): 687–93.

4. O'Callaghan MJ, Harvey JM. Biological predictors and co-morbidity of attention deficit and hyperactivity disorder in extremely low birthweight infants at school. *J Paediatr Child Health* 1997; **33**(6): 491–6.

5. Szatmari P, Saigal S, Rosenbaum P, Campbell D. Psychopathology and adaptive functioning among extremely low-birth-weight children at 8 years of age. *Dev Psychopathol* 1993; **5**(3): 345–57.

6. American Psychiatric Association. *Diagnostic and Statistical Manual of Mental Disorders*, 4th edn. Washington, DC: American Psychiatric Association; 1994.

7. World Health Organization. *International Classification of Diseases and Related Health Problem*, 10th revision. Geneva: World Health Organization; 1992.

8. Botting N, Powls A, Cooke R W, Marlow N. Attention deficit hyperactivity disorders and other psychiatric outcomes in very low birthweight children at 12 years. *J Child Psychol Psychiatry* 1997; **38**(8): 931–41.

9. Elgen I, Sommerfelt K, Markestad T. Population based, controlled study of behavioural problems and psychiatric disorders in low birthweight children at 11 years of age. *Arch Dis Child* 2007; **87**(2): F128–32.

10. Stjernqvist K, Svenningsen NW. Ten-year follow-up of children born before 29 gestational weeks: health, cognitive development, behaviour and school achievement. *Acta Paediatr* 1999; **88**(5): 557–62.

11. Szatmari P, Saigal S, Rosenbaum P, Campbell D, King S. Psychiatric-disorders at 5 years among children with birth-weights less than 1000g – a regional perspective. *Dev Med Child Neurol* 1990; **32**(11): 954–62.

12. Taylor HG, Klein N, Minich NM, Hack M. Middle-school-age outcomes in children with very low birthweight. *Child Dev* 2000; **71**(6): 1495–511.

13. Linnet KM, Wisborg K, Agerbo E, *et al.* Gestational age, birth weight, and the risk of hyperkinetic disorder. *Arch Dis Child* 2006; **91**(8): 655–60.

14. Hultman CM, Torrang A, Tuvblad C, *et al.* Birth weight and attention-deficit/hyperactivity symptoms in childhood and early adolescence: a prospective Swedish twin study. *J Am Acad Child Adolesc Psychiatry*; **46**(3): 370–7.

15. Mick E, Biederman J, Prince J, Fischer MJ, Faraone SV. Impact of low birth weight on attention-deficit hyperactivity disorder. *J Dev Behav Pediatr* 2002; **23**(1): 16–22.

16. Breslau N, Brown GG, DelDotto JE, *et al.* Psychiatric sequelae of low birth weight at 6 years of age. *J Abnorm Child Psychol* 1996; **24**(3): 385–400.

17. Breslau N, Chilcoat HD. Psychiatric sequelae of low birth weight at 11 years of age. *Bio Psychiatry* 2000; **47**(11): 1005–11.

18. Nigg JT, Breslau N. Prenatal smoking exposure, low birth weight, and disruptive behavior disorders. *J Am Acad Child Adolesc Psychiatry* 2007; **46**(3): 362–9.

19. Stefanatos GA, Baron IS. Attention-deficit/hyperactivity disorder: a neuropsychological perspective towards DSM-V. *Neuropsychol Rev* 2007; **17**(1): 5–38.

20. Wolke D. Cognitive and psychological development at 5 1/2 years. Paper presented at the EPICure and the challenge of extreme prematurity, Nottingham; 2003.

21. Elgen I, Lundervold A J, Sommerfelt K. Aspects of inattention in low birth weight children. *Pediatr Neurol* 2004; **30**(2): 92–8.

22. Martel MM, Lucia VC, Nigg JT, Breslau N. Sex differences in the pathway from low birth weight to inattention/hyperactivity. *J Abnorm Child Psychol* 2007; **35**(1): 87–96.

23. Jeyaseelan D, O'Callaghan M, Neulinger K, Shum D, Burns Y. The association between early minor motor difficulties in extreme low birth weight infants and school age attentional difficulties. *Early Hum Dev* 2006; **82**(4): 249–55.

24. Hille ETM, den Ouden AL, Saigal S, *et al.* Behavioural problems in children who weigh 1000 g or less at birth in four countries. *Lancet* 2001; **357**(9269): 1641–3.

25. Horwood LJ, Mogridge N, Darlow BA. Cognitive, educational, and behavioural outcomes at 7 to 8 years in a national very low birthweight cohort. *Arch Dis Child* 1998; **79**(1): F12–20.

26. Sommerfelt K, Ellertsen B, Markestad T. Personality and behaviour in eight-year-old, non-handicapped children with birth weight under 1500 g. *Acta Paediatr* 1993; **82**(10): 723–8.

27. Sommerfelt K, Ellertsen B, Markestad T. Parental factors in cognitive outcome of nonhandicapped low-birth-weight infants. *Arch Dis Child* 1995; **73**(3): F135–42.

28. Stevenson C, Blackburn P, Pharoah P. Longitudinal study of behaviour disorders in low birthweight infants. *Arch Dis Child Fetal Neonatal Ed* 1999; **81**(1): F5–9.

29. Whitfield, MF, Grunau RVE, Holsti L. Extremely premature (< = 800 g) schoolchildren: multiple areas of hidden disability. *Arch Dis Child* 1997; **77**(2): F85–90.

30. McDonald MA, Sigman M, Ungerer JA. Intelligence and behavior problems in 5-year-olds in relation to representational abilities in the 2nd year of life. *J Dev Behav Pediatr* 1989; **10**(2): 86–91.

31. Rickards AL, Kelly EA, Doyle LW, Callanan C. Cognition, academic progress, behavior and self-concept at 14 years of very low birth weight children. *J Dev Behav Pediatr* 2001; **22**(1): 11–18.

32. Rice F, Harold GT, Thapar A. The effect of birth-weight with genetic susceptibility on depressive symptoms in childhood and adolescence. *Eur Child Adolesc Psychiatry* 2006; **15**(7): 383–91.

33. De Groote I, Roeyers H, Warreyn P. Social-communicative abilities in young high-risk preterm children. *J Dev Phys Disabil* 2006; **18**(2): 183–200.

34. Landry SH, Densen SE, Swank PR. Effects of medical risk and socioeconomic status on the rate of change in cognitive and social development for low birth weight children. *J Clin Exp Neuropsychol* 1997; **19**(2): 261–74.

35. Hoy EA, Sykes DH, Bill JM, *et al.* The social competence of very-low-birth-weight children – teacher, peer, and self-perceptions. *J Abnorm Child Psychol* 1992; **20**(2): 123–50.

36. Schothorst PF, van Engeland H. Long-term behavioral sequelae of prematurity. *J Am Acad Child Adolesc Psychiatry* 1996; **35**(2): 175–83.

37. Larsson HJ, Eaton WW, Madsen KM, *et al.* Risk factors for autism: perinatal factors, parental psychiatric history, and socioeconomic status. *Am. J. Epidemiol* 2005; **161**(10): 916–25.

38. Limperopoulos C, Bassan H, Sullivan NR, *et al.* Positive screening for autism in ex-preterm infants: prevalence and risk factors. *Pediatrics* 2008; **121**(4): 758–65.

39. Johnson S, Hollis C, Wolke D, Marlow N. Autistic spectrum symptoms in extremely preterm children at 11 years. *Pediatric Academic Society Meeting* [Abstract, E-PAS2008:634865.7]; 2008.

40. Kuban KC, Allred EN, O'Shea M, *et al.* An algorithm for identifying and classifying cerebral palsy in young children. *J. Pediatr* 2008; **153**(4): 466–72.

41. Kuban KC, O'Shea TM, Allred EN, *et al.* Positive screening on the Modified Checklist for Autism in Toddlers (M-CHAT) in extremely low gestational age newborns. *J. Pediatr* 2009; **154**(4): 535–40.

42. Nadeau L, Boivin M, Tessier R, Lefebvre, F, Robaey P. Mediators of behavioral problems in 7-year-old children born after 24 to 28 weeks of gestation. *J Dev Behav Pediatr* 2001; **22**(1): 1–10.

43. Halpern LF, Brand KL, Malone AF. Parenting stress in mothers of very-low-birth-weight (VLBW) and full-term infants: a function of infant behavioral characteristics and child-rearing attitudes. *J Pediatr Psychol* 2001; **26**(2): 93–104.

44. Singer LT, Salvator A, Guo SY, *et al.* Maternal psychological distress and parenting stress after the birth of a very low-birth-weight infant. *JAMA* 1999; **281**(9): 799–805.

45. Wightman A, Schluchter M, Drotar D, *et al.* Parental protection of extremely low birth weight children at age 8 years. *J Dev Behav Pediatr* 2007; **28**(4): 317–26.

46. Botting N, Powls A, Cooke, RWI, Marlow N. Cognitive and educational outcome of very-low-birthweight children in early adolescence. *Dev Med Child Neurol* 1998; **40**(10): 652–60.

47. Cooke RWI, Abernethy LJ. Cranial magnetic resonance imaging and school performance in very low birth weight infants in adolescence. *Arch Dis Child Fetal Neonatal Ed* 1999; **81**(2): F116–21.

48. Doyle LW, Casalaz D. Outcome at 14 years of extremely low birthweight infants: a regional study. *Arch Dis Child* 2001; **85**(3): F159–64.

49. Ericson A, Kallen B. Very low birthweight boys at the age of 19. *Arch Dis Child Fetal Neonatal Ed* 1998; **78**(3): F171–4.

50. Hack M, Flannery DJ, Schluchter M, *et al.* Outcomes in young adulthood for very-low-birth-weight infants. *N Engl J Med* 2002; **346**(3): 149–57.

51. O'Brien F, Roth S, Stewart A, *et al.* The neurodevelopmental progress of infants less than 33 weeks into adolescence. *Arch Dis Child* 2004; **89**(3): 207–11.

52. Saigal S, Stoskopf B, Streiner D, *et al.* Transition of extremely low-birth-weight infants from adolescence to young adulthood – comparison with normal birth-weight controls. *JAMA* 2006; **295**(6): 667–75.

53. Saigal S, Stoskopf BL, Streiner DL, Burrows E. Physical growth and current health status of infants who were of extremely low birth weight and controls at adolescence. *Pediatrics* 2001; **108**(2): 407–15.

54. Stewart AL, Rifkin L, Amess PN, *et al.* Brain structure and neurocognitive and behavioural function in adolescents who were born very preterm. *Lancet* 1999; **353**(9165): 1653–7.

55. Grunau RE, Whitfield MF, Fay TB. Psychosocial and academic characteristics of extremely low birth weight (<= 800 g) adolescents who are free of major impairment compared with term-born control subjects. *Pediatrics* 2004; **114**(6): E725–32.

56. Healy E. Adolescent mental health consequences of very preterm birth. Unpublished PhD thesis, University of London, London; 2008.

57. Indredavik MS, Vik T, Heyerdahl S, Kulseng S, Brubakk AM. Psychiatric symptoms in low birth weight adolescents, assessed by screening

questionnaires. *Eur Child Adolesc Psychiatry* 2005; **14**(4): 226–36.

58. Levy-Shiff R, Einat G, Hareven D, *et al*. Emotional and behavioral-adjustment in children born prematurely. *J Clin Child Psychol* 1994; **23**(3): 323–33.

59. Saigal S, Pinelli J, Hoult L, Kim MM, Boyle M. Psychopathology and social competencies of adolescents who were extremely low birth weight. *Pediatrics* 2003; **111**(5): 969–75.

60. Indredavik MS, Skranes JS, Vik T, *et al*. Low-birth-weight adolescents: psychiatric symptoms and cerebral MRI abnormalities. *Pediatr Neurol* 2005; **33**(4): 259–66.

61. Indredavik M S, Vik T, Heyerdahl S, *et al*. Psychiatric symptoms and disorders in adolescents with low birth weight. *Arch Dis Child Fetal Neonatal Ed* 2004; **89**(5): F445–50.

62. Nosarti C, Allin MPG, Frangou S, Rifkin L, Murray RM. Decreased caudate volume is associated with hyperactivity in adolescents born very preterm. *Biol Psychiatry* 2005; **57**(6): 661–6.

63. Faraone SV, Biederman J, Mick E. The age-dependent decline of attention deficit hyperactivity disorder: a meta-analysis of follow-up studies. *Psychol Med* 2006; **36**(2): 159–65.

64. Steinhausen HC. Attention-deficit hyperactivity disorder in a life perspective. *Acta Psychiatr Scand* 2003; **107**(5): 321–2.

65. Kulseng S, Jennekens-Schinkel A, Naess P, *et al*. Very-low-birthweight and term small-for-gestational-age adolescents: attention revisited. *Acta Paediatr* 2006; **95**(2): 224–30.

66. Gale CR, Martyn CN. Birth weight and later risk of depression in a national birth cohort. *BJ Psychiatry* 2004; **184**: 28–33.

67. Patton GC, Coffey C, Carlin JB, Olsson CA, Morley R. Prematurity at birth and adolescent depressive disorder. *Br J Psychiatry* 2004; **184**, 446–7.

68. Dahl LB, Kaaresen PI, Tunby J, *et al*. Emotional, behavioral, social, and academic outcomes in adolescents born with very low birth weight. *Pediatrics* 2006; **118**(2): E449–59.

69. Cooke RWI. Health, lifestyle, and quality of life for young adults born very preterm. *Arch Dis Child* 2004; **89**(3): 201–6.

70. Raikkonen K, Pesonen AK, Kajantie E, *et al*. Length of gestation and depressive symptoms at age 60 years. *Br J Psychiatry* 2007; **190**: 469–74.

71. Wals M, Reichart CG, Hillegers MHJ, *et al*. Impact of birth weight and genetic liability on psychopathology in children of bipolar parents. *J Am Acad Child Adolesc Psychiatry* 2003; **42**(9): 1116–21.

72. Phillips DIW. Programming of the stress response: a fundamental mechanism underlying the long-term effects of the fetal environment? *J Intern Med* 2007; **261**(5): 453–60.

73. Laucht M, Esser G, Schmidt MH. Differential development of infants at risk for psychopathology: the moderating role of early maternal responsivity. *Dev Med Child Neurol* 2001; **43**(5): 292–300.

74. Kaffman A, Meaney MJ. Neurodevelopmental sequelae of postnatal maternal care in rodents: clinical and research implications of molecular insights. *J Child Psychol Psychiatry* 2007; **48**(3–4): 224–44.

75. Cnattingius S, Hultman CM, Dahl M, Sparen, P. Very preterm birth, birth trauma, and the risk of anorexia nervosa among girls. *Arch Gen Psychiatry* 1999; **56**(7): 634–8.

76. Feingold E, Sheir-Neiss G, Melnychuk J, Bachrach S, Paul D. Eating disorder symptomatology is not associated with pregnancy and perinatal complications in a cohort of adolescents who were born preterm. *Int J Eat Disord* 2002; **31**(2): 202–9.

77. Johnson A, Bowler U, Yudkin P, *et al*. Health and school performance of teenagers born before 29 weeks gestation. *Arch Dis Child Fetal Neonatal Ed* 2003; **88**(3): 190–8.

78. Bjerager M, Steensberg J, Greisen G. Quality of life among young adults born with very low birthweights. *Acta Paediatr* 1995; **84**(12): 1339–43.

79. Richter LM. Studying adolescence. *Science* 2006; **312**(5782): 1902–5.

80. Cohen SE. Biosocial factors in early infancy as predictors of competence in adolescents who were born prematurely. *J Dev Behav Pediatr* 1995; **16**(1): 36–41.

81. Taylor HG, Minich NM, Klein N, Hack M. Longitudinal outcomes of very low birth weight: neuropsychological findings. *J Int Neuropsychol Soc* 2004; **10**(2): 149–63.

82. Indredavik MS. Mental health and cerebral magnetic resonance imaging in adolescents with low birth weight. Doctoral thesis, Norwegian University of Science and Technology, Faculty of Medicine; 2005.

83. Halvorsen T, Skadberg BT, Eide GE, *et al*. Pulmonary outcome in adolescents of extreme preterm birth: a regional cohort study. *Acta Paediatr* 2004; **93**(10): 1294–300.

84. Hack M. Young adult outcomes of very-low-birth-weight children. *Semin Fetal Neonatal Med* 2006; **11**(2): 127–37.

85. Saigal S, Lambert M, Russ C, Hoult L. Self-esteem of adolescents who were born prematurely. *Pediatrics* 2002; **109**(3): 429–33.

86. de Kleine MJK, den Ouden AL, Kollee LAA, *et al*. Outcome of perinatal care for very preterm infants at 5 years of age: a comparison between 1983 and 1993. *Paediatr Perinatal Epidemiol* 2007; **21**(1): 26–33.

87. Bendersky M, Lewis M. Environmental risk, biological risk, and developmental outcome. *Dev Psychol,* 1994; **30**(4): 484–94.

88. Levy-Shiff R, Einat G, Mogilner MB, Lerman M, Krikler R. Biological and environmental correlates of developmental outcome of prematurely born infants in early adolescence. *J Pediatr Psychol* 1994; **19**(1): 63–78.

89. Giedd JN, Blumenthal J, Jeffries NO, *et al.* Brain development during childhood and adolescence: a longitudinal MRI study. *Nat Neurosci* 1999; **2**(10): 861–3.

90. Giedd JN, Snell JW, Lange N, *et al.* Quantitative magnetic resonance imaging of human brain development: ages 4–18. *Cereb Cortex* 1996; **6**(4): 551–60.

91. Whitaker AH, VanRossem R, Feldman JF, *et al.* Psychiatric outcomes in low-birth-weight children at age 6 years: relation to neonatal cranial ultrasound abnormalities. *Arch Gen Psychiatry* 1997; **54**(9): 847–56.

92. Allin MP, Henderson M, Suckling J, *et al.* (2001). The brains of adults of very low birth weight have altered patterns of grey and white matter organisation. *Schizophr Res* 2001; **49**(1–2): 149.

93. Nosarti C, Giouroukou E, Healy E, *et al.* Grey and white matter distribution in very preterm adolescents mediates neurodevelopmental outcome. *Brain* 2008; **131**(Pt I): 205–17.

94. Kesler SR, Ment LR, Vohr B, *et al.* Volumetric analysis of regional cerebral development in preterm children. *Pediatr Neurol* 2004; **31**(5): 318–25.

95. Martinussen M, Fischl B, Larsson HB, *et al.* Cerebral cortex thickness in 15-year-old adolescents with low birth weight measured by an automated MRI-based method. *Brain* 2005; **128**(Pt II): 2588–96.

96. Peterson BS. Brain imaging studies of the anatomical and functional consequences of preterm birth for human brain development. *Ann NY Acad Sci* 2003; **1008**: 219–37.

97. Reiss AL, Kesler SR, Vohr B, *et al.* Sex differences in cerebral volumes of 8-year-olds born preterm. *J Pediatr* 2004; **145**(2): 242–9.

98. Kesler SR, Vohr B, Schneider KC, *et al.* (2006). Increased temporal lobe gyrification in preterm children. *Neuropsychologia* 2006; **44**(3): 445–53.

99. Kolb B, Gorny G, Soderpalm AHV, Robinson TE. Environmental complexity has different effects on the structure of neurons in the prefrontal cortex versus the parietal cortex or nucleus accumbens. *Synapse* 2003; **48**(3): 149–53.

100. Peterson BS, Vohr B, Staib LH, *et al.* Regional brain volume abnormalities and long-term cognitive outcome in preterm infants. *JAMA* 2000; **284**(15): 1939–47.

101. Nosarti C, Rubia K, Smith AB, *et al.* Altered functional neuroanatomy of response inhibition in adolescent males who were born very preterm. *Dev Med Child Neurol* 2006; **48**(4): 265–71.

102. Carmody DP, Bendersky M, Dunn SM, *et al.* Early risk, attention, and brain activation in adolescents born preterm. *Child Dev* 2006; **77**(2): 384–94.

103. Davis NM, Ford GW, Anderson PJ, Doyle LW. Developmental coordination disorder at 8 years of age in a regional cohort of extremely-low-birthweight or very preterm infants. *Dev Med Child Neurol* 2007; **49**(5): 325–30.

104. Aylward GP. The relationship between environmental risk and developmental outcome. *J Dev Behav Pediatr* **13**(3), 222–9.

105. Dittrichova J, Brichacek V, Mandys F, *et al.* The relationship of early behaviour to later developmental outcome for preterm children. *Inter J Behav Dev* 1996; **19**(3): 517–32.

106. Gross SJ, Mettelman BB, Dye TD, Slagle, TA. Impact of family structure and stability on academic outcome in preterm children at 10 years of age. *J Pediatr* 2001; **138**(2): 169–75.

107. Kalmar M. The course of intellectual development in preterm and fullterm children: an 8-year longitudinal study. *Int J Behav Dev* 1996; **19**(3): 491–516.

108. Rieck M, Arad I, Netzer D. Developmental evaluation of very-low-birthweight infants: Longitudinal and cross-sectional studies. *Int J Behav Dev* 1996; **19**(3): 549–62.

109. Jackson K, Ternestedt B M, Magnuson A, Schollin J. Parental stress and toddler behaviour at age 18 months after pre-term birth. *Acta Paediatr* 2007; **96**(2): 227–32.

110. Cox SM, Hopkins J, Hans SL. Attachment in preterm infants and their mothers: Neonatal risk status and maternal representations. *Infant Ment Health J* 2000; **21**(6): 464–80.

111. Plunkett JW, Meisels SJ, Stiefel GS, Pasick PL, Roloff DW. Patterns of attachment among preterm infants of varying biological risk. *J Am Acad Child Adolesc Psychiatry* 1986; **25**(6): 794–800.

112. Poehlmann J, Fiese BH. (2001). The interaction of maternal and infant vulnerabilities on developing attachment relationships. *Dev Psychopathol* 2001; **13**(1): 1–11.

113. Fava Vizziello G, Calvo V. La perdita della speranza. Efetti della nascita prematura sulla rappresentazione genitoriale e sullo sviluppo dell' attaccamento. *SAGGI* 1997; **23**(1): 15–35.

114. Weiss SJ, Wilson P, Hertenstein MJ, Campos R. The tactile context of a mother's caregiving: implications for attachment of low birth weight infants. *Infant Behav Dev* 2000; **23**(1): 91–111.

115. Brachfeld S, Goldberg S, Sloman J. Parent-infant interaction in free play at 8 and 12 months – effects of prematurity and immaturity. *Infant Behav Dev* 1980; **3**(4), 289–305.

116. Eckerman CO, Hsu HC, Molitor A, Leung EHL, Goldstein RF. Infant arousal in an en-face exchange with a new partner: effects of prematurity and perinatal biological risk. *Dev Psychol* 1999; **35**(1): 282–93.

117. Feldman R. Infant-mother and infant-father synchrony: the coregulation of positive arousal. *Infant Ment Health J* 2003; **24**(1): 1–23.

118. Goldberg S. Premature birth – consequences for the parent-infant relationship. *Am Sci* 1979; **67**(2): 214–20.

119. Mouradian LE, Als H, Coster WJ. Neurobehavioral functioning of healthy preterm infants of varying gestational ages. *J Dev Behav Pediatr* 2000; **21**(6): 408–16.

120. Malatesta CZ, Grigoryev P, Lamb C, Albin M, Culver C. Emotion socialization and expressive development in preterm and full-term infants. *Child Dev* 1986; **57**(2): 316–30.

121. Cohen SE, Beckwith L. Preterm infant interaction with the caregiver in the 1st year of life and competence at age 2. *Child Dev* 1979; **50**(3): 767–76.

122. Feldman R. Parent-infant synchrony and the construction of shared timing; physiological precursors, developmental outcomes, and risk conditions. *J Child Psychol Psychiatry* 2007; **48**(3–4): 329–54.

123. Levy-Shiff R, Sharir H, Mogilner MB. Mother-preterm and Father-preterm infant relationship in the hospital preterm nursery. *Child Dev* 1989; **60**(1): 93–102.

124. Schmucker G, Brisch KH, Kohntop B, *et al*. The influence of prematurity, maternal anxiety, and infants' neurobiological risk on mother-infant interactions. *Infant Ment Health J* 2005; **26**(5): 423–41.

125. Landry SH, Smith KE, Miller-Loncar CL, Swank PR. The relation of change in maternal interactive styles to the developing social competence of full-term and preterm children. *Child Dev* 1998; **69**(1): 105–23.

126. Tu MT, Grunau RE, Petrie-Thomas J, *et al*. Maternal stress and behavior modulate relationships between neonatal stress, attention, and basal cortisol at 8 months in preterm infants. *Dev Psychobiol* 2007; **49**(2): 150–64.

127. Belsky J, Fearon RM. Infant-mother attachment security, contextual risk, and early development: a moderational analysis. *Dev Psychopathol* 2002; **14**(2): 293–310.

128. Finzi-Dottan R, Manor I, Tyano S. ADHD, temperament, and parental style as predictors of the child's attachment patterns. *Child Psychiatry Hum Dev* 2006; **37**(2): 103–14.

129. Graham P, Turk J, Verhulst F. *Child Psychiatry. A Developmental Approach*, 3rd edn. Oxford: Oxford University Press; 1999.

130. Halasz G, Vance ALA. Attention deficit hyperactivity disorder in children: moving forward with divergent perspectives. *Med J Aust* 2002; **177**(10): 554–7.

131. Pinto C, Turton P, Hughes P, White S, Gillberg C. ADHD and infant disorganised attachment: a prospective study of children next-born after stillbirth. *J Atten Disord* 2006; **10**(1): 83–91.

132. Barnett D, Butler CM, Vondra JJ. Atypical patterns of early attachment: discussion and future directions. In: Vondra JJ, Barnett D, eds., *Atypical Attachment in Infancy and Early Childhood Among Children at Developmental Risk*. Monographs of the Society for Research in Child Development, 64(3). Malden, MA: Blackwell Publishing on behalf of the Society for Research in Child Development. 1999; 172–92.

Preterm birth and fetal growth in relation to adult psychopathology

Christina M. Hultman and Chiara Nosarti

Intrauterine and neonatal factors seem to be important in the pathogenesis of childhood and adolescent psychiatric disorders like infantile autism, attention deficit hyperactivity disorder (ADHD), and anorexia nervosa, but also in psychiatric disorders which are not usually seen until late adolescence or adulthood, such as schizophrenia. Being born preterm, with a low birth weight or with indications of fetal growth retardation are among the most robust and replicated perinatal risk factors associated with psychiatric outcome. Additionally, preterm delivery is more common in mothers with schizophrenia, mothers with bipolar disorder, and among women with postpartum psychoses. No consensus has yet been reached concerning the interpretation of the association between preterm birth and psychopathology. In this chapter we report some of the findings and methodological challenges in the field.

Introduction

In studies of preterm birth as a risk factor for development of psychiatric disorders in adulthood, at least four research traditions and paradigms can be identified.

Firstly, during the last 30 years, the evolution of neonatal intensive care has encouraged extensive follow-up studies of very low birth weight (VLBW; < 1500 g) and very preterm infants, investigating developmental, behavioral, and neurological outcome in early childhood (reviewed in Chapters 3, 9, and 11). This has partly occurred due to an increase in survival of very preterm and VLBW babies, the introduction of new medical technology, and improvements in clinical neonatal intensive care (see also Chapters 1 and 2). Consequently, longer periods of follow-up have been facilitated, as has the investigation of diverse cognitive and behavioral deficits in late childhood and early adolescence. Although opinions appear to be divided

concerning the long-term neurodevelopmental outcome of very preterm and VLBW populations, there seems to be a consensus that some of the neurodevelopmental characteristics and traits observed in these groups may be on the causal pathway to the development of psychiatric problems later in life.

Secondly, during the last two decades, an influential research area has emerged, focusing on fetal programing, mostly investigating the association between low birth weight and cardiovascular diseases and diabetes later in life. The "programing hypothesis" suggests that the fetus adapts to undernutrition by permanently changing the development of its organs and metabolism and thereby increasing disease susceptibility later in life [1]. Within this paradigm, the developmental model of the origins of adult diseases has been strongly acknowledged. Recently, efforts have been made to study adult psychiatric outcome in relation to a similar programing hypothesis [2].

Thirdly, in parallel during the last two decades, neurodevelopmental models of schizophrenia have proposed that a brain that is in some way abnormally "set up" as a result of an early insult may start to exhibit functional impairments later in life [3]. This is increasingly viewed as an etiological hypothesis that directs research towards early life. For a number of psychiatric disorders, early hazards in utero and deviant fetal growth have been shown to have a relatively consistent but modest risk-increasing effect [4,5]. Large and psychiatrically well-defined samples drawn from population-based registers have been important in providing support to the hypothesis that maternal, pregnancy, and child characteristics at birth may be associated with the development of psychiatric disorders.

Fourthly, studies of the brain in adolescence and early adulthood following adverse pregnancy outcomes might conceptually link subtle brain changes

Neurodevelopmental Outcomes of Preterm Birth, ed. Chiara Nosarti, Robin M. Murray, and Maureen Hack. Published by Cambridge University Press. © Cambridge University Press 2010.

following preterm birth to psychiatric disorders. Structural and functional imaging studies are important for the understanding of the mechanisms underlying the development of behavioral and psychiatric problems in high-risk individuals, and are reviewed in Chapters 4–8.

These four fertile research areas overlap and converge to still relatively non-specific conclusions about the role of preterm birth in the etiology of psychiatric disorders. The main approach to the investigation of the possible association between pre- and perinatal complications (often collectively termed obstetric complications or OCs) and later psychiatric disorders has been adopted by studies which selected patients with a specific psychiatric diagnosis and then investigated whether patients with this diagnosis were more likely to have experienced obstetric complications than healthy controls. Another type of design consists of cohort studies of individuals who were born very preterm/VLBW who are followed up into adulthood with a psychiatric or more general psychological assessment. In this chapter, we will summarize studies investigating a broad psychological profile as well as selective psychiatric diagnoses in association with very preterm/VLBW birth.

Psychological distress and non-psychotic psychiatric disorders

In childhood, preterm and low birth weight individuals are at increased risk of impaired attention and behavioral abnormalities. Behavioral deficits persist into adolescence and may be secondary to pre- and perinatal brain injury [6–8], as reviewed in Chapter 9. Fewer studies have investigated psychological and psychiatric outcome of preterm and low birth weight individuals in adulthood.

Walshe and colleagues [9] assessed 169 preterm-born 18-year-old individuals and 101 age-matched controls using the Clinical Interview Schedule–Revised (CIS-R), which allows for diagnosis of non-psychotic psychiatric disorders according to the classification criteria set by the International Classification of Diseases (ICD). Results of this study suggested that young adults born very preterm had a threefold likelihood of having a psychiatric diagnosis compared with individuals born at term, with the most commonly occurring diagnoses being mood and anxiety disorders. This study further investigated the role of family history, and found that psychiatric diagnoses were

more common in preterm-born individuals who also had a family psychiatric history. Another UK study by Wiles and colleagues examined with the General Health Questionnaire a large birth cohort from the Aberdeen Children of the 1950s study at age 45–51 years . Individuals born full term but with low birth weight (<2500 g) had an increased likelihood of experiencing psychological distress in later life, after adjustment for potential confounders, including parity, maternal age, gender and IQ (odds ratio [OR] = 1.49, 95% confidence interval [CI] = 1.01–2.20). One standard deviation (SD) decrease in birth weight for gestational age was associated with a 4% increased odds of psychological problems in adulthood (OR = 1.04, 95% CI = 0.97–1.12), indicating a direct association between neonatal complications and adult mental health [10]. A study by Hack and colleagues [11] of 241 20-year-old individuals who were born with VLBW found that VLBW women, but not men, reported significantly more withdrawn behaviors than controls (n = 233) and they were also twice as likely than controls to experience internalizing problems, including anxiety and depression. Interestingly, parents of VLBW women reported a fourfold increase in rates of anxiety and depression in their daughters, as well as an increase in rates of thought and attention problems.

Birth cohort studies have suggested an association between low birth weight/preterm birth and depressive disorder [12–15]. The 26-year-old follow-up of the 1970 British Birth Cohort again used the General Health Questionnaire to study approximately 8000 individuals and showed that women who were born with a low birth weight (< 3000 g) had an increased risk of depression (OR = 1.3, 95% CI = 0.9–1.8), whereas low birth weight men were more likely than controls to have a history of depression (OR = 1.6, 95% CI = 1.1–2.3) [13]. Another UK study examined the association between birth weight and depression in elderly individuals in Hertfordshire [15], and found the opposite gender effect, men and not women with a low birth weight were at increased risk of depression. Data from the longitudinal study of an UK 1958 birth cohort followed up approximately 1000 individuals to age 42 years and studied the effects birth weight for gestational age and weight gain in early childhood may have had on psychological distress in adulthood [12]. Malaise inventory scores were measured at ages 23, 33, and 42 years. Results suggested that psychological distress scores were inversely associated with birth weight and weight gain from birth to the age of 7 years.

A recent study however found that intrauterine growth retardation rather than VLBW may pose a risk for depression from age 18 to 27 years [16]. The results of this investigation were compelling in that they showed that VLBW individuals who were appropriate for gestational age were less likely to report a depression diagnosis than controls (OR = 4.8, 95% CI = 1.3–10.0), whereas only VLBW individuals who were born small for gestational age (SGA) were more likely to report a depression diagnosis than controls (OR = 2.5, 95% CI = 1.0–6.3); in addition the SGA group reported 36.2% higher scores on the depression scale used in the assessment (Beck Depression Inventory). Similar results were reported by Dalziel and colleagues [17], who studied 31-year-old individuals who were born at less than 1900 g: those who were appropriate for gestational age were less likely to report depressive symptoms and experience psychiatric problems than controls. These data suggest that mental health outcome of VLBW individuals may thus be modulated by intrauterine growth patterns, which we will discuss later in this chapter.

However, compared to data regarding cognitive and academic outcome of low birth weight and very preterm young adults, data on mental health outcome is not always consistent. Some groups have in fact reported no differences in self-reported anxiety, depression, or overall well-being between VLBW individuals aged 19–22 years and controls [18], as well as in self-reported mental health [19].

Violent and non-violent suicide attempts

The possible relationship between fetal growth, obstetric complications, and the risk in early adulthood of suicide and attempted suicide in the offspring have only sparsely been studied. Three large population-based studies have essentially confirmed obstetric, neonatal, and maternal risk factors for suicide and attempted suicide in young adults. The focus has been on low birth weight. Mittendorfer-Rutz and colleagues studied 713 370 young adults born in Sweden between 1973 and 1980, identified by data linkage between Swedish registers, and found significantly raised risk of attempted suicide for individuals of short birth length, adjusted for gestational age (hazard ratio [HR] = 1.29, 95% CI = 1.18–1.41); born fourth or higher in birth order (HR = 1.79, 95% CI = 1.62–1.97); born to mothers with a low educational level (HR = 1.36, 95% CI = 1.27–1.46)

(attributable proportion 10.3%); and those who, at time of delivery, had mothers aged 19 years or younger (HR = 2.09, 95% CI = 1.89–2.32). In addition, low birth weight, adjusted for gestational age (HR = 2.23, 95% CI = 1.43–3.46), and having a teenage mother (HR = 2.30, 95% CI = 1.64–3.22) were significantly predictive of both suicide completion and suicide attempt [20].

Similar results were found in a Scottish study using linked data from the Scottish Morbidity Record and Scottish death records on 1 061 830 people followed up for a mean of 25.1 years. Low birth weight (< 2500 g) was independently associated with higher suicide risk in young adults, whereas no statistically significant independent association with gestational age was found [21].

In a Swedish cohort study of 318 953 men, the effect of fetal and childhood growth on suicide attempt both violent and non-violent, between the ages of 18 and 25, was studied [22]. Risk of suicide attempt was increased for men with reduced linear growth across all levels of adult stature. Birth weight in the range of 2500–3000 g was associated with an increase in risk of suicide (HR = 1.36, 95% CI = 1.1–1.7) in relation to the reference category of birth weight of 3500–4000 g. Children with a birth weight below 2500 g had a similar, but non-significant risk increase (HR = 1.25, 95% CI = 0.8–1.9). Preterm birth was not a significant predictor of suicide attempts (week 28–34, HR = 1.32, 95% CI = 0.8–2.35). The authors hypothesized further that violent and non-violent suicide attempts would differentially affect patterns of fetal growth. There were some indications that violent suicide attempts might be related to preterm birth even after adjustment for maternal characteristics. Impulsivity and aggression are well-known features of violent suicidal behavior and are associated with low serotonin levels, which have been reported in preterm-born children [23]. Thus, the data so far seem to indicate that a low birth weight rather than an independent effect of gestational age may be related to risk of suicide in early adulthood.

Anorexia nervosa and bulimia nervosa

Anorexia nervosa, characterized by low body weight, distorted body image, amenorrhea, and an intense fear of gaining weight is etiologically poorly understood [24]. The occurrence of anorexia nervosa has increased over the past ten years among adolescents and young women and it is estimated to occur in 0.5–1% of the population. Preterm birth and low birth weight have been repeatedly associated with increased risks of behavioral problems in childhood, including eating difficulties [25].

In a population-based, case-control study of all live-born girls in Sweden from 1973 to 1984, 781 girls were identified who had been discharged from hospital with a main diagnosis of anorexia at the age of 10–21 years [26]. The mean age of admission was 14.8 years. A three-fold increase in risk was observed among girls born very preterm (before the thirty-third week of gestation). Small for gestational age was reported as being more common among very preterm births than among children with a longer period of gestation. In very preterm births, girls who were SGA faced higher risks (OR = 5.7, 95% CI = 1.1–28.7) than girls with higher birth weight for gestational age (OR = 2.7, 95% CI = 1.2–5.8).

Preterm birth may play a role also in bulimia nervosa defined by food binges, or recurrent episodes of significant overeating. A blind analysis of the obstetric records of a sample of subjects with anorexia nervosa, with bulimia nervosa, and normal subjects was performed in a population birth cohort in Padua, Italy, between 1971 and 1979 [27]. The obstetric complications significantly associated with bulimia nervosa were the following: a low birth weight for gestational age (p = 0.009), placental infarction (p = 0.10), neonatal hyporeactivity (p = 0.005), and early eating difficulties (p = 0.02). The investigators found that being shorter for gestational age significantly differentiated subjects with bulimia nervosa from both those with anorexia nervosa (p = 0.04) and control subjects (p = 0.05).

The possible association between preterm birth and maladaptive eating patterns across infancy, childhood, adolescence, and adulthood merits further investigation using longitudinal designs. The possible underlying biological mechanisms are unknown. The period between birth and term is one of relative malnutrition for the very preterm infant mainly due to acute and chronic illness and poor feed tolerance [27]. Diet of nutrient-enriched formula in the early weeks postpartum has been found to be strongly associated with later growth and development of the very preterm infant [28]. This might put the preterm infant/child at risk for feeding problems that in turn might increase the risk for eating disorders. It has also been proposed that delayed oral-motor development related to subtle brain damage [29], parental reactions to the birth of a very preterm infant with specific feeding problems [30], and early hypothalamic dysfunction [31] might be involved in the etiology of eating disorders. An alternative hypothesis postulates that this risk is mediated by some form of nutritional imprinting. Early environmental effects, i.e., in utero or early postnatal nutrition, may set the level of activity of the appetite system, a type of metabolic imprinting or programing [32].

Of interest are finally studies investigating the effects of maternal eating disorder on perinatal/obstetric complications, which have reported high rates of SGA, preterm [33], and low birth weight babies [34] born to women with an eating disorder diagnosis. The hypothesis of a possible cycle of risk, i.e., a pathway through which a maternal eating disorder increases the risk of eating disorder in the offspring via an increase in obstetric complications or poor nutrition in utero, has also been suggested [24].

Schizophrenia

There is increasing evidence that pregnancy and birth complications may be important risk factors for schizophrenia in the offspring. Early hazards in utero and deviant fetal growth have a relatively consistent but modest risk-increasing effect. Based on meta-analyses, the pooled odds ratio of the effect of exposure to pre- and perinatal factors on the subsequent development of schizophrenia has been estimated to be about 2.0 [4]. Studies from the Nordic countries have used methodologically sound designs and have been important for the development of this research field [35–38]. Specific pathological mechanisms that can serve as an etiological link between complications during the pre- and perinatal period and schizophrenia are yet to be established. The prevailing hypothesis associates prenatal adverse conditions to structural brain damage ("neurodevelopmental approach"), mediated by anoxic damage to the fetal brain, viral infection during pregnancy, insults to cerebral structures critically involved in the control of autonomic responses, or an unspecific fetal stress ("second hit") for children with a genetic predisposition ("first hit").

The study of preterm birth as an independent risk factor for schizophrenia is a fertile research area even if the focus most often has been on low birth weight, fetal growth restriction at birth, and retarded growth postnatally. A vast variation in concepts and sample characteristics, definitions of growth aberrations, and the possibility to control for maternal lifestyle factors still befogs the field and can at best be described as a group of similar risk factors related to being born early or small [4]. It is important to state that most variables thought to mirror a non-optimal fetal growth are coarse "proxies" (i.e., indicators of risks, not casually related to the disorder) of a range of possible pathways. Even quantitative measures like birth weight and head circumference are "proxy" variables that encompass many known and unknown risk factors, possibly interacting with one another to produce a given effect. Low birth weight may be caused by preterm delivery or by intrauterine growth retardation (IUGR). There is an overlap between categories and the proportion of children in the normal population with birth weight below 2500 g not being born preterm or with IUGR is estimated to be only 1%. Over half of the infants with IUGR and about 40% of preterm babies do not have low birth weight [39].

Most studies show a modest to large effect of *low birth weight* for the development of schizophrenia [4,40–43]. The epidemiological study by Jones *et al.* reviewed the psychiatric status of all children born in North Finland in 1966 and showed that low birth weight babies (defined as < 2000 g) were 6.2 times more likely to develop schizophrenia after adjusting for possible confounders such as gender, parental socioeconomic status at birth, maternal depression, and maternal smoking [41]. In an early review Kunugi *et al.* [44] reported a pooled odds ratio of 2.6 (95% CI = 2.0–3.3, p < 0.00001) for schizophrenia associated with a birth weight of less than 2500 g and in the historical and meta-analytic review published by Cannon *et al.* [4], low birth weight was associated with schizophrenia (< 2000 g: fixed pooled estimate 3.9, 95% CI = 1.4–10.8; < 2500 g: fixed pooled estimate 1.7, 95% CI = 1.2–2.3). In a recent large Danish register-based cohort study of 1039 individuals with a diagnosis of schizophrenia, a significant effect of low birth weight was found (< 2500 g: OR = 1.25, 95% CI = 1.04–1.50; < 1999 g: OR = 1.70, 95% CI = 1.09–2.63), which became non-significant in the adjusted model [45].

Preterm birth also seems to be more common among individuals who later develop schizophrenia [4,40–43,45,46]. In the most comprehensive study so far, Byrne *et al.* reported an increased risk of schizophrenia in children with a gestational age of 37 weeks or below (incidence rate ratio [IRR] = 1.51, 95% CI = 1.0–2.2) after adjustment for parental wealth, maternal education, family psychiatric history, parental age, maternal citizenship, and urbanicity of place of birth [45]. Threatened preterm delivery had a slightly higher relative risk (IRR = 2.39, 95% CI = 1.4–4.1). However, in another recent Danish study, no increased risk of schizophrenia was found among preterm children (< 37 week) if they were in the lower 10% of birth

weight. For schizophrenia cases with a family history of psychiatric admission, a significant increased risk was found for prematurity as well as in cases with bipolar disorder, schizoaffective disorder, and unipolar disorder [47].

We have recently studied preterm birth as an independent risk factor for psychiatric disorders in adulthood in a historical population-based cohort design and selected individuals born between 1973 and 2001 (n = 2 686 364), 34 853 of whom were born "very preterm" (before 32 weeks) and 155 634 "moderately preterm" (between 32 and 36 weeks) [48]. Very preterm individuals were more likely to be hospitalized with a diagnosis of psychosis (OR = 3.0) than individuals born between 37 and 41 weeks of gestation. Results further indicated that being born "moderately preterm" increased the risk for psychosis (OR = 1.7), after adjusting for the following risk factors: birth weight for gestational age, Apgar score at 5 minutes, mother's age at delivery, mother's educational level, gender, parity, and maternal family history of at least one psychiatric diagnosis (any). However, our results also suggested that those individuals exposed to obstetric hazards grow up to have an increased risk of psychiatric illness in general, which includes but is not confined to psychosis .

The support for the involvement of *fetal growth restriction* in the etiology of schizophrenia, as indicated by being SGA or a low ponderal index, is mixed [35–37,46,47] and more difficult to interpret. Some studies reporting significant associations might be questioned, as they failed to control for important confounders, such as maternal smoking during pregnancy. In our own series of studies of pre- and perinatal risk factors for psychiatric disorder, we found indications of both retarded and accelerated intrauterine growth in clinical samples of patients with schizophrenia, which were interpreted as being possibly caused by utero-placental insufficiency or intrauterine infections [36]. In a larger population-based registry study this was only confirmed in males [37]. In other studies with a similar design, fetal growth restriction was partly also shown to be a risk factor for infantile autism [49] and anorexia nervosa [26]. Our next step was to use twin designs and to analyze fetal growth within same-sex twin pairs discordant for schizophrenia, which allows matching for gestational age, as well as genetic and environmental factors shared by the twins. Individuals with a birth weight of less than 2300 g faced an almost doubled risk of developing schizophrenia compared to individuals with higher birth weight. Compared with children born at term (≥ 37 gestational weeks), children born preterm (≤ 36 weeks) had a 70% increased risk of developing schizophrenia. There were no statistically significant differences between twins with and without schizophrenia with regard to maternal age, maternal complications during pregnancy, birth year, sex of the child, birth order, or birth place [50]. However, even if this study gave support for both preterm birth and fetal growth restriction as independent risk factors for schizophrenia, the sample was small (only 90 twin pairs discordant for schizophrenia) and we were not able to analyze monozygotic and dizygotic twin pairs separately, in order to investigate genetic or shared environmental factors in relation to the familial mediation of the association between fetal growth restriction and schizophrenia.

An interaction between IUGR and asphyxia has been frequently reported in studies of risk factors for schizophrenia, other neurodevelopmental disorders, and chronic neurological handicaps. The contribution of fetal hypoxia to the development of schizophrenia has been reported to be two to three times greater among children born SGA [4], and hypoxic-ischemic damage and aberrations in fetal growth were the most consistent risk-increasing effects recently confirmed in our Swedish twin study [50]. However, Smith *et al.* showed an independent effect of preterm birth and poor fetal growth [46]. Prematurity, but not poor fetal growth, was associated with earlier age at onset and poorer premorbid functioning in schizophrenia.

In conclusion, preterm birth undoubtedly plays a role in the etiology of schizophrenia, but the strength, the nature, and the overlap between preterm birth, low birth weight, and fetal growth retardation needs further exploration. As described in Chapter 1, the main risk factors for preterm birth include infections, maternal characteristics, socioeconomic status, multiple pregnancies, smoking during pregnancy, ethnicity, family history, and air pollution. Several of these factors are also associated with an increased risk of schizophrenia. Preterm birth may be on the causal pathway between prenatal exposure to bacterial or viral infection, maternal characteristics such as stress during pregnancy, socioeconomic status, substance abuse, urbanization and schizophrenia.

Bipolar disorder

For bipolar disorder, generally no statistically significant association with obstetric complications and characteristics of the pre- and perinatal period has

been found [37,51,52]. In a systematic review of 22 studies, the pooled odds ratio for exposure to obstetric complications and subsequent development of bipolar disorder was 1.01 (95% CI = 0.76–1.35) [52], with a significant effect of low birth weight in a single study [53], but no significance in the pooled odds ratio for low birth weight or SGA. A more recent population-based Danish study [54], which had the advantage of focusing on a more narrow diagnosis of bipolar disorder, found only a trend between the development of bipolar disorder between the ages of 12 and 26 and gestational age < 37 weeks (OR = 1.58, 95% CI = 0.67–3.75) and birth weight < 2500 g and gestational age < 37 weeks (OR = 2.10, 95% CI = 0.86–5.15). For females only, preterm birth was significantly related to bipolar disorder (OR = 2.91, 95% CI = 1.10–7.73). In the cohort of Hack [55] of adult outcomes of very low birth weight children, there was no evidence of major psychiatric disorder. Bipolar disorder was reported more often in individuals born with low birth weight, 2% versus 1% of the normal birth weight controls. The difference was not significantly different, but the number of subjects was relatively small and they had only reached young adulthood at time of testing. In summary, the support for preterm birth as a risk factor for bipolar disorder is not strong, although an association between the two cannot yet be conclusively excluded.

Postpartum psychoses

Psychotic illness starting shortly after childbirth is a relatively rare condition. However, the negative implications of such an illness can be enormous: repeated episodes of psychoses and hospitalization of the mother, increased risk of self-harm or suicide, as well as the rare but tragic occurrences of harm to the newborn infant and infanticide. Are there any indications that giving birth to a child born preterm is associated with a higher risk of postpartum psychosis?

Women developing postpartum psychosis have in some studies shown a higher incidence of preterm delivery compared to controls [56]. In a recent study, we investigated potential maternal and obstetric risk factors for maternal psychoses following childbirth in a national cohort of first-time mothers from 1983 through 2000 (n = 745 596) [57]. Within 90 days after delivery, 892 women (1.2 per 1000 births) were hospitalized due to psychoses. Obstetric and perinatal exposures were: perinatal death (stillbirth or infant death within 7 days), congenital malformations, gestational age (in completed weeks), and birth weight. An increased risk of postpartum psychoses was found when giving birth during gestational week 22–31 (HR = 1.7, 95% CI = 1.0–3.0), but not in gestational week 32–36 in an adjusted model controlling for maternal age, education, cohabitation, diabetes, smoking, and calendar period of birth. Giving birth to a VLBW child was associated with a close to significant risk of postpartum psychoses (HR = 1.7, 95% CI = 0.9–3.1). In contrast, high birth weight (> 4500 g) and being large for gestational age (LGA) decreased the risk by 70–80% and seemed to be protective, especially for first-onset psychosis, distinctly during the postpartum period. Perinatal death and congenital malformations also increased the risk of developing psychosis. After the first 90 days post partum, perinatal death was the only obstetric factor increasing the risk of psychosis. Thus, we concluded that preterm birth seems to be a post partum-specific risk factor for psychosis.

In another Swedish study recently published, a gestational length of < 37 weeks and acute Cesarian section were reported as being the only obstetric complications that were associated with post partum psychosis [58]. An earlier Scandinavian study however found that preterm delivery predicted the best prognosis after postpartum psychosis [59]. Based on the Danish Medical Birth Register and the Danish Psychiatry Central Register, the authors showed that among prognostic and risk factors for readmission after postpartum psychosis, preterm delivery was the only factor associated with a reduced risk of readmission.

Concerning a potential explanatory mechanism, as suggested by previous research [60,61] stressful characteristics of the birth, e.g., perinatal death, might be a triggering factor for post partum psychosis. In light of the evidence reviewed in this section, preterm birth could also be a triggering factor.

Alcohol and drug consumption

The effect of preterm birth on alcohol and drug dependence in adulthood is seemingly contradictory. A recent Swedish registry study of 304 275 men and women born between 1973 and 1975 gives some support for a positive association between obstetric complications and addiction behaviors [62]. Preterm birth and being SGA were both related to increased risk of hospitalizations for mental disorders. Children being born SGA were more prone to be hospitalized for non-dependent abuse of drugs (ICD-9 code 305; OR = 1.30, 95% CI = 1.07–1.58), and those born preterm and SGA were more likely to be hospitalized for drug dependence (ICD-9 code 304; OR = 2.94, 95% CI = 1.30–6.67), after accounting for childhood socioeconomic characteristics. Only 0.4% of the children were born both preterm and SGA, but had an increased overall risk of 42% of being hospitalized for any diagnosis. The authors did not distinguish between childhood and adult hospitalizations, but the admittance for drug dependence diagnoses is likely to have occurred in late adolescence or early adulthood.

Children born preterm have also been reported to use less drug and alcohol compared to controls within a frame of less risk-taking behavior of VLBW children [18,55,63]. A small study of adult characteristics at 31 years of age of 126 individuals born preterm [17], found a lower percent of illicit drug use (p = 0.05) and a tendency for preterm-born individuals not to be heavy drinkers compared with individuals born at term. Thus, the evidence is non-conclusive and future studies exploring the severity of alcohol and drug problems and their continuity over adolescence and adulthood are needed.

One possible explanation of these apparently contradictory results could be the type of drug and alcohol consumption behaviors being measured in different study designs. Whereas Swedish registry studies investigate addiction behaviors leading to hospitalization in large population-based groups, follow-up studies tend to include a much smaller number of subjects and measure recreational behaviors instead. Furthermore, some bias can exist in terms of subjects' admitting to addictive behavior that is not going to be cross-examined.

Mothers with schizophrenia and bipolar disorder

Women with schizophrenia face increased risks of adverse pregnancy outcomes [64–66]: they often smoke, misuse other substances, and are socioeconomically disadvantaged [67]. These variables are well-known risk factors for adverse pregnancy outcomes, and smoking is causally related to fetal growth retardation and possibly also to stillbirth and preterm birth [68]. In several recent population-based studies the increased risks for preterm birth, low birth weight, and infant death in women with schizophrenia persist even after these covariates are controlled for [69]. As an example, we have previously shown that the increased risk for preterm birth among women with schizophrenia decreased from 70% to 40% when maternal factors were controlled for [69]. Women with an episode of schizophrenia during pregnancy had the highest risks (preterm delivery, < 37 gestational weeks, OR = 3.4, 95% CI = 2.1–5.4; low birth weight, < 2500 g, OR = 4.3, 95% CI = 2.9–6.6). Controlling for a high incidence of smoking during pregnancy among women with schizophrenia (51% vs. 24% in the normal population) and other maternal factors (single motherhood, maternal age, parity, maternal education, mothers' country of birth, and pregnancy-induced hypertensive diseases) in a multiple regression model markedly reduced the risk estimates [69]. However, the risks for adverse pregnancy outcomes were generally doubled for women with an episode of schizophrenia during pregnancy compared to women in the control group, even after adjusting for possible confounders.

What might be the causes for the higher risks of preterm birth in women experiencing a psychotic episode during pregnancy? If these women consume antipsychotics or antipsychotics in higher doses during pregnancy, this may partly account for the increased risks. It has been a concern that neuroleptic medication may compromise uterine blood flow, and produce postpartum neonatal sedation and extrapyramidal signs [70]. In a follow-up study of outcome of 215 pregnancies exposed to haloperidol or penfluridol in the first trimester, a higher rate of preterm birth was found compared to unexposed control pregnancies (13.9% vs. 6.9%, p = 0.006) [71]. The rate of congenital anomalies was not increased, but there were indications of fetal growth restriction with a lower median birth weight in full-term infants (3250 g vs. 3415 g, p = 0.004) . A second explanation could be that women with schizophrenia attend antenatal care clinics less frequently [64,72] and have underdiagnosed medical illness [73]. Thirdly, a common familial vulnerability for non-optimal pregnancy outcome might be considered. Schizophrenia is under a high degree of genetic influence and the offspring carries a 10% risk of the disorder [74]. The offspring's risk for adverse pregnancy outcomes if the father has schizophrenia is less known. A recent study by Webb *et al.* [75] found an increased risk for postnatal death among offspring of fathers with schizophrenia. However, the risk was not statistically significant and a meta-analysis by Webb *et al.* [66] indicated a need for evidence concerning the effects of exposure to paternal disorder. Recent data in a cohort of 1 890 550 births in Sweden indicate that not only the offspring of mothers with schizophrenia, but also of fathers with schizophrenia, have an increased

risk of non-optimal birth outcome. However, the association between schizophrenia and preterm delivery is primarily maternal and largely explained by measured environmental factors [76].

To test the hypothesis that infants of women with affective psychosis face increased risks of adverse pregnancy outcomes, we performed a similar study with data from the Swedish Medical Birth Register and the Hospital Discharge Register on 5593 births to mother with affective psychoses and 46 068 control mothers [77]. Births in mothers with affective psychosis had an increased risk of being preterm birth (unadjusted OR = 1.40, 95% CI = 1.23–1.59). The risks were greatest in mothers receiving hospital treatment for affective disorder during pregnancy (OR = 2.67, 95% CI = 1.71–4.17). Affected mothers were approximately twice as likely to have been heavy smokers as controls in our sample. There is a well-established association between smoking and fetal growth restriction [78,79], which is probably accounted for by a reduction in placental blood flow due to vasoconstriction, and reduced oxygen availability due to the formation of carboxyhemoglobin. It is therefore not surprising that controlling for smoking attenuated the association of affective psychosis with all outcomes. However, significant associations for preterm delivery and low birth weight persisted, suggesting that smoking is unlikely to be the sole cause of these outcomes.

The study of preterm birth in parents with psychosis has clinical implications. Even if the fertility rate is lower in psychosis [80], psychiatrists frequently treat women with psychosis who become pregnant. It is therefore important to raise awareness among clinicians of the increased risk of adverse pregnancy outcomes in these women. It is not clear whether the increased risks of adverse pregnancy outcomes result from the effects of the disorder or its treatment, or both. A focus on the mechanisms underlying these associations, including the effects of psychotropic medicines on the developing fetus, is therefore needed.

Possible etiological mechanisms and conclusions

Several studies reviewed in this chapter suggest that VLBW and very preterm birth may be associated with a range of psychiatric outcomes. The effect is generally small and the large number of social and lifestyle-related factors that influence the risk of preterm birth and low birth weight need to be taken into account when considering the possible causal relationship between adverse neonatal events and psychopathology [81]. Further, the association between preterm birth and adverse outcome in adulthood could be explained by maternal or neonatal morbidity commonly associated with preterm birth like prenatal exposure to infection during pregnancy, low Apgar score, and intracranial bleeding. Even if recent studies have valid, non-biased, prospectively collected information from birth records or registers, gestational age encompasses many known and unknown risk factors, possibly interacting with each other to have developmental consequences.

To date, the mechanisms underlying these possible relationships remain unclear, although several studies have indicated that psychiatric morbidity may be partly a consequence of impaired neurodevelopment. Possible etiological mechanisms include the existence of a "critical" period during which alteration in the course of normal development may result in a later susceptibility to psychopathology [82,83]. There are in fact indications that psychiatric disorders and diseases of the nervous system may be relatively more common for admission diagnosis in adolescence and early adulthood for individuals born preterm and those born SGA [84].

Future studies need to have longer follow-up, be population-based, control for confounders, and if possible discuss and create mutually exclusive categories for individuals born preterm, SGA not preterm, and preterm with growth retardation. The link between early environment with adult-life susceptibility to psychiatric disorders might include both mechanisms leading to shorter gestational age as well as those related to slower fetal growth. Long-term follow-up studies suffer from biases introduced by initial cohort selection and attrition. Hospital-based cohorts have often been selected by birth weight rather than gestational age with a likely increased proportion of growth retarded children.

Some investigators have attempted to explain the association between birth weight and depression and psychological distress by hypothesizing that the same adverse environmental mechanisms in utero may be influencing both birth weight and the set point of the hypothalamic–pituitary–adrenal (HPA) axis. Animal studies have described that exposure to stressful events during pregnancy results in rats showing behavior consistent with depression, including sleep abnormalities, a hedonic deficit, greater acquisition of learned helplessness under specific conditions, and increased corticotropin-releasing hormone activity [85]. According to this hypothesis, adverse neonatal events increase individuals' susceptibility to psychological distress and depression. Data from a Swedish psychological conscript assessment in young males in fact suggested an association between increasing birth weight up to 4200 g and stress susceptibility [86].

Moreover, there is evidence from animal data that obstetric complications involving hypoxia may result in alterations in cortical and subcortical gray matter volumes, including the hippocampus [87], which has also been reported to be smaller in individuals with schizophrenia and their first-degree relatives [88], as well as adolescents who were born very preterm [89]. Animal models further indicate that neonatal lesions to the ventral hippocampus/temporal cortex may be associated with behavioral indices consistent with increased mesolimbic dopamine (DA) response to stressful stimuli [90]. This suggests that exposure to obstetric insults results in "sensitized" dopaminergic transmission, which increases the susceptibility to environmental stressors. Early birth insults may therefore be associated with long-lasting alterations in dopaminergic function, such that the set point of this system and its regulation can be permanently modified [91].

Amphetamine sensitization in human subjects has been extensively documented and has been associated with the development of hyperdopaminergic states (for a review see [92]). Some studies have in fact suggested that stress can trigger psychosis in susceptible groups through sensitization-like processes [93]. Dysregulation of brain DA activity is believed to be involved in the pathophysiology of several disorders including schizophrenia, ADHD, substance abuse [94], bipolar disorder [95], as well as in the susceptibility to psychotic illness [96], suggesting differential DA responses may precede psychiatric disorder rather than develop subsequent to onset.

Finally, environmental influences (e.g., gestational age) may interact with genetic factors to contribute to increased susceptibility for psychopathology. Most psychiatric diseases are moderately to highly heritable and genetic factors account for almost half of the liability to have SGA births [97]. A recent study found that brain-derived neurotrophic factor (BDNF) was present in lower levels amongst individuals born with a gestational age < 37 weeks compared to term controls [98]. Brain-derived neurotrophic factor plays a critical role in protecting against the adverse consequences of fetal hypoxia by promoting growth and differentiation of new neurons, hence a dysregulation of neurotrophic signaling may lead to dendritic atrophy and disruption of synaptogensesis in the fetus in response to obstetric complications. A differential BDNF response to birth hypoxia between individuals with schizophrenia and controls suggests that the expression of this critical cell-signaling mechanism may not be associated with increased vulnerability to schizophrenia in the absence of a particular biological risk. In addition, genetic factors may be associated with neurodevelopmental outcome. A recent study investigated the relationship between the val108/158met polymorphism of the catechol-O-methyl transferase (COMT) gene and corpus callosum development in young adults who were born very preterm and found that the met allele was associated with greater growth and more organized microstructure of the corpus callosum [99]. This allele produces a lower-activity form of the enzyme, suggesting that COMT genotype may confer resilience to the effects of perinatal white matter damage in individuals who were born very preterm. It would be therefore important for future studies to disentangle the maternal genetic, fetal genetic, and environmental effects for the study of the relationship between preterm birth and low birth weight and adult psychopathology.

References

1. Barker DJ. The origins of the developmental origins theory. *J Intern Med* 2007; **261**(5): 412–17.

2. St Clair D, Xu M, Wang P, *et al*. Rates of adult schizophrenia following prenatal exposure to the Chinese famine of 1959–1961. *JAMA* 2005; **294**(5): 557–62.

3. Murray RM, Lewis SW. Is schizophrenia a neurodevelopmental disorder? *Br Med J (Clin Res Ed)* 1987; **295**(6600): 681–2.

4. Cannon M, Jones PB, Murray RM. Obstetric complications and schizophrenia: historical and meta-analytic review. *Am J Psychiatry* 2002; **159**(7): 1080–92.

5. Verdoux H. Perinatal risk factors for schizophrenia: how specific are they? *Curr Psychiatry Rep* 2004; **6**(3): 162–7.

6. Abernethy LJ, Palaniappan M, Cooke RW. Quantitative magnetic resonance imaging of the brain in survivors of very low birth weight. *Arch Dis Child* 2002; **87**(4): 279–83.

7. Nosarti C, Allin M, Frangou S, Rifkin L, Murray R. Decreased caudate volume is associated with hyperactivity in adolescents born very preterm. *Biol Psychiatry* 2005; **13**(6): 339.

8. Stewart AL, Rifkin L, Amess PN, *et al*. Brain structure and neurocognitive and behavioural function in adolescents who were born very preterm. *Lancet* 1999; **353**(9165): 1653–7.

9. Walshe M, Rifkin L, Rooney M, *et al*. Psychiatric disorder in young adults born very preterm: role of family history. *Eur Psychiatry* 2008; **23**(7): 527–31.

10. Wiles NJ, Peters TJ, Leon DA, Lewis G. Birth weight and psychological distress at age 45–51 years: results from the Aberdeen Children of the 1950s cohort study. *Br J Psychiatry* 2005; **187**: 21–8.

11. Hack M, Youngstrom EA, Cartar L, *et al*. Behavioral outcomes and evidence of psychopathology among very low birth weight infants at age 20 years. *Pediatrics* 2004; **114**(4): 932–40.

12. Cheung YB, Khoo KS, Karlberg J, Machin D. Association between psychological symptoms in adults and growth in early life: longitudinal follow up study. *BMJ* 2002; **325**(7367): 749.

13. Gale CR, Martyn CN. Birth weight and later risk of depression in a national birth cohort. *Br J Psychiatry* 2004; **184**: 28–33.

14. Patton GC, Coffey C, Carlin JB, Olsson CA, Morley R. Prematurity at birth and adolescent depressive disorder. *Br J Psychiatry* 2004; **184**: 446–7.

15. Thompson C, Syddall H, Rodin I, Osmond C, Barker DJ. Birth weight and the risk of depressive disorder in late life. *Br J Psychiatry* 2001; **179**: 450–5.

16. Raikkonen K, Pesonen AK, Heinonen K, *et al*. Depression in young adults with very low birth weight: the Helsinki study of very-low-birth-weight adults. *Arch Gen Psychiatry* 2008; **65**(3): 290–6.

17. Dalziel SR, Lim VK, Lambert A, *et al*. Psychological functioning and health-related quality of life in adulthood after preterm birth. *Dev Med Child Neurol* 2007; **49**(8): 597–602.

18. Cooke RW. Health, lifestyle, and quality of life for young adults born very preterm. *Arch Dis Child* 2004; **89**(3): 201–6.

19. Bjerager M, Steensberg J, Greisen G. Quality of life among young adults born with very low birthweights. *Acta Paediatr* 1995; **84**(12): 1339–43.

20. Mittendorfer-Rutz E, Rasmussen F, Wasserman D. Restricted fetal growth and adverse maternal psychosocial and socioeconomic conditions as risk factors for suicidal behaviour of offspring: a cohort study. *Lancet* 2004; **364**(9440): 1135–40.

21. Riordan DV, Selvaraj S, Stark C, Gilbert JS. Perinatal circumstances and risk of offspring suicide. Birth cohort study. *Br J Psychiatry* 2006; **189**: 502–7.

22. Mittendorfer-Rutz E, Wasserman D, Rasmussen F. Fetal and childhood growth and the risk of violent and non-violent suicide attempts: a cohort study of 318,953 men. *J Epidemiol Community Health* 2008; **62**(2): 168–73.

23. Luciana M. Cognitive development in children born preterm: implications for theories of brain plasticity following early injury. *Dev Psychopathol* 2003; **15**(4): 1017–47.

24. Bulik CM, Hebebrand J, Keski-Rahkonen A, *et al.* Genetic epidemiology, endophenotypes, and eating disorder classification. *Int J Eat Disord* 2007; **40** Suppl: S52–60.

25. Whitaker AH, Van Rossem R, Feldman JF, *et al.* Psychiatric outcomes in low-birth-weight children at age 6 years: relation to neonatal cranial ultrasound abnormalities. *Arch Gen Psychiatry* 1997; **54**(9): 847–56.

26. Cnattingius S, Hultman CM, Dahl M, Sparen P. Very preterm birth, birth trauma, and the risk of anorexia nervosa among girls. *Arch Gen Psychiatry* 1999; **56**(7): 634–8.

27. Favaro A, Tenconi E, Santonastaso P. Perinatal factors and the risk of developing anorexia nervosa and bulimia nervosa. *Arch Gen Psychiatry* 2006; **63**(1): 82–8.

28. Lucas A, Morley R, Cole TJ. Randomised trial of early diet in preterm babies and later intelligence quotient. *BMJ* 1998; **317**(7171): 1481–7.

29. Mathisen B, Skuse D, Wolke D, Reilly S. Oral-motor dysfunction and failure to thrive among inner-city infants. *Dev Med Child Neurol* 1989; **31**(3): 293–302.

30. Rastam M. Anorexia nervosa in 51 Swedish adolescents: premorbid problems and comorbidity. *J Am Acad Child Adolesc Psychiatry* 1992; **31**(5): 819–29.

31. Sedin G, Bergquist C, Lindgren PG. Ovarian hyperstimulation syndrome in preterm infants. *Pediatr Res* 1985; **19**(6): 548–52.

32. Waterland R, Garza C. Potential mechanisms of metabolic imprinting that lead to chronic disease. *Am J Clin Nutr* 1999; **69**(2): 179–97.

33. Brinch M, Isager T, Tolstrup K. Anorexia nervosa and motherhood: reproduction pattern and mothering behavior of 50 women. *Acta Psychiatr Scand* 1988; **77**(5): 611–17.

34. Micali N, Simonoff E, Treasure J. Risk of adverse perinatal outcomes in women with eating disorders. *Br J Psychiatry* 2007; **190**: 255–9.

35. Dalman C, Allebeck P, Cullberg J, Grunewald C, Koster M. Obstetric complications and the risk of schizophrenia: a longitudinal study of a national birth cohort. *Arch Gen Psychiatry* 1999; **56**(3): 234–40.

36. Hultman CM, Ohman A, Cnattingius S, Wieselgren IM, Lindstrom LH. Prenatal and neonatal risk factors for schizophrenia. *Br J Psychiatry* 1997; **170**: 128–33.

37. Hultman CM, Sparen P, Takei N, Murray RM, Cnattingius S. Prenatal and perinatal risk factors for schizophrenia, affective psychosis, and reactive psychosis of early onset: case-control study. *BMJ* 1999; **318**(7181): 421–6.

38. McNeil TF. Perinatal risk factors and schizophrenia: selective review and methodological concerns. *Epidemiol Rev* 1995; **17**(1): 107–12.

39. Horta BL, Victora CG, Menezes AM, Halpern R, Barros FC. Low birthweight, preterm births and intrauterine growth retardation in relation to maternal smoking. *Paediatr Perinat Epidemiol* 1997; **11**(2): 140–51.

40. Geddes JR, Verdoux H, Takei N, *et al.* Schizophrenia and complications of pregnancy and labor: an individual patient data meta-analysis. *Schizophr Bull* 1999; **25**(3): 413–23.

41. Jones PB, Rantakallio P, Hartikainen AL, Isohanni M, Sipila P. Schizophrenia as a long-term outcome of pregnancy, delivery, and perinatal complications: a 28-year follow-up of the 1966 north Finland general population birth cohort. *Am J Psychiatry* 1998; **155**(3): 355–64.

42. Matsumoto H, Takei N, Saito F, Kachi K, Mori N. The association between obstetric complications and childhood-onset schizophrenia: a replication study. *Psychol Med* 2001; **31**(5): 907–14.

43. Ichiki M, Kunugi H, Takei N, *et al.* Intra-uterine physical growth in schizophrenia: evidence confirming excess of preterm birth. *Psychol Med* 2000; **30**(3): 597–604.

44. Kunugi H, Nanko S, Murray RM. Obstetric complications and schizophrenia: prenatal underdevelopment and subsequent neurodevelopmental impairment. *Br J Psychiatry Suppl* 2001; **40**: s25–9.

45. Byrne M, Agerbo E, Bennedsen B, Eaton WW, Mortensen PB. Obstetric conditions and risk of first admission with schizophrenia: a Danish national register based study. *Schizophr Res* 2007; **97**(1–3): 51–9.

46. Smith GN, Flynn SW, McCarthy N, *et al.* Low birthweight in schizophrenia: prematurity or poor fetal growth? *Schizophr Res* 2001; **47**(2–3): 177–84.

47. Laursen TM, Munk-Olsen T, Nordentoft M, Bo Mortensen P. A comparison of selected risk factors for unipolar depressive disorder, bipolar affective disorder, schizoaffective disorder, and schizophrenia from a danish population-based cohort. *J Clin Psychiatry* 2007; **68**(11): 1673–81.

48. Nosarti C, Hultman CM, Cnattingius S, *et al.* Preterm birth and psychiatric outcome in adolescence and early adulthood: A study using the Swedish National Registers. *Schizophr Res* 2008; **98**(Suppl 1): 76.

49. Hultman CM, Sparen P, Cnattingius S. Perinatal risk factors for infantile autism. *Epidemiology* 2002; **13**(4): 417–23.

50. Nilsson E, Stalberg G, Lichtenstein P, *et al.* Fetal growth restriction and schizophrenia: a Swedish twin study. *Twin Res Hum Genet* 2005; **8**(4): 402–8.

51. Tsuchiya KJ, Byrne M, Mortensen PB. Risk factors in relation to an emergence of bipolar disorder: a systematic review. *Bipolar Disord* 2003; **5**(4): 231–42.

52. Scott J, McNeill Y, Cavanagh J, Cannon M, Murray R. Exposure to obstetric complications and subsequent

development of bipolar disorder: systematic review. *Br J Psychiatry* 2006; **189**: 3–11.

53. Wals M, Reichart CG, Hillegers MH, *et al.* Impact of birth weight and genetic liability on psychopathology in children of bipolar parents. *J Am Acad Child Adolesc Psychiatry* 2003; **42**(9): 1116–21.

54. Ogendahl BK, Agerbo E, Byrne M, *et al.* Indicators of fetal growth and bipolar disorder: a Danish national register-based study. *Psychol Med* 2006; **36**(9): 1219–24.

55. Hack M. Young adult outcomes of very-low-birth-weight children. *Semin Fetal Neonatal Med* 2006; **11**(2): 127–37.

56. Videbech P, Gouliaev G. First admission with puerperal psychosis: 7–14 years of follow-up. *Acta Psychiatr Scand* 1995; **91**(3): 167–73.

57. Valdimarsdottir U, Hultman CM, Harlow B, Cnattingius S, Sparen P. Psychotic illness in first-time mothers with no previous psychiatric hospitalizations: a population-based study. *PLoS Med* 2009; **6**(2): e13 doi:10.1371/journal.pmed.1000013.

58. Nager A, Sundquist K, Ramirez-Leon V, Johansson LM. Obstetric complications and postpartum psychosis: a follow-up study of 1.1 million first-time mothers between 1975 and 2003 in Sweden. *Acta Psychiatr Scand* 2008; **117**(1): 12–19.

59. Terp IM, Engholm G, Moller H, Mortensen PB. A follow-up study of postpartum psychoses: prognosis and risk factors for readmission. *Acta Psychiatr Scand* 1999; **100**(1): 40–6.

60. Kendell RE, Chalmers JC, Platz C. Epidemiology of puerperal psychoses. *Br J Psychiatry* 1987; **150**: 662–73.

61. Kendell RE, Rennie D, Clarke JA, Dean C. The social and obstetric correlates of psychiatric admission in the puerperium. *Psychol Med* 1981; **11**(2): 341–50.

62. Selling KE, Carstensen J, Finnstrom O, Josefsson A, Sydsjo G. Hospitalizations in adolescence and early adulthood among Swedish men and women born preterm or small for gestational age. *Epidemiology* 2008; **19**(1): 63–70.

63. Hack M, Flannery DJ, Schluchter M, *et al.* Outcomes in young adulthood for very-low-birth-weight infants. *N Engl J Med* 2002; **346**(3): 149–57.

64. Bennedsen BE, Mortensen PB, Olesen AV, Henriksen TB, Frydenberg M. Obstetric complications in women with schizophrenia. *Schizophr Res* 2001; **47**(2–3): 167–75.

65. Jablensky AV, Morgan V, Zubrick SR, Bower C, Yellachich LA. Pregnancy, delivery, and neonatal complications in a population cohort of women with schizophrenia and major affective disorders. *Am J Psychiatry* 2005; **162**(1): 79–91.

66. Webb R, Abel K, Pickles A, Appleby L. Mortality in offspring of parents with psychotic disorders: a critical review and meta-analysis. *Am J Psychiatry* 2005; **162**(6): 1045–56.

67. Bennedsen BE, Mortensen PB, Olesen AV, Henriksen TB. Preterm birth and intra-uterine growth retardation among children of women with schizophrenia. *Br J Psychiatry* 1999; **175**: 239–45.

68. Cnattingius S. The epidemiology of smoking during pregnancy: smoking prevalence, maternal characteristics, and pregnancy outcomes. *Nicotine Tob Res* 2004; **6** Suppl 2, S125–40.

69. Nilsson E, Lichtenstein P, Cnattingius S, Murray RM, Hultman CM. Women with schizophrenia: pregnancy outcome and infant death among their offspring. *Schizophr Res* 2002; **58**(2–3): 221–9.

70. Pinkofsky HB. Psychosis during pregnancy: treatment considerations. *Ann Clin Psychiatry* 1997; **9**(3): 175–9.

71. Diav-Citrin O, Shechtman S, Ornoy S, *et al.* Safety of haloperidol and penfluridol in pregnancy: a multicenter, prospective, controlled study. *J Clin Psychiatry* 2005; **66**(3): 317–22.

72. Bagedahl-Strindlund M. Mentally ill mothers and their children. An epidemiological study of antenatal care consumption, obstetric conditions, and neonatal health. *Acta Psychiatr Scand* 1986; **74**(1): 32–40.

73. Jeste DV, Gladsjo JA, Lindamer LA, Lacro JP. Medical comorbidity in schizophrenia. *Schizophr Bull* 1996; **22**(3): 413–30.

74. Lichtenstein P, Bjork C, Hultman CM, *et al.* Recurrence risks for schizophrenia in a Swedish national cohort. *Psychol Med* 2006; **36**(10): 1417–25.

75. Webb RT, Abel KM, Pickles AR, *et al.* Mortality risk among offspring of psychiatric inpatients: a population-based follow-up to early adulthood. *Am J Psychiatry* 2006; **163**(12): 2170–7.

76. Nilsson E, Hultman CM, Cnattingius S, *et al.*. Schizophrenia and offspring's risk for adverse pregnancy outcomes and infant death. *Br J Psychiatry* 2008; **193**(4): 311–5.

77. MacCabe JH, Martinsson L, Lichtenstein P, *et al.* Adverse pregnancy outcomes in mothers with affective psychosis. *Bipolar Disord* 2007; **9**(3): 305–9.

78. Higgins S. Smoking in pregnancy. *Curr Opin Obstet Gynecol* 2002; **14**(2): 145–51.

79. Walsh RA. Effects of maternal smoking on adverse pregnancy outcomes: examination of the criteria of causation. *Hum Biol* 1994; **66**(6): 1059–92.

80. Svensson AC, Lichtenstein P, Sandin S, Hultman CM. Fertility of first-degree relatives of patients with schizophrenia: a three generation perspective. *Schizophr Res* 2007; **91**(1–3): 238–45.

81. Goldenberg RL, Culhane JF, Iams JD, Romero R. Epidemiology and causes of preterm birth. *Lancet* 2008; **371**(9606): 75–84.

82. Jensen FE. The role of glutamate receptor maturation in perinatal seizures and brain injury. *Int J Dev Neurosci* 2002; **20**(3–5): 339–47.

83. Tornhage CJ, Serenius F, Uvnas-Moberg K, Lindberg T. Plasma somatostatin and cholecystokinin levels in preterm infants during their first two years of life. *Pediatr Res* 1997; **41**(6): 902–8.

84. Ekholm B, Ekholm A, Adolfsson R, *et al.* Evaluation of diagnostic procedures in Swedish patients with schizophrenia and related psychoses. *Nord J Psychiatry* 2005; **59**(6): 457–64.

85. Weinstock M. Alterations induced by gestational stress in brain morphology and behaviour of the offspring. *Prog Neurobiol* 2001; **65**(5): 427–51.

86. Nilsson PM, Nyberg P, Ostergren PO. Increased susceptibility to stress at a psychological assessment of stress tolerance is associated with impaired fetal growth. *Int J Epidemiol* 2001; **30**(1): 75–80.

87. Scheepens A, Wassink G, Piersma MJ, Van de Berg WD, Blanco CE. A delayed increase in hippocampal proliferation following global asphyxia in the neonatal rat. *Brain Res Dev Brain Res* 2003; **142**(1): 67–76.

88. Murray RM, Sham P, Van Os J, *et al.* A developmental model for similarities and dissimilarities between schizophrenia and bipolar disorder. *Schizophr Res* 2004; **71**(2–3): 405–16.

89. Nosarti C, Al-Asady MH, Frangou S, *et al.* Adolescents who were born very preterm have decreased brain volumes. *Brain* 2002; **125**(Pt 7): 1616–23.

90. Lipska BK, Jaskiw GE, Weinberger DR. Postpubertal emergence of hyperresponsiveness to stress and to amphetamine after neonatal excitotoxic hippocampal damage: a potential animal model of schizophrenia. *Neuropsychopharmacology* 1993; **9**(1): 67–75.

91. Boksa P, El-Khodor BF. Birth insult interacts with stress at adulthood to alter dopaminergic function in animal models: possible implications for schizophrenia and other disorders. *Neurosci Biobehav Rev* 2003; **27**(1–2): 91–101.

92. Featherstone RE, Kapur S, Fletcher PJ. The amphetamine-induced sensitized state as a model of schizophrenia. *Prog Neuropsychopharmacol Biol Psychiatry* 2007; **31**(8): 1556–71.

93. Myin-Germeys I, Delespaul P, van Os J. Behavioural sensitization to daily life stress in psychosis. *Psychol Med* 2005; **35**(5): 733–41.

94. Nieoullon A, Coquerel A. Dopamine: a key regulator to adapt action, emotion, motivation and cognition. *Curr Opin Neurol* 2003; **16** Suppl 2: S3–9.

95. Berk M, Dodd S, Kauer-Sant'anna M, *et al.* Dopamine dysregulation syndrome: implications for a dopamine hypothesis of bipolar disorder. *Acta Psychiatr Scand Suppl* 2007; (**434**): 41–9.

96. Soliman A, O'Driscoll GA, Pruessner J, *et al.* Stress-induced dopamine release in humans at risk of psychosis: a [(11)C]raclopride PET study. *Neuropsychopharmacology* 2007; **33**(8): 2033–41.

97. Svensson AC, Pawitan Y, Cnattingius S, Reilly M, Lichtenstein P. Familial aggregation of small-for-gestational-age births: the importance of fetal genetic effects. *Am J Obstet Gynecol* 2006; **194**(2): 475–9.

98. Cannon TD, Yolken R, Buka S, Torrey EF. Decreased neurotrophic response to birth hypoxia in the etiology of schizophrenia. *Biol Psychiatry* 2008; **64**(9): 797–802.

99. Allin M, Walshe M, Shaikh M, *et al.* COMT genotype influences corpus callosum development in adolescents born preterm. *Schizophr Res* 2008; **102**(1): 47.

Cognitive and functional outcomes of children born preterm

Betty R. Vohr

Introduction

Advances in contemporary perinatal care including antenatal steroids and neonatal intensive care have resulted in continued improvement in survival of extremely low birth weight (ELBW) (< 1000 g) infants in the 1990s [1,2–4] which has been most significant among infants at the limits of viability (23–24 weeks and < 750 g) birth weight [2,4–8]. Approximately 40 000 ELBW infants (1% of the live births) are born annually in the United States. The goal of healthcare professionals in neonatal intensive care units (NICUs) caring for these vulnerable preterm infants is not only to assure survival, but to continually improve the neonatal and long-term neurodevelopmental outcomes of these high-risk infants. Data from the National Institute of Child Health and Human Development (NICHD) Neonatal Network indicate survival rates for ELBW infants 501–750 g improved from 41% to 55%, and for ELBW infants 750–1000 g from 81% to 86% between 1990–1 and 1997–2000 [7]. However, the number of infants with serious neonatal complications including intraventricular hemorrhage (IVH), bronchopulmonary dysplasia (BPD), and necrotizing enterocolitis (NEC), also increased during the study period. Concurrent with the increase in the total number of ELBW infant survivors, and the number of survivors with serious neonatal morbidities, there has been an increase in the total number of infants with a spectrum of post-discharge adverse neurodevelopmental outcomes requiring long-term support and intervention services. Perinatologists and neonatologists need to have current outcomes information available to guide the decision-making and parental counseling process. The outcomes with the greatest long-term impact on the child and family are the cognitive, neurosensory, neurological, and functional impairments that are identified after discharge from the NICU [9–18].

Cognitive impairment is by far the most common disability identified among ELBW survivors [12,19–21]. This chapter will review the early cognitive and functional outcomes of high-risk ELBW infants born since 1990, assess whether rates of post-discharge adverse cognitive sequelae are increasing, remaining stable, or decreasing, and review the multiple factors contributing to cognitive outcomes.

Developmental/cognitive outcomes of children born preterm

Cognitive outcome and developmental outcome are sometimes used interchangeably when describing the outcomes of young children. In very young infants and toddlers, it is common to describe development, whereas in children 3 years and older, the term cognition or intelligence is used. Cognitive development refers to how children think and gain understanding of the world around them as influenced by genetics, the child's central nervous system function, exposure to insults, and environment. Areas of cognitive development include information processing, language development, reasoning, memory, and intelligence.

Assessment of cognitive development in the first three years of life is dependent upon the child's motor skills, memory (object permanence), symbolic language (early gestures), and early receptive and expressive language. The Bayley Scales of Infant Development II (BSID-II, Bayley II) [22] combines receptive language, expressive language, and cognitive skills into a mental developmental index. The Bayley II has been the most commonly reported test for infants, toddlers, and preschoolers from 4 months to 36 months of age and provides information in both cognitive (the Mental Developmental Index [MDI]) and motor (the Psychomotor Developmental Index [PDI]) domains. The Bayley II is being replaced by the Bayley Scales of

Infant and Toddler Development III (BSID-III, Bayley III) Bayley III [23], which has separate scales for cognition, language, and motor skills. The language scale is subdivided into receptive and expressive language subscales and the motor scale is subdivided into gross motor and fine motor subscales. It is expected that investigators will begin reporting the Bayley III cognitive index in the near future.

Challenges encountered in conducting a study to evaluate the developmental/cognitive outcomes of low birth weight infants are multiple. The high-risk ELBW population is extremely heterogeneous relative to the spectrum of neonatal characteristics, the severity of perinatal and neonatal morbidities, post-discharge morbidities, and post-discharge environment. In addition, the child's cognitive skills and functional skills become more complex with increasing age and subtle or higher executive function skills and learning disabilities that are identified in the older child cannot, for the most part, be recognized in the toddler. Cognitive outcomes are also impacted by the quality of the child's hearing, vision, neurological status, functional status, and behavior.

As part of the conceptual model of the development of cognition, not only multiple biomedical factors but a multitude of social and demographic factors interact and impact on cognitive outcome. The effects of sociodemographic factors including higher maternal education, higher family income, private health insurance, and access to early intervention services, have been clearly shown to impact on the cognitive development of preterm infants [24–27] (see also Chapter 17). In addition, outcomes may differ by age of assessment. Some children improve in their cognitive development with increasing age, some remain unchanged and some worsen [27–29].

Effects of year of birth

One of the major challenges of long-term outcome studies is that perinatal and neonatal interventions continue to evolve over time so that the findings of a 5, 10, or 20 year follow-up of a cohort may have limited current clinical significances. Nonetheless, significant changes have occurred in perinatal and neonatal care in the past 40 years resulting in increased survival of very preterm infants, who, in turn, are at increased risk of major neonatal morbidities [19,30,31].

Several studies have shown improvements in the outcomes of extremely premature infants over a period of time [29,32–34] and some studies suggest

that rates of impairments may be increasing [35,36]. Mean survival of infants < 27 weeks' gestation from a series of cohorts of infants born between 1970 and 1992 was 30%, and 14% of the survivors were mentally retarded [33]. Although the rates of children with disabilities remained relatively unchanged among the centers between 1970 and 1992, the prevalence of children with disabilities increased because of the increased survival rates. In contrast, a large NICHD Network study [21] compared the outcomes of infants < 1000 g born during three more recent epochs (1993–4, 1995–6, and 1997–8) and identified improving Bayley MDI scores. Multivariate analyses to determine changes in the use of medical interventions during the study period, and which medical interventions predict improved outcomes, revealed that antenatal steroids were associated with a decreased risk of a PDI < 70 and cerebral palsy (CP) whereas postnatal steroids were associated with an increased risk of moderate to severe CP, low Bayley MDI, low Bayley PDI, and increased neurodevelopmental impairment [21].

Another challenge in comparing published reports of outcomes of extremely preterm infants is the denominator used in calculating the percentage of adverse post-discharge outcomes. The denominator can be a live fetus upon arrival of the mother at the hospital, live births, infants admitted to the NICU, infant survivors of the NICU, or children presenting for follow-up assessment. In many studies the statistical analyses are based on the number of infants admitted to the NICU or the number of infants discharged from the NICU. A significant percentage of live 22- to 24-week fetuses, however, die during labor or in the delivery suite [2]. As an example, if two infants of 22 weeks' gestation survive and one has a major neonatal morbidity and one does not during a 12-month period, the center may report that 50% of 22-week survivors have a good outcome. However, if in the course of the year, 100 mothers arrived with a live 22-week fetus, the percentage with a "good outcome" would be 1% (see also Chapter 12 for methodological considerations).

Finally it is well documented that center differences exist for neonatal and post-discharge outcomes including MDI [37–41]. A multicenter NICHD Network study which examined center differences identified that the mean 18–22 months' corrected age (CA) Bayley MDI at centers ranged from a low of 70±17 to a high of 83±15. Differences in MDI scores at centers persisted even after adjusting for demographics and antenatal interventions suggesting unmeasured differences in neonatal practices and post-discharge family and environmental factors affect outcomes. All of these factors contribute to the challenge of conducting post-discharge outcomes studies to assess the effects of antenatal and neonatal interventions on cognitive outcomes.

Cognitive assessments in the first three years

Outcome studies in the first two to three years of life reported by the NICHD Neonatal Research Network have used a composite outcome termed neurodevelopmental impairment (NDI) which is derived from Bayley MDI and PDI scores, vision, hearing, and neurological status. A diagnosis of NDI is made if any of the following are present: moderate to severe CP, bilateral blindness (vision worse than 20/200 or no useful vision in either eye) or bilateral hearing impairment (requiring amplification in both ears), Bayley Scales of Infant Development II MDI or PDI < 70. Although this chapter will focus on cognitive and functional outcomes of preterm infants, these outcomes will be related to neuromotor and neurosensory outcomes and NDI.

Cognitive assessments in preschool and school-age children

Although much has been written about the capacity of preterm infants to recover or gain skills with increasing age, there is increasing evidence of an increased incidence of cognitive and functional disability at school age [32,42–45]. The following tests are often used to assess children 3 years and older.

The Stanford-Binet Intelligence Scale – fourth edition [46], the Wechsler Preschool and Primary Scale of Intelligence – third edition [47], the Woodcock–Johnson Psycho–Educational Battery–Revised [48], the Differential Ability Scales [49], and the McCarthy Scales of Children's Abilities [50] are all tests of cognitive/developmental ability and provide an IQ as well as subtests which permit a limited assessment of strengths and weaknesses in specific areas of learning. Because of the limitations of IQ, it is becoming more acceptable to evaluate a child's performance on a battery of tests which include visual perceptual skills [51,52], speech and language skills [53–56], cognition [46–50], fine and gross motor function [57–60], and kindergarten readiness [61–64].

Functional outcomes

The newest practical and clinically relevant approach to evaluating a child is to provide information on functional skills in daily living and healthcare status [65–67]. Functional assessment is the process of determining a child's ability to perform the tasks of daily living and to fulfill the social roles expected of a physically and emotionally healthy person of the same age and culture [68]. For children, the tasks include feeding, dressing, bathing, maintaining continence, mobility, communication, play, and social interaction [69]. The social roles expected include involvement with peers and attending school.

In 1980, a model of pathophysiology, impairment, disability, and handicap for comprehensively assessing health status in individuals with musculoskeletal disabilities was developed for the World Health Organization (WHO) [70]. In this model, pathophysiology reflects cellular injury or dysfunction (e.g., hypoxemia), impairment is the consequence at the organ level (e.g., parenchymal brain injury), disability occurs at a person level (e.g., difficulty with self-care, mobility, and/or communication) and handicap occurs at a societal level (e.g., special education resources, family support, respite, limited opportunities). The National Center for Medical Rehabilitation Research (NCMRR) expanded the WHO model to include functional limitations and social limitations [71] and more recently in 2001 the WHO revised the above-described 1980 International Classification of Impairments, Disabilities and Handicaps (ICIDH) and introduced the International Classification of Functioning, Disability and Health known as ICF which includes health and health-related domains described from the perspective of the body, the individual, and society [72]. Four functional outcome measures are currently available: the Pediatric Evaluation of Disability Inventory (PEDI) for children 6 months to 7.5 years [73], the Functional Independence Measure for Children (WeeFIM) [67] for children with and without disabilities through age 8 years, the Vineland Adaptive Behavior Scale (VABS) [66] for children from birth to 18 years, and the Battelle Developmental Inventory for children age 0–8 years [65].

Factors impacting on childhood outcomes

Factors contributing to the outcome of premature infants include the characteristics of the intrauterine

Table 11.1 Spectrum of factors contributing to cognitive and functional outcomes of VLBW infants

Intrauterine environment	Infection, smoking, hypertension, medications, multiple birth
Extreme prematurity	The immature brain, altered brain development
Neonatal morbidities and characteristics	IVH, PVL, BPD, NEC, sepsis, ROP, gender
Perinatal and neonatal interventions	Antenatal cortiosteroids, surfactant, assisted ventilation, antibiotics, indomethacin, postnatal cortiosteroids, nutrition and growth
Post-discharge environment	Maternal education, family income, health insurance, early intervention services
Post-discharge healthcare needs	Chronic lung disease recurrent hospitalization
Comorbidities	Cerebral palsy, vision impairment, hearing impairment, congenital anomalies

IVH = intraventricular hemorrhage;
PVL = periventricular leukomalacia;
BPD = bronchopulmonary dysplasia;
NEC = necrotizing enterocolitis;
ROP = retinopathy of prematurity.

environment, extreme prematurity, neonatal characteristics and morbidities, neonatal interventions, the post-discharge environment, post-discharge healthcare needs, and comorbidities (Table 11.1).

The intrauterine environment

Characteristics of the intrauterine environment which have been shown to be associated with increased risk of neonatal and long-term morbidities include maternal infection, drug exposure, smoking, and multiple gestation [74–79]. Inflammatory mechanisms are known to be associated with preterm birth and neonatal morbidities. Two maternal complications associated with inflammation and infection, chorioamnionitis and prolonged rupture of membranes, are associated with the development of periventricular leukomalacia (PVL). In one report [77] examining the association between histological chorioamnionitis and PVL, severe inflammation in the umbilical cord was observed in 53% of infants with PVL and 32% without PVL (p < 0.05). Periventricular leukomalacia is strongly associated with an increased rate of CP and associated morbidities [80].

Multiples accounted for 3% of all births in the USA in 2002 [81,82] and rates range from 8% to 28% of admissions of infants < 1500 g to NICHD Neonatal Research Network NICUs [12]. Although recent population data indicate that the higher-order multiple rates have plateaued, there were 6898 sets of triplets, 434 sets of quadruplets, and 69 sets of quintuplets born in the United States in 2002, accounting for 3% of all births [83]. These pregnancies are often complicated by increased maternal complications, preterm delivery, perinatal complications, and intrauterine growth restriction [75,84]. There is evidence for increased rates of adverse neurodevelopmental outcomes among multiples [85].

Extreme prematurity

In addition to the effects of antenatal, perinatal, and neonatal factors potentially causing brain injury, the stage of brain development at the time of birth, and the subsequent brain development and organization in an extrauterine environment all impact on the subsequent development of cognition and functional skills [86].

Advances in perinatal and neonatal care have contributed to an increased number of ELBW infants < 750 g and very preterm infants of 22–25 weeks' gestation surviving [2,19,87,88]. Infants born between 22 and 25 weeks of gestation are medically fragile and vulnerable, with immature organ systems. Their skin is gelatinous, and they breathe through terminal bronchioles because the alveoli have not yet formed [89]. Active brain development occurs during the second and third trimesters, with neurogenesis, neuronal migration, maturation, apoptosis, and synaptogenesis [12]. Infants are at extremely high risk for brain injury during this period of active brain maturation, from hypoxia, ischemia, undernutrition, and sepsis, which start a cascade of events that increase the risk of brain hemorrhage, white matter injury, PVL, ventriculomegaly, poor brain growth, and subsequent neurodevelopmental impairment. The immaturity of the brain at 22–25 weeks of gestation increases the extremely preterm infant's vulnerability to insult during the prolonged stay in a NICU [90–92].

Concerns regarding cognitive outcomes are often centered on the lowest birth weight infants < 750 g and the most immature infants with an estimated gestational age of less than 25 weeks. These infants continue to survive in increasing numbers and are at greatest risk of major neonatal morbidities including BPD, IVH, sepsis, NEC, and ROP. Although there are occasional reports of a survivor at 22 weeks' gestation, the American Academy of Pediatrics does not recommend resuscitation of infants less than or equal to 22 weeks' gestation [93].

Outcomes for infants < 1000 g and < 25 weeks' gestation born during two time periods, epoch 1 (January 1993 to December 1996) and epoch 2 (July 1996 to December 1999), at NICHD Neonatal Network centers were compared to assess the effects of interventions on outcomes at 18–22 months' CA [6]. During epoch 2 there were higher percents of Cesarian section delivery, prenatal antibiotic use, prenatal corticosteroid use and surfactant administration. However, the prevalence of an MDI < 70 appeared to worsen over time and was 40% during epoch 1 and 47% during epoch 2 (p = 0.06). For infants with a gestational age of ≤ 23 weeks, 38% had an MDI < 70 during epoch 1 and 52% during epoch two. Multivariate analyses to predict Bayley MDI < 70 demonstrated that only 2 factors (higher birth weight and epoch 1 versus epoch 2) were protective, whereas male gender, IVH grade 3–4, late-onset sepsis, and less than a high school education for the mother were associated with an MDI < 70. These findings once again demonstrate the importance of examining the effects of both biological and environmental factors on cognitive outcomes.

A second multicenter NICHD Neonatal Network study [5] examined the 18–22 month outcomes of a cohort of infants both ELBW (≤ 750 g) and extremely preterm (≤ 24 weeks) (n = 244) with an additional risk factor of a 1 minute Apgar score ≤ 3. Forty-six percent had an MDI < 70 and 60% had NDI. Remarkably 33% had an MDI ≥ 85 at 18 months' CA, considered average for age. Factors associated with an MDI < 70 were grade 3–4 IVH, PVL, male gender, black race, and Medicaid insurance (i.e., a state administered healthcare program), whereas residing in a two-parent household was associated with an MDI > 70. After separating the infants by week of gestation, 43% of 24-week infants and 51% of ≤ 23-week infants had an MDI < 70.

De Groote et al. published a population-based study of 92 infants ≤ 26 weeks evaluated at 3 years of age [94]. Cognitive and disability outcomes were reported for infants ≤ 24 weeks, 25 weeks and 26 weeks. Among the infants evaluated, 20% of infants ≤ 24 weeks, 30% of infants of 25 weeks, and 31% of infants of 26 weeks' gestation had a Bayley MDI < 70. Outcomes were also reported as disability rates for the three gestational age groups. No overall disability was defined as Bayley scores > 70, and no neuromotor or sensory impairment. Severe disability was defined as one or more severe impairments and the remainder were classified as intermediate disability. Overall, 58% of the children discharged alive had a disability, and 32% were categorized as severe. Among those infants discharged alive, the number with no disability were 1 (100%) at 23 weeks, 3 (27%) at 24 weeks, 12 (39%) at 25 weeks, and 22 (42%) at 26 weeks. The authors then addressed the issue of the denominator in calculating disability rates which can be successfully addressed in a population-based study. The following rates for "no disability" were calculated for the entire cohort with four different denominators: all recorded births (15%), all live births (22%), all NICU admissions (25%), and all infants discharged alive (40%). The rates of "no disability" for infants discharged are important quality indicators for a NICU; however, it is the percent based on the earlier denominators that are needed when providing antenatal counseling about neurodevelopmental outcomes to families who arrive in labor with a live fetus of 22–26 weeks' gestation.

Neonatal morbidities and characteristics

Extremely low birth weight infants have increased rates of high acuity neonatal morbidities including IVH, PVL, sepsis, NEC, and BPD [6,10,19,95,96]. They may experience prolonged periods of weeks to months of a need for hyperalimentation, assisted ventilation, and intensive care hospitalization. The following section will review neonatal characteristics and morbidities that are associated with poor neurodevelopmental outcomes. Table 11.2 summarizes several cohort studies of ELBW infants which have investigated the effects of specific neonatal morbidities.

IVH and PVL

Brain injury which occurs in association with severe grade 3–4 IVH, PVL, ventriculomegaly, or white matter injury has consistently been demonstrated to be associated with poor developmental and neuromotor outcomes. In a number of large cohort studies of ELBW infants grade 3–4 IVH and PVL have been independently associated with NDI at 18–22 months of age after adjusting for known confounders, and, in fact, the majority of neonates with these findings do develop neurological sequelae [19]. In the international multicenter outcome study of ELBW infants reported by Schmidt et al. [10], outcomes of infants were analyzed by types of neonatal morbidity. Within the cohort, 194 infants had a brain injury defined as the presence of any of the following: echodense intraparenchymal lesions, PVL, porencephalic cysts, ventriculomegaly with or without IVH, and IVH grades 3 and 4. Serial ultrasounds were obtained. Among infants with brain injury 42% had an MDI < 70 compared with 23% of infants who had no evidence of brain injury (Table 11.2). Infants with brain injury also had increased rates of CP (36% versus 6.7%), deafness (2.9 versus 2.2%) and blindness (2.9 versus 1.6%) compared to infants with no brain injury.

However, in one large multicenter cohort study of ELBW children who had a completely normal neurological assessment at 18–22 months, 14% had a history of grade 3–4 IVH and 3% had a history of PVL identified by cranial ultrasound [17]. Intraventricular hemorrhage is most frequently identified on cranial ultrasound in the first week of life and a late head ultrasound at 36 weeks' gestation may not show evidence of a prior bleed. Therefore, a clear description of the timing of head ultrasounds is important in evaluating a report of the rate of IVH. In addition, white matter injury, which is clearly related to subsequent CP and cognitive impairments, is often not identified by cranial ultrasound. More tertiary centers are recognizing the importance of obtaining a 36-week magnetic resonance imaging (MRI) scan as a more optimal predictor of white matter injury.

Laptook et al. [99] reported that in a large cohort of ELBW infants with at least two normal neonatal cranial ultrasounds and no abnormal ultrasound, 25.3% had a Bayley MDI score < 70 and 9.4% had a diagnosis of CP at 18–22 months' CA. Magnetic resonance imaging data were not obtained on this cohort. Biological factors independently associated with increased risk of low MDI with a normal cranial ultrasound were male gender, multiple births, lower birth weight, pneumothorax, and longer duration of ventilation. Risk of a low Bayley MDI score was associated with sociodemographic factors including non-white race, lower maternal education, and public health insurance. A number of investigators have reported that neonatal MRI is superior to cranial ultrasound in identifying white matter injury and is a better predictor of CP at 18 and 30 months of age [100,101].

Bronchopulmonary dysplasia (BPD)

The majority of ELBW infants are discharged with a diagnosis of BPD, a chronic lung disease defined according to duration of oxygen dependence. In the past, although outcomes of infants with BPD have tended to be poorer than those without BPD, there was a spectrum of outcomes for children with the diagnosis. The National Institute of Health (NIH) developed disease severity criteria for BPD that include mild (need for supplemental O_2 for $\geq$ 28 days, but not at 36 weeks' postmenstrual age [PMA] or discharge), moderate (supplemental O_2 for $\geq$ 28 days plus treatment with < 30% O_2 at 36 weeks' PMA), or severe (supplemental $O_2 \geq$ 28 days plus $\geq$ 30% O_2 and/or positive pressure at 36 weeks' PMA). These were further validated by the NICHD Network [96]. As reported, the frequency of mild, moderate and severe BPD was 30.3%, 30.2%, and 16.4% of ELBW infants, respectively with a diagnosis of BPD. When assessed at 18–22 months of age, the incidence of a Bayley MDI < 70 increased significantly for children with increasing severity of BPD (no BPD: 21%, mild: 25.6%, moderate: 35.1% and severe BPD: 49.8%, $p < 0.0001$ for trend) respectively [96] (Table 11.2).

Schmidt et al. [10] reported the rate of low cognitive function at 18 months' CA in ELBW children with BPD defined as a need for supplemental oxygen at 36 weeks who participated in the International Indomethacin Trial (Table 11.2). Four-hundred–and-nine infants (45%) developed BPD. Children with BPD were more likely to have an MDI < 70 (36% versus 19%), CP (17% versus 9.3%), deafness (3.5% versus 1.4%), and blindness (1.9% versus 1.8%) compared with ELBW children with no BPD. The rate of low MDI for children with BPD is consistent with the moderate severity BPD group of ELBW children in the NICHD Neonatal Network study [96].

Bronchopulmonary dysplasia severity has also been related to the number of days of assisted ventilation. Among a cohort of ELBW infants born from 1995 to 1998, 89% received mechanical ventilation on the first day of life [18]. The median duration of ventilation was 18 days, with 7%, 1.3%, and 0.3% ventilated for $\geq$ 60, $\geq$ 90, and $\geq$ 120 days, respectively. As ventilation exceeded 28 days, the incidence of CP and neurodevelopmental impairment progressively increased [18]. The mean MDI score fell with increasing duration of ventilation from 89±16 for children with no ventilation to 52.6±6 for children with $\geq$ 120 days of ventilation. The percentage of children with an MDI < 70 at 18–22 months' CA was 14% for infants with no ventilation and increased to 61%, 85%, and 100% for infants with $\geq$ 60, $\geq$ 90, and $\geq$ 120 days of ventilation, respectively. Type

Table 11.2 Cognitive scores at 18–36 months' CA for infants < 1000 g born in the 1990s related to neonatal risk factor

Weight	Sample size	Subgroup sample N	DOB	Age	MDI < 70 Comparison group	MDI < 70 Subgroups	Country	Author
≤ 26 weeks	92, of whom 77 received full assessments	≤ 24 w 10 25 w 27 26 w 40	1999–2000	3 y	Gender analyses Male 30% female 27%	≤ 24 w 20% 25 w 30% 26 w 31%	Belgium	De Groote et al. [94]
< 1000 g Brain injury[a] ROP BPD	910	194 brain injury 21% 89 Severe ROP 10% 409 BPD 45%	1996–8	18 m	No brain injury 23% No ROP 25% No BPD 19%	Brain injury 42% ROP 49% BPD 36%	International	Schmidt et al. [10]
< 1000 g BPD	4866	None 1124 Mild 1473 Mod 1471 Severe 798	1993–2001	18 m		No BPD 21% Mild 25.6% Mod 35.1% Severe 49.8%	United States	Ehrenkranz et al. [96]
< 1000 g NEC	2948	118	1995–8	18 m	No NEC 31%	Medical 37% Surgical 44%	United States	Hintz et al. [97]
< 1000 g Culture + sepsis	6093	None 2161 Clinical 1538 Sepsis 1922 Sepsis ± NEC 279 Meningitis ± sepsis 193	1993–2001	18 m	No sepsis 22%	Clinical 33% Sepsis 37% Sepsis + NEC 42% Meningitis ± sepsis 38%	United States	Stoll et al. [95]
< 1000 g	1739[b] 1860	Normal neuro 1340 Hemiplegia 39 Diplegia 107 Triplegia 16 Quadriplegia 73 Hypotonic CP 25 Monoplegia 10 Abnormal other 129	1995–8	18 m	Normal neuro 21%	Hemiplegia 41% Diplegia 69% Triplegia 63% Quadriplegia 96% Hypotonic CP 84% Monoplegia 45% Abnormal other 50%	United States	Vohr et al. [17]
< 1000 g anomalies	3632	185	1998–2000	18 m	No anomalies 20%	51%	United States	Walden et al. [98]

[a] brain injury was defined as the presence of any of the following: echodense intraparenchymal lesions, periventricular leukomalacia, porencephalic cysts, ventriculomegaly with or without intraventricular hemorrhage, and intraventricular hemorrhages of grade 3 and 4.

[b] with Bayley MDI score.

of ventilation has been evaluated relative to outcome. Although one early trial suggested that high-frequency oscillatory ventilation (HFOV) may increase neurodevelopmental abnormalities, more recent studies found no difference in outcome between HFOV and conventional ventilation [15,102].

Necrotizing enterocolitis (NEC)

Necrotizing enterocolitis is the most common gastrointestinal emergency, affecting approximately 10–15% of preterm infants with a birth weight < 1500 g. Necrotizing enterocolitis is also classified by levels of severity ranging from none to mild to surgical. Infants with NEC defined as Modified Bell's classification stage IIA or greater were included in a multicenter study[97]. In a cohort of 2498 ELBW infants born from 1995 to 1998 [97] (Table 11.2), increased severity of NEC was associated with longer duration of hospitalization and increased mortality. At 18–22 months' CA, infants who had surgically managed NEC had higher rates of MDI < 70, PDI < 70, and NDI (44%, 37%, and 57%, respectively) than those managed medically (37%, 25%, and 44%) or those without NEC (31%, 19%, and 40%) [97]. Regression analyses showed that surgical NEC was an independent risk factor for MDI < 70 (OR = 1.61, 95% CI = 1.05–2.50). Surgical NEC was also an independent predictor for PDI < 70 and NDI, and was associated with significantly greater growth failure at 18 months. The strong association of NEC with poor outcome may reflect the fact that the sickest infants are the ones who need the surgical intervention. These infants are also more likely to have infections and postsurgical complications.

Sepsis

Extremely low birth weight infants are at risk of both early-onset (≤ 72 hours) and late-onset (> 72 hours) sepsis. Rates of infection increase with decreasing birth weight and gestational age. Several studies have suggested an association between sepsis and cerebral white matter damage and CP [103–106]. One report identified a fourfold increase in CP among very low birth weight (VLBW) infants with a history of neonatal sepsis compared to infants with no neonatal infection [107]. Sixty-five percent of ELBW infants in a NICHD Neonatal Network study had at least one infection during their hospitalization in a NICU including 32% with sepsis alone, 5% with sepsis and NEC, and 3% with meningitis with or without sepsis [95]. In addition, 25% of the infants studied had indications of clinical infection

treated with antibiotics for ≥ 5 days but negative cultures. At 18–22 months' CA, infants in each of these infection groups including those with clinical infection had increased rates of neurodevelopmental abnormalities, including low Bayley MDI scores, low PDI scores, CP, and vision impairment, compared with uninfected infants (Table 11.2). A Bayley score < 70 was found in 22% of children with no history of infection, 33% of children with a history of clinical infection, 37% with sepsis alone, 42% with a history of sepsis plus NEC, and 38% with a history of meningitis with or without sepsis. All components of the NDI were higher in the sepsis groups including clinical sepsis. The rates of NDI were 29% of children with no history of infection, 43% of children with a history of clinical infection, 48% with a history of sepsis alone, 53% for a history of sepsis plus NEC, and 48% with a history of meningitis with or without sepsis. Children in all infection groups had evidence of poor head circumference growth (< tenth percentile) at 18 months' CA. In multivariate analyses, after adjusting for confounders, children in all infection groups remained at increased risk of MDI < 70, PDI < 70, CP, and NDI.

Gender

Premature males are at a significantly increased risk of neonatal death, in-hospital morbidity [108–113] and poor neurodevelopmental outcomes [15,19,20,31,114–116] compared with premature female infants. Within a cohort of 7288 inborn VLBW infants admitted to NICHD Neonatal Network Centers between 1991 and 1993, boys were less likely to survive (22% versus 15%), and had lower Apgar scores and higher rates of intubation, BPD, and IVH [111]. Although separate cognitive scores for males and females are often not reported in outcome studies of preterm infants, beneficial effects of female gender are consistently identified in multivariate analyses adjusting for known confounders. The neonatal and post-discharge neurodevelopmental outcomes at 18–22 months' CA were evaluated in a more recent large cohort of 2762 ELBW boys and 2634 ELBW girls < 28 weeks' gestation and < 1000 g birth weight born January 1, 1997 to December 31, 2000 [117]. Girls were more likely to survive (1761[66.9%]) than boys (1610 [58.3%]) and boys were more likely to have BPD, IVH grade 3–4 and ROP ≥ 3 and "plus disease". Boys were significantly more likely to have an MDI < 70 (41.9% versus 27.1% for girls) and have moderate to severe CP, low Bayley PDI and NDI. Multivariate analyses adjusting for multiple confounders confirmed the independent effects of male gender on MDI < 70 and NDI. Laptook *et al.* [99] reported that ELBW male infants with a normal head ultrasound were also more likely to have CP and a Bayley MDI < 70 than female ELBW infants. Effects of gender continue to be observed at school age. Persistent gender effects were reported in a large cohort of infants < 26 weeks' gestation born in the United Kingdom and Ireland in 1995 and evaluated at 6 years of age [15]. Mean cognitive scores for girls were 87±17 compared with 77±20 boys for with a mean difference of 10 points. Gender effects remained significant after removing the children with physical disability. Similar female advantage was observed on subscale scores of the Kaufman Assessment Battery for Children [118].

An analysis of gender within the cohort of the Multicenter Randomized Indomethacin rates of IVH Prevention Trial showed differential male effects of indomethacin. Treated boys but not girls had a more significant reduction in rates of IVH and more improved verbal scores at 3–8 years than untreated boys [119]. Multivariate analysis at age 8 years of this cohort [11] to predict cognitive and achievement test scores showed that male gender was associated with lower reading recognition and reading comprehension scores. Although greater neonatal illness severity in males appears to be a likely predictor of subsequent higher rates of neurodevelopmental impairment, effects of male gender on adverse outcome persist after adjusting for confounding neonatal morbidities [12,15].

Recent studies suggest that the developing brain of preterm boys differs from that of girls [120]. Preterm subjects with a birth weight 600–1250 g enrolled in the Randomized Indomethacin IVH Prevention Trial and matched term controls had MRIs and cognitive assessments completed at 8 years of age. The preterm subjects had significantly lower cerebral gray matter volumes and cerebral white matter volumes compared to controls. However, for white matter there was a significant group-by-gender interaction. Whereas girls in the preterm group had cerebral White Matter volumes similar to control girls, preterm boys had cerebral WM reductions when compared to control boys. Additional analyses were completed to determine if the MRI findings were related to cognitive test scores in the cohort at 4½ years or 8 years. The GM to total brain volume ratios correlated with cognitive measures in girls but not in boys. These findings suggest that the preterm brain of boys may be particularly vulnerable to injury and may be an explanation of some of the gender differences observed in neurodevelopmental outcomes.

Perinatal and neonatal interventions

Antenatal steroids and surfactant

Antenatal steroids and surfactant have been shown to significantly improve survival and decrease the incidence of IVH and respiratory distress syndrome in preterm infants [19,121]. In multivariate analyses, antenatal steroids are consistently the only antenatal intervention contributing to decreased rates of NDI [19]. Beneficial effects of surfactant administration to decrease the risk of respiratory distress, and use of antenatal antibiotics and management of nosocomial infection to reduce neonatal infection rate [95] have been well documented, and these medications are currently considered standard of care for VLBW infants.

Postnatal steroids

After initial reports indicated the beneficial effects of postnatal steroids for ventilator-dependent infants, administration to premature infants became almost universal for chronic lung disease (CLD). This changed to significantly limited use after Yeh *et al.* [122,123] reported the negative effects of dexamethasone therapy at 2 years of age for infants with birth weights of 500–1999 grams born between 1992 and 1995 participating in a randomized trial for the prevention of CLD. Although dexamethasone reduced the incidence of CLD, infants exposed to dexamethasone had higher rates of neuromotor dysfunction (25 of 63 [39.7%] versus 12 of 70 [17.1%]) compared to placebo controls. There were no effects of dexamethasone on MDI at 2 years of age [123]. Ninety-two percent (146 of 159 survivors) were reevaluated at 8 years of age. In addition, to the persistence of poorer motor skills in the dexamethasone group, the children had lower full-scale IQ (78±15 versus 84±13), verbal IQ (84±13 versus 88±12), and performance IQ scores (76.5±15 versus 84.5±13) compared to controls. Children exposed to dexamethasone also had evidence of poorer scores on verbal comprehension, perceptual organization, freedom from distractibility, and processing speed. In addition, the mean head circumference (49.8±3 versus 50.2 cm; p = 0.04) and height (122.8±7 versus 126±6 cm; p = 0.03) were significantly lower for the dexamethasone group compared to the controls. This is worrisome since the association of subnormal head size with poor cognitive outcome is well established in preterm infants [124]. More troubling is the report of an association between dexamethasone administration for CLD and decreased cerebral cortical gray matter [125], which suggests a potential deleterious effect of dexamethasone on neonatal brain and subsequent neurodevelopmental outcome.

Indomethacin

Since IVH is a significant predictor of adverse neurodevelopmental outcome, prevention of IVH in premature infants is an important goal in neonatology. Administration of low-dose prophylactic indomethacin has been shown to reduce the incidence and severity of IVH. In the Multicenter Indomethacin IVH Prevention Trial, indomethacin lowered the rate of any grade IVH from 18 % to 12% and severe IVH from 5% to 1% compared to placebo in premature infants weighing 600–1250 g (p = 0.03) [126]. However, when neurodevelopmental outcome was assessed, no difference in the incidence of CP was seen between the two study groups at 3 years or 4.5 years of age. Mean Stanford-Binet IQ scores did not differ between the treatment groups at the 3-year assessment. There were, however, trends favoring indomethacin in a categorical analysis of Wechsler Preschool and Primary Scale of Intelligence–Revised scores at 4.5 years [127,128]. Indomethacin was not associated with school-age outcomes at 8 years in the same cohort. Severe IVH and PVL/ventriculomegaly, and maternal education < 12 years were significantly associated with less optimal cognitive, academic, behavioral, and functional assessments [11]. The contrast between neonatal findings and subsequent cognitive test scores and neurological findings illustrates the disconnect between neonatal and long-term outcomes. Comparable results of a beneficial effect of prophylactic indomethacin on reducing IVH, but no differences in NDI at 2 years of age were obtained in a second multicenter trial of ELBW infants [129]. Schmidt *et al.* [129] reported a reduction of severe grade 3–4 IVH from 13% to 9% and a reduction of patent ductus arteriosus from 50% to 24%. No effects were identified, however, in rates of MDI < 70 (27% and 26%) between the intervention and control groups respectively at 2 years of age.

Nutrition and growth in the NICU

Good growth throughout infancy and childhood is a reflection of both adequate nutrition intake and physical well-being. Extremely low birth weight infants may have restricted intake nutrition during the neonatal period due to concerns about inability to tolerate enteral feedings, general illness severity (BPD, IVH, NEC, and sepsis), and the risk of metabolic acidosis. In addition, preterm infants have low energy stores and an increased metabolic rate. The initial loss of weight following birth generally results in a slowing of growth velocity compared with intrauterine growth of a fetus of similar gestational age [130].

A number of studies have shown that the majority of VLBW infants in a NICU develop growth restriction with parameters below the 10th percentile by 36 weeks, postconceptional age or time of discharge from the NICU [112,130–135], and many remain small into childhood and adolescence [136,137]. As part of an NICHD Neonatal Network study, Ehrenkranz *et al.* divided the in-hospital growth velocity of a cohort of ELBW infants into quartiles. The incidence of CP, Bayley MDI score < 70, Bayley PDI score < 70, and NDI at 18–22 months' CA increased with decreasing growth velocity, and was highest in the lowest growth velocity quartile. In fact, multivariate analyses showed that in-hospital lowest quartile weight gain velocity was independently associated with increased rates of NDI (OR = 2.53, 95% CI = 1.27– 5.03). After PVL, lowest quartile weight gain velocity was the strongest predictor of NDI [137].

The American Academy of Pediatrics Committee on Nutrition (AAP-CON) recognizes the importance of providing adequate nutrition for premature infants and recommends supplying sufficient nutrients to approximate the rate of growth and composition of weight gain for a normal fetus at the same PMA [138,139]. Despite these recommendations, deficits in growth frequently occur. A recent Cochrane review [140] suggests that higher protein intake accelerates weight gain in low birth weight neonates cared for in a NICU. It is known that poor intrauterine and extrauterine head growth in VLBW infants is associated with lower Bayley MDI scores at 15–20 months [141,142] and lower verbal and performance IQ, receptive and expressive language, and academic abilities at school age [124]. In addition, higher energy intake during the first 10 days of life in small-for-gestational age infants has been correlated with head circumference "catch-up" growth and higher IQ later in life [143].

One easy way to implement cost-effective nutritional intervention in the NICU for premature infants is human milk. Beneficial effects of human milk have been demonstrated for term, near-term, and ELBW infants, including improved cognitive skills [137,144–152], behavior ratings [153–155] and decreased rates of infection [156–161]. Improved cognitive performance has been related to the presence of long-chain

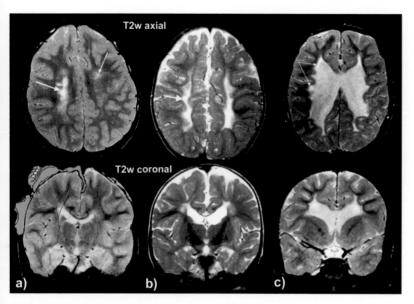

Fig. 3.3. Morphology–function in periventricular leukomalacia with respect to motor tracts/CP. Magnetic resonance imaging of three 6-year-old children with different degrees of periventricular leukomalacia (the bottom images are in coronal orientation in the domain of the motor tracks). Images are displayed in radiological view (Right = Left, Left = Right). (a) A very mild and asymmetrical form with periventricular gliosis only, which affects only the right side (thick arrow) of the motor tracts, on the left only frontal involvement is seen (thin arrow), thus gives rise to **unilateral spastic CP** on the left. (b) Mild PVL, again characterized by gliosis (arrow), but more symmetrical and affecting both motor tracts, thus causes **mild, leg-dominated BS-CP**. (c) Severe PVL with gliosis (arrows) and tissue loss, affecting, thus, motor tracts on both sides **severely and causes spastic CP** not only affecting legs but also trunk, arms, and face (usually also associated with cognitive problems and visual deficits, see Fig. 3.4).

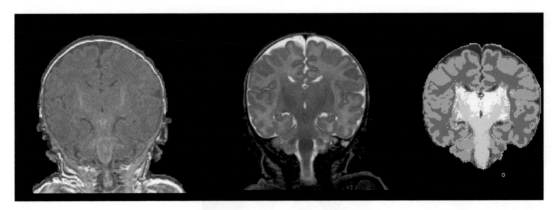

Fig. 4.2. An example of image segmentation for quantitative volumetric analysis. The image on the left is a coronal T1-weighted image. The image in the center is the corresponding T2-weighted image. The image on the right is the segmentation map derived from these MR images. Blue represents CSF, gray is gray matter, red is unmyelinated white matter, white is basal ganglia and thalamus, and yellow is myelinated white matter. This map can be used to determine relative volumes (in cm^3) of these different tissue types.

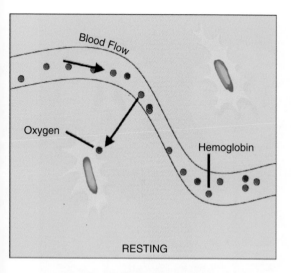

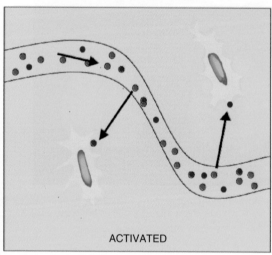

Fig. 7.1. Blood-oxygen-level-dependent contrast in magnetic resonance images: upon metabolic activation, oxygen is extracted by the cells, thereby increasing the level of deoxyhemoglobin in the blood. This is compensated for by an increase in blood flow in the vicinity of the active cells, leading to an increase in oxyhemoglobin and an increase in signal.

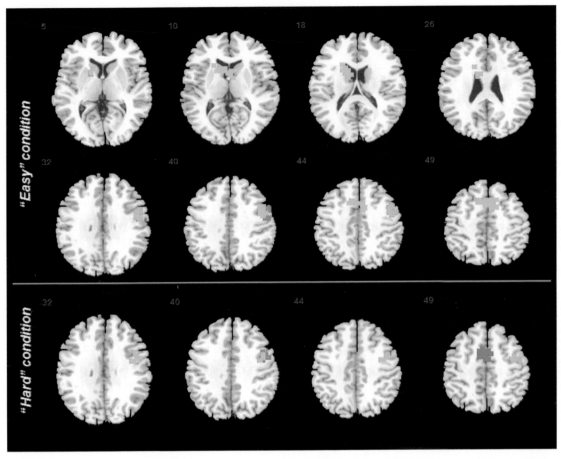

Fig. 7.3. Two-dimensional representative slices are presented for group data with activations displayed on a template image. Numbers indicate z coordinate in standard Talairach space. Brain regions with decreased (yellow) and increased (blue) activation in VPT participants compared with controls during "easy" and "hard" letter trials (adapted from [54]).

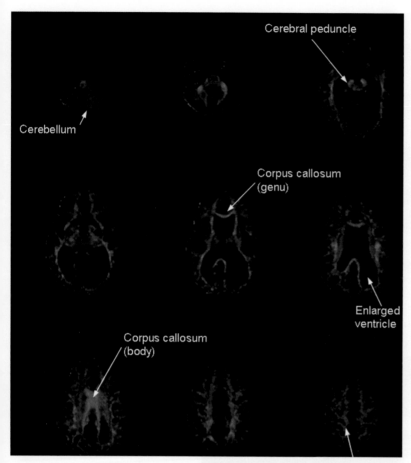

Fig. 8.1. Selected axial cross-sections through the brain of a VPT individual, with color-coding indicating the main orientation of fibers. Red fibers (e.g., corpus callosum) traverse left–right in the plane of the image. Green fibers run antero-posteriorly in the plane of the image. Blue fibers run perpendicular to the plane of the image. This scan is of an 18-year-old female, born at 26 gestational weeks. Enlargement of the lateral ventricles is prominent (University College Hospital London and Institute of Psychiatry Preterm Birth Follow-Up Study).

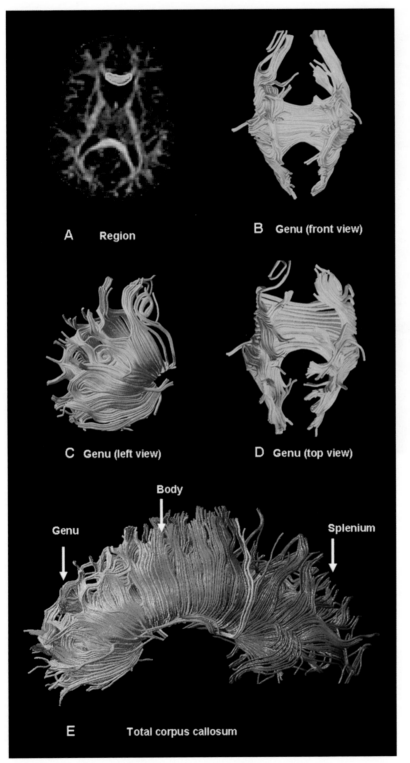

A   Region

B   Genu (front view)

C   Genu (left view)

D   Genu (top view)

Body

Genu

Splenium

E   Total corpus callosum

Fig. 8.2. Tractographic reconstruction of the genu of the corpus callosum. (A) A sample region of interest for tracking the genu is shown in yellow on this single axial slice from the FA map of a single (healthy control) subject. Only one slice is shown, for clarity, but typically the region of interest might extend over several axial slices. Tracts passing through this region are shown in three-dimensional views: (B) from the front; (C) from the left side; (D) from the top. (E) Reconstruction of tracts passing through the whole corpus callosum: genu (yellow); body (green); splenium (red).

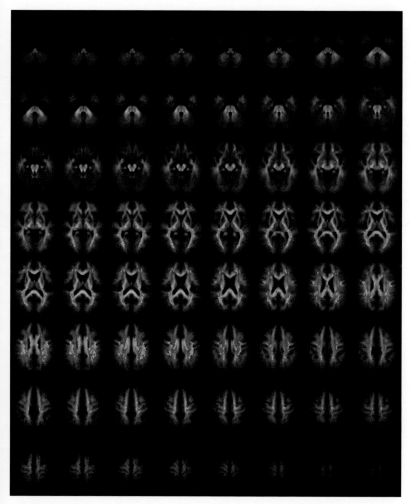

Fig. 8.3. Results of an "optimized VBM" group analysis of FA comparing preterm and term-born adults, using SPM2 (Wellcome Department of Imaging Neurosciences, University College London, UK) and XBAM (Institute of Psychiatry, London, UK: www.brainmap.co.uk/). Serial axial sections are shown, displayed on an FA template. This is the result of a comparison between a group of VPT individuals (born before 33 weeks' gestation) (n = 87) and a group born at term (n = 49), at mean age 19.13 years (range 17–22 years) and 18.54 years (range 17–22 years), respectively. Blue areas indicate significantly lower FA in the preterm group (p = 0.0075); red areas indicate higher FA in the preterm group.

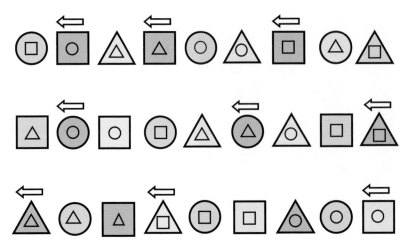

Fig. 15.2. The Contingency Naming Test. In trial 1 children are requested to name the colors of the shape, and in trial 2 the outside shape. In trial 3, the color of the shape is named if the internal and external shapes match, and otherwise the outside shape is named. The same contingency applies for trial 4, except in this trial the rule is reversed for those shapes with a backward arrow.

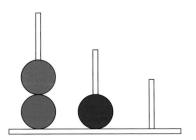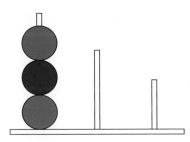

Fig. 15.3. The Tower of London (TOL). The object of the TOL is to move the balls on the pegs from a starting position (left diagram) to achieve a specific configuration (right diagram) following certain rules. In this item the child is allowed 5 moves.

poly-unsaturated fatty acids (LC-PUFA; arachidonic and docosahexaenoic) found in human milk but not bovine milk. A recent study reported that breast milk given to ELBW infants during their stay in the NICU was associated with improved Bayley MDI scores at 18 and 30 months' CA. The total volume of breast milk during hospitalization was calculated for 1035 ELBW infants who participated in the NICHD Neonatal Research Network Glutamine Trial [162]. In the multiple-regression analysis that adjusted for variables typically associated with poor outcomes, increased breast milk ingestion was independently associated with improved neurodevelopmental outcome. For each 10-ml/(kg day) increase in breast milk ingestion, the Bayley MDI score increased by 0.53 points (p = 0.0002), PDI by 0.63 points (p < 0.0001), and Behavior Rating Scale percentile score by 0.82 points (p = 0.0025) [162,163].

Post-discharge environment

Although a disadvantaged environment is well known to be associated with higher rates of cognitive impairment [164], children from high socioeconomic backgrounds still have approximately a 10 point reduction in IQ compared to term controls. Learning disabilities are also seen in higher rates among ELBW children, regardless of socioeconomic background and IQ. When examining predictors of outcomes, environmental factors, including maternal education, maternal IQ, family income, health insurance, and exposure to intervention services, have all been shown to impact on cognitive outcome (see also Chapter 17).

Post-discharge healthcare needs

After discharge, infants are at increased risk of continued complex medical morbidities including CLD requiring home oxygen or ventilator management, gastrointestinal reflux disease, poor feeding, and growth failure. Special healthcare needs which present themselves in the NICU may persist and increase with increasing age. Hack et al. [165] evaluated a cohort of ELBW infants born in 1992–5 at 8 years of age. Compared to age- and gender- matched controls, ELBW children had more asthma requiring therapy (21% versus 9%), took more regular prescribed medications (37% versus 19%), were hospitalized more often after the neonatal period for conditions still present (23% versus 6%), received some type of specialized services such as physical therapy or occupational therapy (31% versus 3%), and had an individualized education plan (39% versus 9%). The ELBW infants also had higher rates of CP (14% versus

none) and low IQ < 70 (15% versus 2%). Of the ELBW children who saw a physician regularly for a chronic condition, 20% saw their pediatrician, 11% an ophthalmologist, 7% an orthopedist, 6% a neurologist, 3% a pulmonologist, 3% an audiologist, and 21% other specialists. Twenty-one of the children had both CP and asthma.

Hack et al. [165] also compared functional outcomes including activities of daily living at 8 years of age between ELBW and normal birth weight children. The ELBW children were reported to have more difficulty feeding themselves (6% versus none), walking (8% versus none), communicating (22% versus 7%), socializing (7% versus 1%), dressing self (13% versus none), bathing (9% versus none), and using the toilet (10% versus none). Since children with neurodevelopmental impairments often have associated chronic medical conditions, more emphasis needs to be focused on examining components of medical sequelae and functional outcomes associated with prematurity other than traditional neurodevelopmental and sensory outcomes, and their effects on cognitive potential.

Comorbidities

Cerebral palsy

Between 8% and 15% of VLBW infants have a diagnosis of CP ranging in severity from mild to severe. The most frequent diagnosis in the preterm infant is spastic diplegia. Preterm infants of 18–22 months' CA with CP have associated low Bayley PDI and MDI scores. A cohort of ELBW infants participating in the NICHD Neonatal Network studies were categorized by neurological status and type of CP at 18–24 months' CA [17] (Table 11.3). One hundred percent of the children with quadriplegia had a PDI < 70 (not shown) and 96% had an MDI < 70. In contrast 41% of children with hemiplegia had an MDI < 70. A significant proportion of children with a CP diagnosis had Bayley MDI scores, however, that were average to low average (70–115), ranging from 23 of 39 (59.0%) with hemiplegia, 33 of 107 (30.8%) with diplegia, 6 of 16 (37.5%) with triplegia, and only 3 of 73 (4.1%) of children with quadriplegia. The majority of children (78.6%) with a normal neurological examination had an IQ score within 2 standard deviations of the mean, compared with only 4.1% of children with spastic quadriplegia. Although children with CP had lower scores than children with a normal neurological examination, there was a significant amount of IQ score variability by type of CP

Table 11.3 Bayley II MDI scores at 18–22 months' corrected age for infants < 1000 g related to neurological abnormalities at 18–22 months' corrected age

Category MDI score	Normal Neurological Exam	Neurological Abnormal Other	Mono-plegia	Hemi-plegia	Diplegia	Triplegia	Quadri-plegia	Hypotonic CP
Subgroup N	1340	129	10	39	107	16	73	28
> 85	49.2%	20.2%	20%	33.4%	17.8%	31.3%	2.7%	12%
70–84	29.4%	34.9%	30%	25.6%	13.1%	6.3%	1.4%	4%
50–69	19.1%	31%	40%	25.6%	37.4%	37.5%	16.4%	24%
< 50	2.3%	14%	10%	15.4%	31.8%	25%	79.5%	60%

Adapted from [17].

and within type of CP, which leads to the importance of assessing functional skills in children with CP.

Functional outcome in the children in this cohort was assessed using the Gross Motor Functional Classification System (GMFCS)) [166–169]. The scoring system ranges from a gross motor skill level of 0 for normal (child walks 10 steps independently) to 5 (unable to maintain antigravity of head/trunk). A score of 3–5 described as moderate to severe CP was found in 76.1% of children with quadriplegia, 31.3% with triplegia, 7.8% with diplegia, and 11.4% with hemiplegia. These findings highlight the importance of performing a comprehensive assessment including the type of CP (number of limbs involved), functional status of the child, and Bayley scores when providing counseling to families regarding cognitive and functional potential.

Msall *et al.* [170] assessed functional skills at 52 months of a cohort of ELBW infants. Fully functional ELBW children free of neurodevelopmental impairments were compared to children with CP and mental retardation (IQ < 68) (Table 11.4). The findings indicate that ELBW survivors at 52 months of age regardless of neurocognitive status remain relatively functional in daily living skills. Children with CP are impacted more in skills requiring motor function, whereas children with mental retardation were impacted more in expressive language and toileting skills.

Vision impairment and retinopathy of prematurity (ROP)

Retinopathy of prematurity remains a common neonatal morbidity and the most common cause of subsequent vision impairments among ELBW infants. Severe threshold ROP occurred in 6% of survivors with a birth weight < 1251 g in the CRYO-ROP multicenter study.

Infants with threshold ROP were the most immature and medically unstable among the cohort. The children were initially evaluated at 5.5 years of age, with acuity testing and a neurodevelopmental functional assessment with the WeeFIM. Rates of severe disability increased from 3.7% for those children with no ROP to 19.7% for those with threshold ROP [171]. A subgroup of the children with threshold ROP was reevaluated at 8 years of age [172]. Overall, 70% of children with an unfavorable vision outcome and 56% with a favorable outcome had a neurodevelopmental, behavioral, or learning disorder. Although rates of neurodevelopmental impairment were high for both groups of children with a history of threshold ROP, it was the children with vision impairment at 8 years who were more likely to have multiple morbidities [172]. The children with unfavorable vision status at 8 years had more developmental disability (57% versus 22%), special education services (63% versus 27%), below grade level academic performance (39% versus 15.8%), and CP (84% versus 48%), compared to the children with a favorable vision outcome. In a recent cohort of ELBW children born in 1996–7 and seen at 5 years of age, 10% had astigmatism, 2% had hypermetropia, 4% had amblyopia, 2% had unilateral amaurosis, and 1% had bilateral amaurosis [173].

The neurodevelopmental outcome of a recent cohort of ELBW infants enrolled in the Schmidt *et al.* [10] study between 1996 and 1998, and diagnosed with severe ROP defined as unilateral or bilateral ROP of stages 4 and 5, was assessed at 18 months' CA. Of the children with severe neonatal ROP, 10% died, 24% had CP, 49% an MDI < 70, 3.8% were deaf and 15% were blind.

Hearing impairment

Congenital hearing loss, which is identified at a rate of 2–3 per/1000 newborns, is the most frequently

Table 11.4 Functional skills of ELBW children at 52 months of age

Functional skill	Non impaired	Cerebral palsy	Mental retardation
N	118	7	15
Walks 30.5 meters	100%	71%	100%
Talks in sentences	100%	100%	93%
Toilets self	100%	71%	93%
Able to use both hands for activities of daily living	100%	71%	100%
Understands simple commands	100%	100%	100%

Adapted from [170].

occurring birth defect. Approximately 15% of infants with permanent hearing loss are NICU graduates [174,175].

Newborns with hearing loss who do not receive early intervention for language development steadily fall behind hearing peers with increasing age in language, cognitive performance, and social skills [176–178]. Extremely low birth weight infants have the disadvantage of prolonged neonatal hospitalization, later onset of early intervention, increased rates of respiratory disease and middle ear effusion, and increased rates of neurodevelopmental comorbidities. Universal hearing screening in NICUs in the United States has led to earlier diagnosis and intervention and improved language skills [178–181]. Studies in the 1990s have reported rates of hearing loss requiring amplification ranging from 1% to 9% [173,182]. Hearing loss requiring amplification is more likely to occur in conjunction with other neonatal morbidities including sepsis [95], NEC [97], BPD, brain injury, and ROP [10].

Congenital anomalies

Most follow-up studies exclude infants with major congenital anomalies from their study sample. The neurodevelopmental outcomes of ELBW infants with anomalies are needed, however, both for counseling parents regarding outcomes and for facilitation of appropriate support and intervention services. The cognitive outcomes of ELBW infants with major anomalies were evaluated in a large cohort of ELBW infants cared for in NICHD Neonatal Network centers [98] (Table 11.2). Mean MDI and PDI scores at the 18- to 22-month follow-up were significantly lower in the anomaly group than in the control group: 68 versus 79, p < 0.001 and 71 versus 83, p < 0.001, respectively. In addition, a greater percentage of children in the anomaly group had MDI scores < 70 (57% versus 31%) and PDI scores < 70 (48% versus 20%),

moderate to severe CP (18% versus 6%), and NDI (65% versus 37%). Regression models adjusting for confounders indicated that infants with severe anomalies had nearly twice the risk of having MDI or PDI scores below 70 compared to ELBW infants without anomalies [98].

Combined neonatal morbidities

Neonatal morbidities associated with adverse outcomes and interventions in the neonatal unit do not occur in isolation, resulting in the need for multivariate analyses to confirm independent effects of predictors. Rates of neurodevelopmental impairment determined at 18 months' CA in the children who participated in the Schmidt et al. [10] trial were analyzed relative to the presence of no neonatal morbidity, one morbidity, two morbidities, and three neonatal morbidities. Morbidities analyzed included BPD, severe brain injury, and severe ROP. For the entire cohort the NDI rate was 35%. However, for children with no morbidities, one morbidity, two morbidities, and three morbidities, the NDI rates were 18%, 42%, 78%, and 88% respectively. These analyses are important, since they provide insight into the differences in NDI rates that may be reported in outcome studies, depending on the definition of the study cohort or subgroups of the cohort. The NDI rate of the children with three neonatal morbidities was almost five times the rate of children with no history of neonatal morbidities.

Early school-age outcomes

Reports of outcomes of extremely preterm infants at school age fairly consistently demonstrate an increased prevalence of cognitive impairment and poor academic achievement [183–185]. Since many studies of school-age outcomes report on a cohort which includes children with neuromotor and sensory abnormalities, it is not unexpected that a significant proportion of the children have poor academic achievement. Although ELBW survivors who are neurologically intact and have average intelligence do better than ELBW children with comorbidities, they also have evidence of less optimal academic achievement when compared with full-term controls of the same age.

Grunau et al. [186] addressed the issue of neurodevelopmental confounders in a study which evaluated cognition in a cohort of preterm children ≤ 800 g with normal intelligence and no neurosensory impairments at 8–9 years of age. The ELBW children were at significantly increased risk of learning disabilities in a number of domains, despite the fact that their mean full-scale IQ was 99.3±11 (normal range). Their IQ, however, was significantly lower than the IQ of the full-term controls IQ (117.3±13). In addition, whereas only 13% of comparison children met criteria for a learning disability in one or more areas, 65% of ELBW children met criteria. Primary areas of disability were written output, arithmetic, and reading. This finding demonstrates that normal intelligence, independently, does not predict academic success. The cohort was largely middle-class white, negating the argument that learning disabilities at school age among former ELBW infants are predominantly among the socioeconomically disadvantaged.

Table 11.5 compares the findings of seven early school-age outcome studies of cohorts that include children with and without neurodevelopmental impairments and the full range of intelligence. Rates of cognitive and achievement deficiencies at early school age have been reported to increase with decreasing birth weight. Hack et al. [43] compared the outcomes of infants with a birth weight < 750 g to infants 750–1499 g and full-term classroom-matched children at 8 years of age, and demonstrated increasing rates of retardation (21%, 8%, and 2%) and placement in special education (45%, 25%, and 14%) with decreasing birth weight, respectively [43]. The children < 750 g had increased rates of below normal performance in cognitive function, academic skills, visual motor skills, gross motor skills, adaptive functioning, and behavior. Multivariate analyses identified severe cranial ultrasound abnormality as a predictor of both mental retardation and CP.

Horwood et al. [187] reported on the outcomes of 298 VLBW survivors from a national birth cohort of New Zealand children born in 1986 at 7–8 years of age. The cohort was divided into infants < 1000 g and 1000–1499 g. The children < 1000 g had the highest rates of below average IQ (Wechsler Intelligence Scale for Children Revised [WSC-R] IQ of < 85) compared to the children 1000–1499 g and controls (25% versus 21% versus 11%, respectively). A need for any form of special education service was also highest in the children < 1000 g compared to the two comparison groups with rates of 27%, 23%, and 9%, respectively.

Vohr et al. evaluated VLBW (600–1250 g) infants who participated in the longitudinal follow-up of the Indomethacin Trial at 3, 4.5, 6, and 8 years of age [11]. Improvement in cognitive and language test scores was observed between 3 and 8 years for children who did not have evidence of severe neonatal brain damage. Severe IVH, PVL, and ventriculomegaly were significantly associated with poor school-age outcomes based on a battery of cognitive, academic, behavioral, and functional assessments [11]. In multivariate analyses, maternal education < 12 years also contributed to poor school-age outcomes. Improvement in cognitive test scores was associated with higher maternal education, two-parent household, and early intervention services if the mother had less than a twelfth grade education.

Marlow et al. [189] reported on a cohort of immature ELBW < 26 weeks' gestation infants evaluated at 6 years of age who were born in the United Kingdom and Ireland in 1995 and enrolled in the EPICure Study. Within this contemporary cohort, 60% received antenatal steroids and 84% received surfactant. Seventy-eight percent of the survivors were evaluated and compared to classmates born at full term. Among these extremely preterm infants, neonatal survival to discharge was: 1% among those born at 22 weeks of gestation, 11% at 23 weeks, 26% at 24 weeks, and 44% at 25 weeks. Disability in this study was defined in the following categories: mild disability as neurological signs with minimal functional consequences or impairments such as squints or refractive errors; moderate disability was defined as reasonable independence, ambulatory CP, an IQ 2–3 standard deviations (SD) below the mean, hearing loss corrected with amplification, and vision impairment without blindness; severe disability was defined as a child highly dependent on caregivers and included non-ambulatory CP, IQ more than 3 SD below the mean, and profound sensorineural hearing loss or blindness. The rates of survival with no evidence of any disability at 6 years of age were: none for infants born at 22 weeks of gestation, 1% at 23 weeks, 3% at 24 weeks, and 8% at 25 weeks.

The study of Anderson et al. [188] evaluated ELBW children born in 1991–2 at 8 years of age and compared

Table 11.5 Cognitive scores at early school age of infants born < 1250 g

Weight	Sample size	DOB	Age	Mean IQ	IQ < 70	Special Education	Country	Author
<750 g	<750 g 68 750–1499 g 65 Term 61	1982–6	6–7 y	<750 g 87 750–1499 g 93 Term 100	<750 g 21% 750–1499 g 8% Term 2%	<750 g 45% 750–1499 g 25% Term 14%	United States	Hack (Hack, et al. [43])
<1000 g	298 VLBW <1000 g 77 1000–1499 g 221 Controls 1092	1986	7–8 y	NA	IQ < 85 <1000 25% 1000–1499 g 21% Control 11%	<1000 g 27% 1000–1499 g 23% Controls 9%	New Zealand	Horwood et al. [87]
<1250 g	384	1989–92	8 y	Indo – IVH 93.2 Saline – IVH 92.5 Indo + IVH 80.5 Saline + IVH 86.2	Indo – IVH 8% Saline – IVH 8% Indo + IVH 40% Saline + IVH 21%	Indo + IVH 79% Saline + IVH 62% Indo – IVH 49% Saline – IVH 47%	United States	Vohr et al. [11]
<1000 g	298	1991–2	8 y	Preterm 95.5 Term 104.9	–9.4 pts –8.8 pts ad. Neuro.[a]	Preterm 38.7% Term 21.5%	Australia	Anderson et al. [188]
<1000 g	219 ELBW 118 ELBW NS[b] Term Controls	1992–1995	8 y	Preterm 87.7 Control 99.8	ELBW 15% ELBW NS 7% Controls 2%	ELBW 48% ELBW NS 41% Controls 12%	United States	Hack et al. [165]
<1000 g <26 w	241	1995	6 y	Preterm girl 82.1 Preterm boy 77.1 Control girl 105.5 Control boy 105.9	Overall 21% 23 w 25% 24 w 27% 25 w 17% Controls 1%	204 Mainstream 34 Special School 3 Mainstream + resource	Great Britain Ireland	Marlow et al. [15]
<1000 g	172	1996–7	5 y	Full cohort 96 AGA < 27 w 96 SGA < 27 w 89	All 9%	19% minor disability 20% major disability 52% received some therapy	Finland	Mikkola et al. [173]

[a]Difference excluding subjects with neurological adversity.
[b]NS Neurosensory intact; excludes children with CP, blind or deaf.
AGA = appropriate for gestational age; NA = not assessed; SGA = small for gestational age.

cognitive outcomes to term children. Although, the IQ of the preterm children was in the normal range (95.5 compared with 104.9 for term controls), it remained 8.8 points lower than controls, after adjusting for neurosensory morbidities, and 7.6 points lower after adjusting for social and environmental confounders. Hack *et al.* [165] evaluated a cohort of 219 ELBW children (92%) of survivors born 1992–5 at 8 years of age and compared their outcomes with term classmate-matched controls. In addition, an analysis was made of the outcomes of the ELBW subgroup with no neurosensory impairments (CP, blind or deaf). Rates of an IQ < 70 on the Kaufman Assessment Battery for Children were 15%, 7%, and 2%, and rates of special education supports were 48%, 41%, and 12% for the total ELBW group, the ELBW sensory intact group and the controls, respectively. The rates of any compensatory dependence need for chronic conditions for more than 12 months duration were 48%, 40%, and 23% for the total ELBW group, the ELBW sensory intact group, and the controls, respectively. Overall 76% of the ELBW children, 72% of the neurosensory intact, and 42% of the controls were identified with a chronic condition in 1 of 3 domains on the Questionnaire for Identifying Children with Chronic Conditions (QUICCC). Their report indicates that ELBW survivors at early school age are at extremely high risk of serious chronic conditions not otherwise reported in standard follow-up studies.

The most recent birth year (1996–7) study by Mikkola *et al.* [173] reported on the outcomes at 5 years of age of a regional cohort of ELBW infants born in Finland. This cohort had only a 9% rate of IQ < 70, however, 19% of the children were classified as having a minor disability, 20% a major disability and 52% were receiving some type of therapy. Factors associated with lower IQ were IVH grade 3–4, male gender, multiparity, multiple pregnancies, vaginal delivery, and no antenatal steroids. Higher social class and each birth weight increment of 100 g were associated with a higher IQ.

These data suggest that there may be different trajectories of development among the heterogeneous group of preterm children. In one cohort of 203 VLBW infants evaluated longitudinally and serially from 1 to 6 years of age, cluster analysis was done to identify distinct developmental profiles [27]. Five clusters of cognitive development between 1 and 6 years of age were identified: average IQ remains stable, average IQ becomes low average, average IQ becomes below average, very low IQ remains low average, and low IQ (> 2 SD below the mean) remains stable. The cluster that remained stable with average IQ had less biomedical risk and the highest maternal education, whereas the stable low IQ cluster had the greatest biomedical risk and the children were most likely to have an abnormal neurological examination at 1 year of age. Developmental trajectories may continue to change past 6 years of age. Hack *et al.* [165] reported that rates of cognitive impairment defined as a 20-month MDI or 8-year Kaufman Assessment Battery for Children < 70 dropped from 39% at 20 months' CA to 16% at 8 years in a cohort of ELBW infants.

Bronchopulmonary dysplasia has been shown to have continued effects on cognition and academic performance in VLBW children at 8 years of age. Short *et al.* [190] reported that children with BPD were more likely to have an IQ < 70 (20% versus 11% versus 3%) and require special education services (54% versus 37% versus 25%) than VLBW children without BPD and term control children, respectively. In addition, IQ scores worsened with increasing severity of BPD. Children with BPD treated with postnatal steroids had even lower IQ scores (72.8 versus 84.8) and a greater need for special education services (78% versus 48%) compared to children with BPD who were not treated with postnatal steroids.

Another important factor which has been shown to have persistent effects on IQ and academic achievement at 6.8 years of age in a cohort of infants < 1500 g at birth is subnormal head size [191]. Current improvements in nutritional management in NICUs and limited use of postnatal steroids may limit the detrimental effects on brain growth in contemporary cohorts.

In summary, effects of ELBW persist throughout childhood and early school age. Multiple biological factors, interventions, comorbidities, and environmental factors mediate the development of cognitive, functional, and academic skills. A determination of whether cognitive outcomes of ELBW infants born in the 1990s are improving, staying the same, or getting worse is complex, and is complicated by the heterogeneous characteristics of the population, including gestational ages ranging from 22 to 28 weeks or higher, and a spectrum of serious neonatal morbidities including IVH, BPD, NEC, sepsis, and ROP. It is troubling that the recent NICHD Neonatal Network publication of Fanaroff *et al.* [7] indicates increasing rates of major neonatal morbidities among ELBW survivors born in the 1990s.

Outcome studies analyzing for effects of specific neonatal morbidities clearly demonstrate the range of effects on cognitive outcomes of ELBW infants (Table 11.2 and Table 11.3). The comparison with term controls brings home the degree of impact on cognition among ELBW survivors, compared to the general population. Add comorbidities to the picture and we can appreciate the approximate 50% need of education support services for ELBW survivors.

Although there is some evidence of improving cognition and language with increasing age, and some improvement reported in studies by year of birth, this may not extend to the most immature infants at the limits of viability. It is, however, apparent that ELBW infants benefit not only from comprehensive perinatal and neonatal intensive care but from post-discharge appropriate comprehensive medical management, behavioral and therapeutic support services, intervention services, and education services that foster optimal development for ELBW survivors, regardless of degree of disability.

References

1. Gilstrap LC, Christensen R, Clewell WH, *et al.* Effect of conticosteroids for fetal maturation on perinatal outcome: NIH Consensus Development Panel on the Effect of Corticosteroids for Fetal Maturation on Perinatal Outcomes. *JAMA* 1995; **273**: 413–18.

2. El-Metwally D, Vohr B, Tucker R. Survival and neonatal morbidity at the limits of viability in the mid 1990s: 22 to 25 weeks. *J Pediatr* 2000; **137**: 616–22.

3. Fanaroff AA, Hack M, Walsh MC. The NICHD neonatal research network: changes in practice and outcomes during the first 15 years. *Semin Perinatol* 2003; **27**: 281–7.

4. Hintz SR, Poole WK, Wright LL., *et al* . Changes in mortality and morbidities among infants born at less than 25 weeks during the post-surfactant era. *Arch Dis Child Fetal Neonatal Ed* 2005; **90**: F128–33.

5. Shankaran S, Johnson Y, Langer JC, *et al.* Outcome of extremely-low-birth-weight infants at highest risk: gestational age < or =24 weeks, birth weight < or =750 g, and 1-minute Apgar < or =3. *Am J Obstet Gynecol* 2004; **191**: 1084–91.

6. Hintz SR, Kendrick DE, Vohr BR, Poole WK, Higgins RD. Changes in neurodevelopmental outcomes at 18 to 22 months' corrected age among infants of less than 25 weeks' gestational age born in 1993–1999. *Pediatrics* 2005; **115**: 1645–51.

7. Fanaroff AA, Stoll BJ, Wright LL, *et al.* Trends in neonatal morbidity and mortality for very low birthweight infants. *Am J Obstet Gynecol* 2007; **196**: 147.e1–8.

8. Hamilton BE, Minino AM, Martin JA, *et al.* Annual summary of vital statistics: 2005. *Pediatrics* 2007; **119**: 345–60.

9. Taylor HG, Klein N, Minich NM, Hack M. Middle-school-age outcomes in children with very low birthweight. *Child Dev* 2000; **71**: 1495–511.

10. Schmidt B, Asztalos EV, Roberts RS, *et al.* Impact of bronchopulmonary dysplasia, brain injury, and severe retinopathy on the outcome of extremely low-birth-weight infants at 18 months: results from the trial of indomethacin prophylaxis in preterms. *JAMA* 2003; **289**: 1124–9.

11. Vohr BR, Allan WC, Westerveld M, *et al.* School-age outcomes of very low birth weight infants in the indomethacin intraventricular hemorrhage prevention trial. *Pediatrics* 2003; **111**: e340–6.

12. Vohr BR, Wright LL, Dusick AM, *et al.* Center differences and outcomes of extremely low birth weight infants. *Pediatrics* 2004; **113**: 781–9.

13. Doyle LW, Anderson PJ. Improved neurosensory outcome at 8 years of age of extremely low birthweight children born in Victoria over three distinct eras. *Arch Dis Child Fetal Neonatal Ed* 2005; **90**: F484–8.

14. Litt J, Taylor HG, Klein N, Hack M. Learning disabilities in children with very low birthweight: prevalence, neuropsychological correlates, and educational interventions. *J Learn Disabil* 2005; **38**: 130–41.

15. Marlow N, Wolke D, Bracewell MA, Samara M. Neurologic and developmental disability at six years of age after extremely preterm birth. *N Engl J Med* 2005; **352**: 9–19.

16. Sherlock RL, Anderson PJ, Doyle LW. Neurodevelopmental sequelae of intraventricular haemorrhage at 8 years of age in a regional cohort of ELBW/very preterm infants. *Early Hum Dev* 2005; **81**: 909–16.

17. Vohr BR, Msall ME, Wilson D, *et al.* Spectrum of gross motor function in extremely low birth weight children with cerebral palsy at 18 months of age. *Pediatrics* 2005; **116**: 123–9.

18. Walsh MC, Morris BH, Wrage LA, *et al.* Extremely low birthweight neonates with protracted ventilation: mortality and 18-month neurodevelopmental outcomes. *J Pediatr* 2005; **146**: 798–804.

19. Vohr BR, Wright LL, Dusick AM,*et al.* Neurodevelopmental and functional outcomes of extremely low birth weight infants in the National Institute of Child Health and Human Developmental Neonatal Research Network, 1993–1994. *Pediatrics* 2000; **105**: 1216–26.

20. Wood NS, Marlow N, Costeloe K, Gibson AT, Wilkinson AR. Neurologic and developmental

disability after extremely preterm birth. EPICure Study Group. *N Engl J Med* 2000; **343**: 378–84.

21. Vohr BR, Wright LL, Poole WK, McDonald SA. Neurodevelopmental outcomes of extremely low birth weight infants <32 weeks' gestation between 1993 and 1998. *Pediatrics* 2005; **116**: 635–43.

22. Bayley N. *Bayley Scales of Infant Development,* 2nd edn. San Antonio, TX: The Psychological Corporation; 1993.

23. Bayley N. *Bayley Scales of Infant and Toddler Development,* 3rd edn. San Antonio, TX: PsychCorp; 2006.

24. Escalona SK. Babies at double hazard: early development of infants at biologic and social risk. *Pediatrics* 1982; **70**: 670–6.

25. Hack M, Breslau N. Very low birth weight infants: effects of brain growth during infancy on intelligence quotient at 3 years of age. *Pediatrics* 1986; **77**: 196–202.

26. Hunt JV, Cooper BA, Tooley WH. Very low birth weight infants at 8 and 11 years of age: role of neonatal illness and family status. *Pediatrics* 1988; **82**: 596–603.

27. Koller H, Lawson K, Rose SA, Wallace I, McCarton, C. Patterns of cognitive development in very low birth weight children during the first six years of life. *Pediatrics* 1997; **99**: 383–9.

28. Ment LR, Vohr B, Allan W, *et al.* Change in cognitive function over time in very low-birth-weight infants. *JAMA* 2003; **289**: 705–11.

29. Wilson-Costello D, Friedman H, Minich N, *et al.* Improved neurodevelopmental outcomes for extremely low birth weight infants in 2000–2002. *Pediatrics* 2007; **119**: 37–45.

30. Piecuch RE, Leonard CH, Cooper BA, *et al.* Outcome of infants born at 24–26 weeks' gestation: II. Neurodevelopmental outcome. *Obstet Gynecol* 1997; **90**: 809–14.

31. Hack M, Wilson-Costello D, Friedman H, *et al.* Neurodevelopment and predictors of outcomes of children with birth weights of less than 1000 g: 1992–1995. *Arch Pediatr Adolesc Med* 2000; **154**: 725–31.

32. Hack M, Friedman H, Fanaroff AA. Outcomes of extremely low birth weight infants. *Pediatrics* 1996; **98**: 931–7.

33. Lorenz JM, Wooliever DE, Jetton JR, Paneth N. A quantitative review of mortality and developmental disability in extremely premature newborns. *Arch Pediatr Adolesc Med* 1998; **152**: 425–35.

34. Jacobs SE, O'Brien K, Inwood S, Kelly EN, Whyte HE. Outcome of infants 23–26 weeks' gestation pre and post surfactant. *Acta Paediatr* 2000; **89**: 959–65.

35. Emsley HC, Wardle SP, Sims DG, Chiswick ML, D'Souza SW. Increased survival and deteriorating developmental outcome in 23 to 25 week old gestation infants, 1990–4 compared with 1984–9. *Arch Dis Child Fetal Neonatal Ed* 1998; **78**: F99–104.

36. Hack M, Fanaroff AA. Outcomes of children of extremely low birthweight and gestational age in the 1990's. *Early Hum Dev* 1999; **53**: 193–218.

37. Bednarek FJ, Weisberger S, Richardson DK, *et al.* Variations in blood transfusions among newborn intensive care units. SNAP II Study Group. *J Pediatr* 1998; **133**: 601–7.

38. Lee SK, Chan K, Ohlson A, *et al.* Canadian NICU Network. Variations in treatment decisions and outcomes of infants <25 weeks gestation: evidence from Canada. *Pediatr Res* 1999; **45**(4) Part 2 of 2: 247A.

39. Richardson DK, Shah BL, Frantz I D, 3rd, *et al.* Perinatal risk and severity of illness in newborns at 6 neonatal intensive care units. *Am J Public Health* 1999; **89**: 511–16.

40. Horbar JD, Rogowski J, Plsek PE, *et al.* Collaborative quality improvement for neonatal intensive care. NIC/Q Project Investigators of the Vermont Oxford Network. *Pediatrics* 2001; **107**: 14–22.

41. Synnes AR, Chien LY, Peliowski A, Baboolal R, Lee SK. Variations in intraventricular hemorrhage incidence rates among Canadian neonatal intensive care units. *J Pediatr* 2001; **138**: 525–31.

42. Grogaard JB, Lindstrom DP, Parker RA, Culley B, Stahlman MT. Increased survival rate in very low birth weight infants (1500 grams or less): no association with increased incidence of handicaps. *J Pediatr* 1990; **117**: 139–46.

43. Hack M, Taylor HG, Klein N, *et al.* School-age outcomes in children with birth weights under 750 g. *N Engl J Med* 1994; **331**: 753–9.

44. Msall ME, Buck GM, Rogers BT, *et al.* Multivariate risks among extremely premature infants. *J Perinatol* 1994; **14**: 41–7.

45. La Pine TR, Jackson JC, Bennett FC. Outcome of infants weighing less than 800 grams at birth: 15 years' experience. *Pediatrics* 1995; **96**: 479–83.

46. Thorndike RI, Hagan EP, Sattler JM. *Stanford-Binet Intelligence Scale,* 4th edn. Chicago, IL: Riverside Publishing; 1986.

47. Wechsler D. *Manual for the Wechsler Intelligence Scale for Children,* 3rd edn. San Antonio, TX: The Psychological Corporation; 1991.

48. Woodcock RW, Johnson MB. *Woodcock-Johnson Psycho-Educational Battery-Revised,* Allen, TX: DLM Teaching Resources; 1989.

49. Elliott CD. *Differential Ability Scales. Introductory and Technical Handbook.* New York, NY: The Psychological Corporation; 1990.

50. McCarthy D. *Manual for the McCarthy Scales of Children's Abilities.* New York, NY: The Psychological Corporation; 1972.

51. Colarusso RH, Mamill D. *Motor-Free Visual Perception Test Manual*. Los Angeles, CA: Western Psychological Services; 1972.

52. Beery K. *Developmental Test of Visual Motor Integration*, 4th edn. Parsippany, NJ: Modern Curriculum Press; 1997.

53. Dunn LM Dunn LM. *PPVT: Peabody Picture Vocabulary Test-Revised Form*. Circle Pines, MN: American Guidance Service; 1981.

54. Hendrick DL, Prather M, Tobin AR. *Sequenced Inventory of Communication Development (SICD) Revised Edition*. Austin, TX: Pro-ed; 1984.

55. Zimmerman IL, Steiner V, Pond R. *Preschool Language Scale*, 3rd edn. San Antonio, TX: The Psychological Corporation; 1992.

56. Coplan J. *Early Language Milestone Scale*, 2nd edn. Austin, TX: Pro-ed; 1993.

57. Bruininks R. *Bruininks-Oseretsky Test of Motor Proficiency*. Circle Pines, MN: American Guidance Service; 1978.

58. Folio MR, Fewell RR. *Peabody Developmental Motor Scales and Activity Cards*. Allen, TX: Developmental Learning Materials Resource; 1983.

59. Harrison P, Kaufman AS, Kaufman NL, *et al. Early Screening Profiles (ESP)*. Circle Pines, MN: American Guidance Service; 1990.

60. Palisano RJ. Validity of goal attainment scaling in infants with motor delays. *Phys Ther* 1993; **73**: 651–8; discussion 658–60.

61. Larson SL, Vitali GJ. *Kindergarten Readiness Test (KRT)* East Aura, NY: Slosson Educational Publication; 1988.

62. Miller LJ. *Miller Assessment for Preschoolers (MAP)*. San Antonio, TX: The Psychological Corporation; 1998.

63. Ireton H. *Child Development Inventory*. Minneapolis, MN: Behavior Science Systems; 1992.

64. Nehring AD, Nehring EM, Bruni JR, *et al. Learning Accomplishment Profile – Diagnostic (LAP-D) Standardized Assessment – 1992 Revision and Standardization*. Lewisville, NC: Kaplan Press, Examiner's Manual; 1992.

65. Newborg J, Stock JR, Wnek L. *Battelle Developmental Inventory and Recalibrated Technical Data and Norms: Examiner's Manual*. Allen, TX: DLM, LINC Associates; 1984.

66. Sparrow S, Balla D, Cicchetti D. *Vineland Adaptive Behavior Scales: Interview Edition, Survey Form Manual. A Revision of the Vineland Social Maturity Scale by E. A. Doll*. Circle Pines, MN: American Guidance Service; 1984.

67. Msall ME, Digaudio K, Duffy LC, *et al.* WeeFIM. Normative sample of an instrument for tracking functional independence in children. *Clin Pediatr (Phila)* 1994; **33**: 431–8.

68. Msall ME. Functional assessment in neurodevelopmental disabilities. In: Capute AJ, Accardo P J, eds. *Developmental Disabilities in Infancy and Children*, 2nd edn. Baltimore, MD: Paul Brookes Publishing. 1997; 371–92.

69. Granger CV, Seltzer GB, Fishbein CF. (eds.) *Primary Care of the Functionally Disabled: Assessment and Management*. Philadelphia, PA: J.B. Lippincott Company; 1987.

70. World Health Organization. *International Classification of Impairments, Disabilities and Handicaps: A Manual of Classification Relating to the Consequences of Disease*. Geneva, Switzerland: World Health Organization; 1980.

71. National Advisory Board on Medical Rehabilitation Research. *Report and Plan for Medical Rehabilitation Research (NIH Publication No. 93–3509)*. Bethesda, MD: National Center for Medical Rehabilitation Research; 1993.

72. World Health Organization. *International Classification of Functioning, Disability and Health*. Geneva: World Health Organization; 2001.

73. Haley SM, Coster WJ, Ludlow LH, *et al. Pediatric Evaluation of Disability Inventory (PEDI), Version I, Development, Standardization and Administration Manual*. Boston, MA: New England Medical Center-PEDI Research Group; 1992.

74. Allan WC, Vohr B, Makuch RW, Katz KH, Ment LR. Antecedents of cerebral palsy in a multicenter trial of indomethacin for intraventricular hemorrhage. *Arch Pediatr Adolesc Med* 1997; **151**: 580–5.

75. Donovan E F, Ehrenkranz R A, Shankaran S, *et al.* Outcomes of very low birth weight twins cared for in the National Institute of Child Health and Human Development Neonatal Research Network's intensive care units. *Am J Obstet Gynecol* 1998; **179**: 742–9.

76. Dexter S C, Malee M P, Pinar H, *et al.* Influence of chorioamnionitis on developmental outcome in very low birth weight infants. *Obstet Gynecol* 1999; **94**: 267–73.

77. Wharton KN, Pinar H, Stonestreet BS, *et al*. Severe umbilical cord inflammation-a predictor of periventricular leukomalacia in very low birth weight infants. *Early Hum Dev* 2004; **77**: 77–87.

78. Bada HS, Das A, Bauer CR, *et al.* Low birth weight and preterm births: etiologic fraction attributable to prenatal drug exposure. *J Perinatol* 2005; **25**: 631–7.

79. Blondel B, Macfarlane A, Gissler M, Breart G, Zeitlin J. Preterm birth and multiple pregnancy in European countries participating in the PERISTAT project. *BJOG* 2006; **113**: 528–35.

80. Perlman JM. White matter injury in the preterm infant: an important determination of abnormal neurodevelopment outcome. *Early Hum Dev* 1998; **53**: 99–120.

81. Hamilton BE, Martin JA, Ventura SJ, Sutton PD, Menacker F. Births: preliminary data for 2004. *Natl Vital Stat Rep* 2005; **54:** 1–17.

82. Martin JA, Kochanek KD, Strobino DM, Guyer B, Macdorman MF. Annual summary of vital statistics – 2003. *Pediatrics* 2005; **115:** 619–34.

83. Martin JA, Hamilton BE, Sutton PD, *et al.* Births: final data for 2002. *Natl Vital Stat Rep* 2003; **52:** 1–113.

84. Barrett JF. Delivery of the term twin. *Best Pract Res Clin Obstet Gynaecol* 2004; **18:** 625–30.

85. Pharoah PO. Neurological outcome in twins. *Semin Neonatol* 2002; **7:** 223–30.

86. Ferriero DM. Neonatal brain injury. *N Engl J Med* 2004; **351:** 1985–95.

87. Hack M, Fanaroff AA. Outcomes of extremely-low-birth-weight infants between 1982 and 1988. *N Engl J Med* 1989; **321:** 1642–7.

88. Allen MC, Donohue PK, Dusman AE. The limit of viability – neonatal outcome of infants born at 22 to 25 weeks' gestation. *N Engl J Med* 1993; **329:** 1597–601.

89. Vohr BR, Allen M. Extreme prematurity – the continuing dilemma. *N Engl J Med* 2005; **352:** 71–2.

90. Ferrara TB, Couser RJ, Hoekstra RE. Side effects and long-term follow-up of corticosteroid therapy in very low birthweight infants with bronchopulmonary dysplasia. *J Perinatol* 1990; **10:** 137–42.

91. Huttenlocher PR. Morphometric study of human cerebral cortex development. *Neuropsychologia* 1990; **28:** 517–27.

92. Huttenlocher PR, Dabholkar AS. Regional differences in synaptogenesis in human cerebral cortex. *J Comp Neurol* 1997; **387:** 167–78.

93. MacDonald H. Perinatal care at the threshold of viability. *Pediatrics* 2002; **110:** 1024–7.

94. De Groote I, Vanhaesebrouck P, Bruneel E, *et al.* Outcome at 3 years of age in a population-based cohort of extremely preterm infants. *Obstet Gynecol* 2007; **110:** 855–64.

95. Stoll BJ, Hansen NI, Adams-Chapman I, *et al.* Neurodevelopmental and growth impairment among extremely low-birth-weight infants with neonatal infection. *JAMA* 2004; **292:** 2357–65.

96. Ehrenkranz RA, Walsh MC, Vohr BR, *et al.* Validation of the National Institutes of Health consensus definition of bronchopulmonary dysplasia. *Pediatrics* 2005; **116:** 1353–60.

97. Hintz SR, Kendrick DE, Stoll BJ, *et al.* Neurodevelopmental and growth outcomes of extremely low birth weight infants after necrotizing enterocolitis. *Pediatrics* 2005; **115:** 696–703.

98. Walden R, Taylor S, Hansen N, *et al.* Major congenital anomalies place ELBW infants at higher risk for poor growth and developmental outcomes. *Pediatrics* 2007; **120:** e1512–19.

99. Laptook AR, O'Shea TM, Shankaran S, Bhaskar B. Adverse neurodevelopmental outcomes among extremely low birth weight infants with a normal head ultrasound: prevalence and antecedents. *Pediatrics* 2005; **115:** 673–80.

100. Mirmiran M, Barnes PD, Keller K, *et al.* Neonatal brain magnetic resonance imaging before discharge is better than serial cranial ultrasound in predicting cerebral palsy in very low birth weight preterm infants. *Pediatrics* 2004; **114:** 992–8.

101. Woodward LJ, Anderson PJ, Austin NC, Howard K, Inder TE. Neonatal MRI to predict neurodevelopmental outcomes in preterm infants. *N Engl J Med* 2006; **355:** 685–94.

102. Henderson-Smart DJ, Bhuta T, Cools F, Offringa M. Elective high frequency oscillatory ventilation versus conventional ventilation for acute pulmonary dysfunction in preterm infants. *Cochrane Database Syst Rev* 2003; (4): CD000104.

103. Papile LA, Burstein J, Burstein R, Koffler H. Incidence and evolution of subependymal and intraventricular hemorrhage: a study of infants with birth weights less than 1,500 gm. *J Pediatr* 1978; **92:** 529–34.

104. Chamnanvanakij S, Margraf LR, Burns D, Perlman JM. Apoptosis and white matter injury in preterm infants. *Pediatr Dev Pathol* 2002; **5:** 184–9.

105. Shalak L, Perlman JM. Hemorrhagic-ischemic cerebral injury in the preterm infant: current concepts. *Clin Perinatol* 2002; **29:** 745–63.

106. Perlman JM. Summary proceedings from the neurology group on hypoxic-ischemic encephalopathy. *Pediatrics* 2006; **117:** S28–33.

107. Wheater M, Rennie JM. Perinatal infection is an important risk factor for cerebral palsy in very-low-birthweight infants. *Dev Med Child Neurol* 2000; **42:** 364–7.

108. Brothwood M, Wolke D, Gamsu H, Benson J, Cooper D. Prognosis of the very low birthweight baby in relation to gender. *Arch Dis Child* 1986, **61:** 559–64.

109. Hoffman EL, Bennett FC. Birth weight less than 800 grams: changing outcomes and influences of gender and gestation number. *Pediatrics* 1990; **86:** 27–34.

110. Tyson JE, Younes N, Verter J, Wright LL. Viability, morbidity, and resource use among newborns of 501- to 800-g birth weight. National Institute of Child Health and Human Development Neonatal Research Network. *JAMA* 1996; **276:** 1645–51.

111. Stevenson DK, Verter J, Fanaroff AA, *et al.* Sex differences in outcomes of very low birthweight infants: the newborn male disadvantage. *Arch Dis Child Fetal Neonatal Ed* 2000; **83:** F182–5.

112. Lemons JA, Bauer CR, Oh W, *et al.* Very low birth weight outcomes of the National Institute of Child health and human development neonatal research network, January 1995 through December 1996. NICHD Neonatal Research Network. *Pediatrics* 2001; **107:** E1.

113. Elsmen E, Hansen Pupp I, Hellstrom-Westas L. Preterm male infants need more initial respiratory and circulatory support than female infants. *Acta Paediatr* 2004; **93:** 529–33.

114. Msall ME, Buck GM, Rogers BT, *et al.* Predictors of mortality, morbidity, and disability in a cohort of infants < or = 28 weeks' gestation. *Clin Pediatr (Phila)* 1993; **32:** 521–7.

115. Hindmarsh G J, O' Callaghan MJ, Mohay HA, Rogers YM. Gender differences in cognitive abilities at 2 years in ELBW infants. Extremely low birth weight. *Early Hum Dev* 2000; **60:** 115–22.

116. Hoekstra RE, Ferrara TB, Couser RJ, Payne NR, Connett JE. Survival and long-term neurodevelopmental outcome of extremely premature infants born at 23–26 weeks' gestational age at a tertiary center. *Pediatrics* 2004; **113:** e1–6.

117. Hintz SR, Kendrick DE, Vohr BR, Kenneth Poole W, Higgins RD, For the Nichd Neonatal Research, Networks. Gender differences in neurodevelopmental outcomes among extremely preterm, extremely-low-birthweight infants. *Acta Paediatr* 2006; **95:** 1239–48.

118. Kaufman A, Kaufman N. *Kaufman Assessment Battery for Children (K-ABC).* Circle Pines, MN: American Guidance Service; 1983.

119. Ment LR, Vohr BR, Makuch RW, *et al.* Prevention of intraventricular hemorrhage by indomethacin in male preterm infants. *J Pediatr* 2004; **145:** 832–4.

120. Reiss AL, Kesler SR, Vohr B, *et al.* Sex differences in cerebral volumes of 8-year-olds born preterm. *J Pediatr* 2004; **145:** 242–9.

121. Wright LL, Horbar JD, Gunkel H, *et al.* Evidence from multicenter networks on the current use and effectiveness of antenatal corticosteroids in low birth weight infants. *Am J Obstet Gynecol* 1995; **173:** 263–9.

122. Yeh TF, Lin YJ, Hsieh WS, *et al.* Early postnatal dexamethasone therapy for the prevention of chronic lung disease in preterm infants with respiratory distress syndrome: a multicenter clinical trial. *Pediatrics* 1997; **100:** E3.

123. Yeh TF, Lin YJ, Huang CC, *et al.* Early dexamethasone therapy in preterm infants: a follow-up study. *Pediatrics* 1998; **101:** E7.

124. Hack M, Breslau N, Weissman B, *et al.* Effect of very low birth weight and subnormal head size on cognitive abilities at school age. *N Engl J Med* 1991; **325:** 231–7.

125. Murphy BP, Inder TE, Huppi PS, *et al.* Impaired cerebral cortical gray matter growth after treatment with dexamethasone for neonatal chronic lung disease. *Pediatrics* 2001; **107:** 217–21.

126. Ment LR, Oh W, Ehrenkranz RA, *et al.* Low-dose indomethacin and prevention of intraventricular hemorrhage: a multicenter randomized trial. *Pediatrics* 1994; **93:** 543–50.

127. Ment LR, Vohr B, Oh W, *et al.* Neurodevelopmental outcome at 36 months' corrected age of preterm infants in the Multicenter Indomethacin Intraventricular Hemorrhage Prevention Trial. *Pediatrics* 1996; **98:** 714–18.

128. Ment LR, Vohr B, Allan W, *et al.* Outcome of children in the indomethacin intraventricular hemorrhage prevention trial. *Pediatrics* 2000; **105:** 485–91.

129. Schmidt B, Davis P, Moddemann D, *et al.* Long-term effects of indomethacin prophylaxis in extremely-low-birth-weight infants. *N Engl J Med* 2001; **344:** 1966–72.

130. Ehrenkranz RA, Younes N, Lemons JA, *et al.* Longitudinal growth of hospitalized very low birth weight infants. *Pediatrics* 1999; **104:** 280–9.

131. Ehrenkranz RA. Growth outcomes of very low-birth weight infants in the newborn intensive care unit. *Clin Perinatol* 2000; **27:** 325–45.

132. Steward DK, Pridham KF. Growth patterns of extremely low-birth-weight hospitalized preterm infants. *J Obstet Gynecol Neonatal Nurs* 2002; **31:** 57–65.

133. Clark R H, Thomas P, Peabody J. Extrauterine growth restriction remains a serious problem in prematurely born neonates. *Pediatrics* 2003; **111:** 986–90.

134. Dusick A M, Poindexter BB, Ehrenkranz RA, Lemons JA . Growth failure in the preterm infant: can we catch up? *Semin Perinatol* 2003; **27:** 302–10.

135. Poindexter BB, Langer JC, Dusick AM, Ehrenkranz RA. Early provision of parenteral amino acids in extremely low birth weight infants: relation to growth and neurodevelopmental outcome. *J Pediatr* 2006; **148:** 300–5.

136. Hack M, Schluchter M, Cartar L, *et al.* Growth of very low birth weight infants to age 20 years. *Pediatrics* 2003; **112:** e30–8.

137. Ehrenkranz RA, Dusick AM, Vohr B R, *et al.* Growth in the neonatal intensive care unit influences neurodevelopmental and growth outcomes of extremely low birth weight infants. *Pediatrics* 2006; **117:** 1253–61.

138. Tsang RC, Uauy R, Koletzko B, Zlotkin SH. (eds.) *Nutritional Needs of the Preterm Infant. Scientific Basis and Practical Guidelines.* Baltimore, MD: Williams & Wilkins; 1993.

139. American Academy of Pediatrics, Committee on Nutrition. Nutritional needs of the preterm infant In: *Pediatric Nutrition Handbook*, 5th edn. Elk Grove Village: American Academy of Pediatrics. 2004; 23–53.

140. Premji SS, Fenton TR, Sauve RS. Higher versus lower protein intake in formula-fed low birth weight infants. *Cochrane Database Syst Rev* 2006; (1): CD003959.

141. Gross SJ, Oehler JM, Eckerman CO. Head growth and developmental outcome in very low-birth-weight infants. *Pediatrics* 1983; **71**: 70–5.

142. Hack M, Breslau N, Fanaroff AA. Differential effects of intrauterine and postnatal brain growth failure in infants of very low birth weight. *Am J Dis Child* 1989; **143**: 63–8.

143. Brandt I, Sticker EJ, Lentze MJ. Catch-up growth of head circumference of very low birth weight, small for gestational age preterm infants and mental development to adulthood. *J Pediatr* 2003; **142**: 463–8.

144. Lucas A, Gore SM, Cole TJ, et al. Multicentre trial on feeding low birthweight infants: effects of diet on early growth. *Arch Dis Child* 1984; **59**: 722–30.

145. Pollock JI. Mother's choice to provide breast milk and developmental outcome. *Arch Dis Child* 1989; **64**: 763–4.

146. Jacobson SW, Jacobson JL, Dobbing J, Beijers RJ W. Breastfeeding and intelligence. *Lancet* 1992; **339**: 926.

147. Lucas A, Morley R, Cole TJ, Lister G, Leeson-Payne C. Breast milk and subsequent intelligence quotient in children born preterm. *Lancet* 1992; **339**: 261–4.

148. Lucas A, Morley R, Cole TJ, Gore SM. A randomised multicentre study of human milk versus formula and later development in preterm infants. *Arch Dis Child Fetal Neonatal Ed* 1994; **70**: F141–6.

149. Gale CR, Martyn CN. Breastfeeding, dummy use, and adult intelligence. *Lancet* 1996; **347**: 1072–5.

150. Lucas A, Fewtrell MS, Morley R, et al. Randomized outcome trial of human milk fortification and developmental outcome in preterm infants. *Am J Clin Nutr* 1996; **64**: 142–51.

151. Lucas A, Morley R, Cole TJ. Randomised trial of early diet in preterm babies and later intelligence quotient. *BMJ* 1998; **317**: 1481–7.

152. Horwood LJ, Darlow BA, Mogridge N. Breast milk feeding and cognitive ability at 7–8 years. *Arch Dis Child Fetal Neonatal Ed* 2001; **84**: F23–7.

153. Ooylan LM, Hart S, Porter KB, Driskell JA. Vitamin B-6 content of breast milk and neonatal behavioral functioning. *J Am Diet Assoc* 2002; **102**: 1433–8.

154. Hart S, Boylan LM, Carroll S, Musick YA, Lampe RM. Brief report: breast-fed one-week-olds demonstrate superior neurobehavioral organization. *J Pediatr Psychol* 2003; **28**: 529–34.

155. Horne RS, Parslow PM, Ferens D, Watts AM, Adamson TM. Comparison of evoked arousability in breast and formula fed infants. *Arch Dis Child* 2004; **89**: 22–5.

156. Frank AL, Taber LH, Glezen WP, et al. Breast-feeding and respiratory virus infection. *Pediatrics* 1982; **70**: 239–45.

157. Savilahti E, Jarvenpaa AL, Raiha NC. Serum immunoglobulins in preterm infants: comparison of human milk and formula feeding. *Pediatrics* 1983; **72**: 312–16.

158. Howie PW, Forsyth JS, Ogston SA, Clark A, Florey CD. Protective effect of breast feeding against infection. *BMJ* 1990; **300**: 11–16.

159. Covert RF, Barman N, Domanico RS, Singh JK. Prior enteral nutrition with human milk protects against intestinal perforation in infants who develop necrotizing enterocolitis. *Pediatr Res* 1995; **37**: 305A.

160. Hylander MA, Strobino DM, Dhanireddy R. Human milk feedings and infection among very low birth weight infants. *Pediatrics* 1998; **102**: E38.

161. Bier J, Oliver TL, Ferguson A, Vohr BR. Human milk reduces outpatient infections in very low birth weight infants. *Pediatr Res* 1999; **45**: 120A.

162. Vohr BR, Poindexter BB, Dusick AM, et al. Beneficial effects of breast milk in the neonatal intensive care unit on the developmental outcome of extremely low birth weight infants at 18 months of age. *Pediatrics* 2006; **118**: e115–23.

163. Vohr BR, Dusick AM, Mc Kinley LT, Langer J. Effects of human milk (HM) in the NICU on the developmental outcome and growth of ELBW infants at 30 months of age. *Pediatr Res* 2005; **57**: 146.

164. Hack M, Klein NK, Taylor HG. Long-term developmental outcomes of low birth weight infants. *Future Child* 1995; **5**: 176–96.

165. Hack M, Taylor HG, Drotar D, et al. Chronic conditions, functional limitations, and special health care needs of school-aged children born with extremely low-birth-weight in the 1990s. *JAMA* 2005; **294**: 318–25.

166. Russell DJ, Rosenbaum PL, Cadman DT, et al. The gross motor function measure: a means to evaluate the effects of physical therapy. *Dev Med Child Neurol* 1989; **31**: 341–52.

167. Palisano R, Rosenbaum P, Walter S, et al. Development and reliability of a system to classify gross motor function in children with cerebral palsy. *Dev Med Child Neurol* 1997; **39**: 214–23.

168. Russell DJ, Avery LM, Rosenbaum P, et al. Improved scaling of the gross motor function measure for children with cerebral palsy: Evidence of reliability and validity. *Phys Ther* 2000; **80**: 873–85.

169. Russell DJ, Avery LM, Rosenbaum PL, *et al. Gross Motor Function Measure (GMFM-66 & GMFM-88) User's Manual.* London, UK: Mackeith Press; 2002.

170. Msall ME, Rogers BT, Buck GM, *et al.* Functional status of extremely preterm infants at kindergarten entry. *Dev Med Child Neurol* 1993; **35**: 312–20.

171. Msall ME, Phelps DL, Digaudio KM, *et al.* Severity of neonatal retinopathy of prematurity is predictive of neurodevelopmental functional outcome at age 5.5 years. Behalf of the Cryotherapy for Retinopathy of Prematurity Cooperative Group. *Pediatrics* 2000; **106**: 998–1005.

172. Msall ME, Phelps DL, Hardy RJ, *et al.* Educational and social competencies at 8 years in children with threshold retinopathy of prematurity in the CRYO-ROP multicenter study. *Pediatrics* 2004; **113**: 790–9.

173. Mikkola K, Ritari N, Tommiska V, *et al.* Neurodevelopmental outcome at 5 years of age of a national cohort of extremely low birth weight infants who were born in 1996–1997. *Pediatrics* 2005; **116**: 1391–400.

174. Roizen NJ. Etiology of hearing loss in children. Nongenetic causes. *Pediatr Clin North Am* 1999; **46**: 49–64.

175. Hille ET, Van Straaten HI, Verkerk PH. Prevalence and independent risk factors for hearing loss in NICU infants. *Acta Paediatr* 2007; **96**: 1155–8.

176. Apuzzo ML Yoshinaga-Itano C. Early identification of infants with significant hearing loss and the Minnesota Child Development Inventory. *Semin Hear* 1995; **16**: 124–37.

177. Calderon R, Bargones J, Sidman S. Characteristics of hearing families and their young deaf and hard of hearing children. Early intervention follow-up. *Am Ann Deaf* 1998; **143**: 347–62.

178. Yoshinaga-Itano C, Sedey AL, Coulter DK, Mehl AL. Language of early- and later-identified children with hearing loss. *Pediatrics* 1998; **102**: 1161–71.

179. Yoshinaga-Itano C. The social-emotional ramifications of universal newborn hearing screening: early identification and intervention of children who are deaf or hard of hearing. In: *Proceedings of the Second International Pediatric Conference: A Sound Foundation Through Early Amplification.* Retrieved June 27, 2005 from: www.phonak.com/professional/informationpool/proceedings2001.htm.

180. Yoshinaga-Itano C. Early intervention after universal neonatal hearing screening: impact on outcomes. *Ment Retard Dev Disabil Res Rev* 2003; **9**: 252–66.

181. Yoshinaga-Itano C. From screening to early identification and intervention: discovering predictors to successful outcomes for children with significant hearing loss. *J Deaf Stud Deaf Educ* 2003; **8**: 11–30.

182. Doyle LW, Cheung MM, Ford GW, *et al.* Birth weight <1501 g and respiratory health at age 14. *Arch Dis Child* 2001; **84**: 40–4.

183. Whitfield MF, Eckstein Grunau RV, Holsti L. Extremely premature (≤ 800 g) school-children: multiple areas of hidden disability. *Arch Dis Child* 1997; **77**: P85–90.

184. Taylor HG, Klein N, Hack M. School-age consequences of birth weight less than 750 g: a review and update. *Dev Neuropsychol* 2000; **17**: 289–321.

185. Saigal S, Den Ouden L, Wolke D, *et al.* School-age outcomes in children who were extremely low birth weight from four international population-based cohorts. *Pediatrics* 2003; **112**: 943–50.

186. Grunau RE, Whitfield MF, Davis C. Pattern of learning disabilities in children with extremely low birth weight and broadly average intelligence. *Arch Pediatr Adolesc Med* 2002; **156**: 615–20.

187. Horwood LJ, Mogridge N, Darlow BA. Cognitive, educational, and behavioural outcomes at 7 to 8 years in a national very low birthweight cohort. *Arch Dis Child Fetal Neonatal Ed* 1998; **79**: F12–20.

188. Anderson P, Doyle LW. Neurobehavioral outcomes of school-age children born extremely low birth weight or very preterm in the 1990s. *JAMA* 2003; **289**: 3264–72.

189. Marlow N, Hennessy EM, Bracewell MA, Wolke D. Motor and executive function at 6 years of age after extremely preterm birth. *Pediatrics* 2007; **120**: 793–804.

190. Short EJ, Klein NK, Lewis BA, *et al.* Cognitive and academic consequences of bronchopulmonary dysplasia and very low birth weight: 8-year-old outcomes. *Pediatrics* 2003; **112**: e359.

191. Peterson J, Taylor HG, Minich N, Klein N, Hack M. Subnormal head circumference in very low birth weight children: neonatal correlates and school-age consequences. *Early Hum Dev* 2006; **82**: 325–34.

Chapter 12

Methodological considerations in neurodevelopmental outcome studies of infants born prematurely

Glen P. Aylward

Introduction

It is established that infants born preterm are at increased risk for a variety of later developmental and health problems when compared to their full-term counterparts [1]. These problems include central nervous system (CNS), sensory, motor, cognitive, learning, behavioral, socio-emotional, quality of life, and health concerns [2]. While morbidity is greatest for infants born at the earliest gestational ages, more preterm infants are born closer to term (i.e., 32–36 weeks' gestational age) and these so-called late preterm infants also experience more problems than their full-term peers. However, reported outcomes are based on group probabilities, leaving the outcome of an individual infant less clear.

Numerous biological and environmental factors affect outcomes in addition to birth weight and gestational age. These influences, which are a source of variability, span the pre-, peri-, and postnatal periods and beyond. Among the multiple factors associated with a biological risk condition such as very low birth weight (VLBW, < 1500 g) or extremely low gestational age are: (1) severity of medical complications during the neonatal course (admission status, response to medical interventions, types of medical procedures, duration of hospitalization); (2) sociodemographic factors (socioeconomic status [SES], social support, ethnicity, maternal physical and mental health, environmental exposures to positive and negative experiences); and (3) subsequent illness (rehospitalizations, need for supplemental oxygen, other chronic conditions)[1,3].

Neurodevelopmental outcome, the focus of this chapter, is increasingly used as the benchmark to determine efficacy of medical interventions or the consequences of being born early [4]. Unfortunately, long-term follow-up studies of neurodevelopmental outcome are infrequent, due to increased subject dropout and cost, the long-standing bias that neurodevelopmental data are not as precise as biochemical or radiographic measurements, discrepancies caused by mediating and moderating background variables such as the home environment and family socioeconomic status, and the extended time frame required to complete longitudinal outcome assessments [2,4]. Nonetheless, long-term follow-up is critical in order to identify possible negative effects that prematurity, a medical intervention, or a standard of care might have on the child that are not obvious in the first years of life. The need for extended follow-up for identification of later problems is clearly demonstrated in the use of postnatal steroids for the treatment of chronic lung disease, where there were immediate positive effects, but negative consequences that became obvious later[5].

In addition to the earlier emphasis on major disabilities (moderate/severe mental retardation, cerebral palsy, sensory impairments [visual/auditory], and epilepsy), interest has shifted to the evaluation of more subtle, high-prevalence/low-severity dysfunctions. These include learning disabilities, attention deficit hyperactivity disorders (ADHD), behavioral problems, low average to borderline intelligence, specific neuropsychological deficits (such as poor visual motor integration and deficits in spatial relations), language disorders, and executive dysfunction. Moreover, many children who were born prematurely experience concomitant problems in more than one outcome area (e.g., a combination of executive dysfunction, ADHD, and a learning disability). The combination of multiple, less severe problems works in a more subtle, synergistic

Neurodevelopmental Outcomes of Preterm Birth, ed. Chiara Nosarti, Robin M. Murray, and Maureen Hack. Published by Cambridge University Press. © Cambridge University Press 2010.

fashion to create functional difficulties that potentially are as disabling as some of the major disabilities [1].

While major disabilities (found in 15–20% of those born VLBW and 20–25% in those born extremely low birth weight [ELBW, < 1000 g]) are often identified early during infancy, high-prevalence/low-severity dysfunctions (found in 50–70% of very premature infants) become more obvious as the child grows older, further underscoring the need for prolonged follow-up. At present there are no good predictors of these more subtle problems that can be identified during infancy or preschool age. Moreover, it is extremely difficult to determine whether developmental problems identified during infancy are transient and the result of continuing recovery or catch-up from the negative effects of prematurity, or if they reflect the emergence of a more permanent deficit[6,7].

However, neurodevelopmental follow-up studies often contain methodological flaws that compromise findings. Approximately 15 years ago, we undertook a meta-analysis of 80 follow-up studies published over the preceding decade [8] and pooled outcome results of 4006 infants < 2500 g, and 1568 controls. Eleven major problems were identified in these low birth weight (LBW) follow-up studies. These were: inadequate description of the subject population, the perinatal course not considered, single-hospital samples, lack of appropriate comparison groups, excessively high dropout, no assessment or control for environment, too short duration of follow-up, global or vague outcome measures, variability in diagnostic criteria, inclusion of severely handicapped children in the computation of mean scores, and lack of consensus on correction for prematurity. Similar problems have been cited in more recent reviews [2,9,10] with the inclusion of several recurrent issues: (1) use of gestational age versus birth weight, (2) changes in test instruments, (3) use of neuropsychological "batteries," (4) changes in medical procedures (e.g., surfactant, steroids, ventilation), (5) environmental issues, and (6) the need to include quality-of-life measures. Comparability across studies is further reduced because of a lack of central focus or framework for actual data collection due to the diversity of purposes for follow-up.

Contemporary methodological problems can be distilled into four broad areas: (1) conceptualization/design issues (cause–effect inferences, mediators/moderators, selection of control groups), (2) subject populations (consideration of birth weight and gestational age, use of broad, geographically representative groups, comparable age cohorts), (3) procedural issues (measurement of confounding variables, correction for prematurity, consideration of biological risk issues), and (4) measurement/outcome (lack of a developmental "gold standard," consideration of the Flynn effect [mean IQ scores increase approximately 0.5 point per year], duration of follow-up, comparability of tests, inclusion/exclusion of children with major handicap)[3,8,11].

These problems can dramatically bias interpretation of rates of disability in certain conditions (e.g., ELBW) or how the efficacy of an intervention is gauged. Methodological problems may also affect how certain biological or environmental variables are viewed. More specifically, these problems could determine whether certain variables are considered a *resource* (would yield a positive benefit in the presence or absence of a stressor; e.g. early intervention would help both preterm and full-term infants), a *protective factor* (protective only in the presence of adversity; e.g., center-based preschool is beneficial only in children from lower SES households), a *risk factor* (negatively influences outcome regardless of presence or absence of adversity; e.g., severe intraventricular hemorrhage – IVH), or a *vulnerability factor* (will produce poor outcome only in presence of adversity; e.g., LBW [< 2500 g] and low SES)[12]. Rose *et al.* [12]. indicate that if a variable significantly promotes or impairs the likelihood of a positive outcome in the presence of a stressor, then the variable operates under either protective or vulnerability mechanisms. If the variable promotes or impairs the possibility of achieving a positive outcome regardless of the presence or absence of a stressor, then it operates by means of resource or risk mechanisms.

Conceptualization and design issues

Cause–effect inferences

Outcome studies of infants born preterm involve longitudinal developmental pathways that contain both risk and protective factors. Explanatory links in the relationship between a predictor variable such as ELBW and outcome often involve mediators and moderators. In addition, the "natural" epidemiology of a condition, treatment, or testing may change and therefore differentially affect relationships or prediction rules in different cohorts.

Therefore, cause–effect inferences must be tempered by alternative explanations of observed effects that could be produced by confounding influences. These "antecedent confounders" [13] need to be adjusted in the analyses or balanced by matching. The predominant, albeit simplistic, conceptualization in many follow-up studies is that a condition (e.g., ELBW) leads to a certain type of cognitive or neuropsychological outcome. However, as stated previously, multiple factors are associated with a condition such as ELBW. In fact, some investigators suggest that birth weight is best conceptualized as a marker of concomitant factors that influence outcome. Moreover, various studies have shown that front-end factors that influence outcome vary, depending on time of assessment, type of early risk factor, and type of outcome measured (neurological, cognitive, motor, educational, health-related quality of life [HRQL], social). Hence there are issues at both the front (antecedent) and outcome end. The type of research is more complex than a direct, main-effect, A→ B model [3].

Measurement error that causes spurious correlations will add much uncertainty to a predictive model. Special care must be taken to identify and assess potential confounds, and measures selected to represent confounds must be reliable and valid in and of themselves, because measurement error in the control variables will negatively influence any inferences that can be drawn. For example, a portion of the variance will be attributed to the more reliable predictor simply because it was measured more accurately; conversely, even if a confounding variable is very influential, its impact will be underestimated if it is measured inaccurately.

In general, unreliable measurement on the front end of a follow-up study may produce a Type II error (indicating there is no difference when one actually exists). Poor measurement of a confounding outcome variable may increase variability and produce spurious correlations or a Type I error (assuming there is a difference when one does not exist). Type II error is a particular problem when investigators fail to detect sub-clinical behavioral or developmental deficits because of insensitive test instruments [14].

It is also important to distinguish between moderator and mediator variables. A moderator is a variable that affects the direction or magnitude of a relation between the predictor and the dependent or outcome variable [12,15]. It essentially describes conditions under which two variables are associated. The aforementioned risk, protective, vulnerability, and resource factors can be considered moderators. For example, if one were interested in the relationship between IVH and neurological status at age 2 years, and the data indicate that the relationship is more robust in the presence of periventricular leukomalacia (PVL), then PVL would be a moderator.

A mediator accounts for the relation between a predictor and the outcome or criterion measure [12,15]. It is the generative mechanism through which a specific independent variable is able to influence the dependent (outcome) variable of interest. Stated differently, a mediator accounts for the intervening process that helps explain the association between two variables. For example, assume that a relationship between ELBW and verbal function at age 3 years exists, but when the environment is controlled, this relationship becomes non-significant. Therefore a third variable (in this case, environment) might account for or explain the relationship between ELBW and verbal function. A mediator also suggests a causal model, even though the follow-up data are not experimental – it presumes a direction of influence [12]. Mediator mechanisms typically are proposed only after an A→ B effect has been established in the literature; if there is no relationship to begin with, there is nothing to mediate.

Four statistical criteria must be met to support a mediational model: (1) the predictor variable (e.g., gestational age) is significantly associated with the criterion outcome variable (e.g., Bayley, Mental Developmental Index [MDI] at age 3 years); (2) the predictor variable is significantly associated with the mediator (environment); (3) the mediator is significantly associated with the outcome variable, after controlling for the predictor (environment→ MDI, controlling for gestational age); and (4) the previously significant predictor→ outcome relationship is markedly diminished when the mediator is controlled [12,15].

Both mediating and moderating (confounding) variables can alter the attributable influence of a particular perinatal variable on outcome. Interpretation of this influence depends on a prior categorization of which variables theoretically are expected to function as mediators and which as moderators. Treatment of a mediator as a confounding variable may lead to the incorrect inference of a spurious correlation or a Type II error [14]. Both may be tested by adding a control variable to the multivariate analysis. Selection of control variables should be determined both on a conceptual basis and by univariate correlations that indicate at least a weak relationship between a variable and the outcome measure of interest. In essence, the same variable could be a mediator, moderator, or both, depending on the research question that is posed.

Control groups

When inferences are made regarding the outcome of infants with a specific condition (e.g., very low gestational age) or those receiving a particular medical intervention, these infants should be compared to some other group to make such inferences meaningful. "Control" groups are used in randomized controlled trials, while "comparison" groups are those utilized with naturally occurring investigations. Nonetheless, both terms are often used interchangeably. Traditionally, in studies of infants born prematurely a full-term control group is used, drawn from similar geographic and social circumstances. However, choice of the type of comparison group depends upon the purpose of the study and the hypotheses being tested [3]. For example, when considering the incidence of disability in infants born at < 750 g, use of a full-term comparison group might not be very informative. A comparison group of infants with birth weights between 751 and 1000 g, or another from 1001 to 1499 g, drawn from the same population, could be more appropriate, depending on the questions posed. Determination of a control group when evaluating the efficacy of a new procedure is more straightforward in that randomization would be employed [3].

In the case of extremely premature infants, within-in-group comparisons could be employed, based on arrays of medical/biologic pre- and perinatal factors, or contrasts between those who have done well on a particular outcome measure versus those who have not. Sample stratification can be used when it is anticipated that a high degree of confound exists between a particular perinatal variable and one or more background variables. This has been successfully accomplished in studies where medical risk and biological risk are dichotomized (high/low), thereby yielding four possible stratifications. "Oversampling" of infants manifesting a condition under consideration that occurs less frequently (e.g., grade 4 IVH) also assists in comparisons and decreases the possibility of Type II errors. However, oversampling may be misleading if one was to consider the impact of the risk factor on the overall population [3].

The issue of a control or comparison group is critical for long-term outcomes, due to temporal changes. For example, if one was to follow a group of individuals < 28 weeks' gestational age born in 1990, it is reasonable to surmise that much has changed medically, environmentally, and educationally, when compared to a more contemporary sample. However, if a comparison group was identified at the outset as well, these individuals could be compared to those born very preterm, the assumption being that except for key variables, the age-related changes in medical care, environment, and education should be comparable across both groups. One could not, however, make assumptions about relations between being born very prematurely and outcome at 17 years if only the target population was followed [3,11].

Analyses of outcomes in target and control groups are critical as well. Correlations between medical/biological risk factors (e.g., bronchopulmonary dysplasia) and outcomes (e.g. IQ) are frequently used, but correlations are subject to a restriction of range, and similar, or homogeneous, scores tend to produce low correlations [3]. Correlations typically are employed to obtain a general impression of associations among variables, and because cause–effect relationships cannot be assumed in "naturally occurring" conditions that are not experimentally manipulated. When describing neurodevelopmental outcomes in those born prematurely, interest is in *ranges* of scores, versus *exact* scores. Correlations assume the existence of a level of precision in measurement that is not achieved in psychological tests, measurement of environmental variables, or values of many biomedical variables. As a result, more innovative ways to look at data are necessary. Cluster analysis [16,17] is well suited to this type of research, enabling identification of homogeneous subsets of children with similar developmental patterns over time (e.g., stable, declining, improving). Developmental epidemiological approaches are also very promising in follow-up studies [3]. Here, interest is on differences in proportions of cases rather than differences in means or variance accounted for. As a result, epidemiological approaches yield qualitatively different information regarding relationships among risk factors and developmental outcome, using measures such as risk ratios or odds ratios. Receiver operating characteristic (ROC) curves enable evaluation of the accuracy of a variable or group of variables in predicting outcome. While regression analyses are useful, they can be problematic when multicollinearity exists, due to highly correlated predictor variables, if there is much missing data, or when many correlated outcome variables are measured. If moderate to high correlations exist among predictors, meaningful associations between a single predictor and outcome variables can be obscured. Path analysis, structural equation modeling (SEM), and growth curve analyses are attractive possibilities, particularly when repeated measures are involved (i.e., the same children are followed longitudinally). Structured equation modeling allows simultaneous testing of interdependent associations between predictors and dependent variables [18].

Growth curve analysis allows evaluation of developmental trajectories, versus simple outcomes, and is an exciting possibility in neurodevelopmental outcome studies [19]. For example, in a reanalysis of the Infant Health and Development Program, the relation of covariates (e.g., maternal age, maternal education) to outcome were found to vary over time, and in relation to developmental trajectories [19]. More specifically, change was modeled over time, versus taking repeated cross-sectional comparisons of the data. Covariates were associated with developmental trajectories, and the intervention group displayed accelerated development over the first 3 years, then cessation after intervention was terminated. The control group, however, demonstrated an initial lag followed by "catch-up," accelerated development in rate of IQ change between 3 and 8 years. This finding would be obscured using typical cross-sectional analyses. Moreover, such data are critical in addressing the nagging problem of whether children who are born prematurely are displaying a developmental lag or a more persistent deficit in neurodevelopmental outcomes, and clarifying if and when decline in cognitive function occurs.

Subject populations

Birth weight and gestational age

Prematurity reflects biological immaturity for extrauterine life, and is the major influence on mortality and morbidity [2]. Birth weight essentially is a proxy for prematurity. Prior to the 1990s infants were primarily grouped by birth weight versus gestational age because of the uncertainty of the obstetric estimation of gestational age and the questionable utility of the postnatal assessment, particularly in very small infants [20]. However, fetal ultrasound has improved gestational age estimation, and gestational age is a stronger determinant of organ/system maturation and viability than is birth weight. In fact, prenatal ultrasound studies at < 20 weeks' gestation are more accurate than postnatal estimates of gestational age (95% confidence interval [CI] = ± 3–5 days) [2]. Unfortunately, mothers of many infants at risk are not given ultrasounds because of lack of adequate prenatal care. Moreover, infants of very or extremely low birth weight may be: (1)

extremely premature babies (gestational age) with appropriate-for-gestational-age (AGA) birth weights, (2) less premature babies with small-for-gestational-age (SGA) (< tenth percentile) birth weights, or (3) older preterm and term infants with extreme SGA birth weights. This distinction is necessary because the ultimate survival and outcome of infants included in these groups can vary markedly. Therefore, *both* birth weight and gestational age should be considered in outcome studies, with particular care taken to insure that only AGA infants are included in specific birth weight categories if this is the benchmark used for grouping subjects [1,3]. Moreover, the range of weights in any birth weight category makes this measure less precise than gestational age. With regard to prematurity, < 28 weeks is considered extremely premature, < 32 weeks very premature, 33–36 weeks moderately premature, and < 37 weeks, premature [2]. Depending on sample size, a breakdown by weeks of gestational age or several week gestational age groupings is recommended .

Representative samples

A recent National Institute of Child Health and Human Development (NICHD) workshop on follow-up care of high-risk infants [21] underscored the need to improve standardization and comparability of methodology and data collection in outcome studies. Small, single-hospital samples may yield data with limited applicability because of the variations in routine medical care at different centers. For example, the incidence of cerebral palsy can vary fourfold between different neonatal intensive care units (NICUs), and outcomes may differ in terms of whether the NICU is located in a hospital with a training program (marker for teaching hospital) and the volume of babies admitted (proxy for experience) [9]. While use of control groups drawn from the same hospital population can minimize this effect to some degree, pooling data from a geographically defined sample is more appropriate. Geographically defined studies are sounder because the numbers are larger, inferences are more secure, and hospital selection bias is minimized. Regional data, or those derived from nation-wide collaborative networks, are most useful and generalizable. However, some population-based studies such as the Netherlands' Project On Preterm and Small for Gestational Age Infants study have reported higher levels of impairment than have center-based studies.

Multicenter networks enable assessment of low-incidence neonatal issues such as asphyxia or PVL, and allow for adequate sample sizes for hypothesis-driven studies. As Vohr *et al.*[21] indicate, the downside is that protocols must be standardized (methodology, measurements, recruitment), adequate and comparable follow-up rates are necessary across centers (despite diverse SES populations, cultures, and languages), agreement as to the critical study population for enrollment is required, and comparable control infants must be identified and enrolled. Several large multicenter networks include the NICHD Research Follow-up Network (16 centers), the Vermont Oxford Network (> 400 centers), and the Canadian Neonatal Network (17 centers). The importance of proper selection of the patient population cannot be underestimated, as the incidence of any outcome is strongly dependent on the "denominator" (i.e., study population) [22].

Age cohort

The age cohort is important due to rapidly evolving changes in medical interventions. For example, 30- to 40-year-old data on asphyxia obtained from the National Perinatal Collaborative Study have been important historically, but have reduced relevance today. In terms of contemporary long-term follow-up, by the time school-age data on a particular cohort are collected and analyzed, practice changes in treatment may have occurred (e.g., assisted ventilation in the delivery room, surfactant, and prenatal steroids). This argues for clear delineation of medical practices at the time of enrollment in follow-up studies and timely data analyses [2].

This dilemma can be ameliorated to some degree by the use of aforementioned SEM, path analysis, and growth curve analysis which enable determination of the relationship among events (mediators and moderators) and among events and developmental trajectories. This would be particularly helpful in long-term follow-up and could be applicable to different birth cohorts. For example, relationships among certain variables and trajectories (such as SES and language or brain reorganization over time) should be relatively constant over age cohorts, although the incidence of certain insults could be reduced due to changes in medical procedures. Long-term data could then be useful to identify relationships and perhaps elucidate continuities that would also be applicable to more contemporary samples [1].

Subject loss

Subject loss can bias the estimation of rate of handicap in follow-up studies [10]. There is some debate with regard to profiles of study participants who do drop out of follow-up. Dropout rates as high as 40–50% have been reported over the first year in indigent populations. Risk for dropout increases in larger, less sick babies, those from lower SES households, babies born to single, young mothers, and those not born at a tertiary care hospital. Caretakers of infants with identified problems or disabilities are more compliant with regard to follow-up attendance[23], thereby potentially inflating rates of disability in samples with a high dropout rate. Subject loss of 10% per year should be anticipated, this arguing for power analyses to secure ample sample sizes. Recommended retention rates for early childhood is 90%, 80% for school age, and 70% for middle school [21]. Higher rates of subject loss are often reported among lower SES control children than in their counterparts born prematurely, and control or comparison groups routinely have a 10–20% greater dropout rate than study children. In addition, the utility of other potentially useful data such as those provided by home health visitors, primary care physicians, and parent report should be explored as a means of reducing subject loss and providing much needed information [21]. At minimum, comparison of children who dropped out and those who continue in the follow-up program on background and outcome measures obtained prior to discontinuation (if available) is critical so as to prevent bias in data. If control groups are not identified at the time of enrollment, investigators can randomly select a classmate of the same gender, ethnicity, and age. This would help to control for SES, educational environment, neighborhood, and similar factors [21].

Environmental factors

The social, ethnic, and educational backgrounds of mothers and fathers will also influence the prevalence of disabilities. In our original meta-analysis [8], the Hollingshead Index [23] was used in approximately one third of the meta-analytic studies, while maternal education was the most frequently used single marker variable. However, many children born prematurely are exposed to both biological and environmental risk and this combination is sometimes referred to as "double jeopardy" or "double hazard." Here, non-optimal biological and environmental risks work synergistically to affect later functioning [24]. However, there is a ceiling effect in which a severe biological risk will minimize environmental influences. Stated differently, the sickest infants are least responsive to environmental influences [24] (see also Chapter 17).

It appears that SES (maternal education and occupational status) may be an insufficient marker for environmental quality. Quantification of family income is also a significant component of the overall determination of SES [25]. Social support, which includes tangible components (e.g., housing) and more intangible components (attitudes, encouragement), should also be considered. The environment involves both *process* (proximal aspects experienced most directly; e.g. mother–infant interaction) and *status* features (distal and broader, involving aspects experienced more indirectly; e.g., social class, neighborhood). Process or proximal environmental variables are more predictive early on; status or distal factors are more predictive later. Environmental effects become increasingly apparent between 18 and 36 months, with 24 months being cited frequently. Environmental variables tend to influence verbal, academic, and general cognitive outcome while medical/biologic factors are more strongly related to neurological, neuropsychological, motor, and perceptual-performance function [24,26]. Medical/biologic factors tend to determine whether or not a developmental problem occurs, but environmental factors temper or exacerbate the degree of problem[27].

Negative components of the environment have a synergistic or additive effect on infants who are biologically vulnerable vis-à-vis the transactional [28] or "risk-route" models [29]. Procedurally, infants can be stratified on some environmental measure (e.g., by quartiles), or environmental effects can be partialled out in statistical procedures. If possible, process and status aspects need to be measured. Because of the changing complexity and composition of contemporary environments, more recently developed, valid measures that are comparable across studies and administered quickly should be employed.

There is a more direct association between a given perinatal condition and early outcome. However, as indicated earlier, our ability to detect more subtle problems increases with the use of more detailed, sophisticated tests at later ages – it is at these ages that environment (particularly status factors) exerts a stronger influence. Moreover, certain aspects of the environment mediate or moderate the effects of other environmental variables on outcome, depending on the child's age [30]. The effects of SES are mediated or moderated by characteristics specific to the child, family characteristics and external support systems [25]. For example, relations between family income and parent education could depend on cofactors such as number of siblings in the household, single parenting, or minority status. Mediating models involve the process through which SES operates to influence children's development; moderational models address the conditions in which the process operates. Both are complementary.

Ethnicity and SES should be considered markers of a myriad of associated environmental risk factors. Socioeconomic status will have an impact on a child's well-being at multiple levels, including access to material and social services, family, and neighborhood. There is wide variability in what children experience within a given SES level; these experiences are by no means homogeneous. Socioeconomic status also involves "capital": financial, human (e.g., education), and social [31]. Socioeconomic status indicators may also perform differently across different cultural groups. This underscores the point made earlier that uncorrected regression can underestimate environmental effects when errors in measuring the environment exist. Actual timing and duration of non-optimal environmental influences such as poverty are often overlooked, although there is no doubt that persistent exposure to such negative influences will have significant long-term effects.

Correction for prematurity

Correction for prematurity continues to be a significant issue. This is a highly common practice that is based on rather weak scientific evidence. The general consensus, though not unanimous, is that correction should occur, arguably up to 2 years of age. However, some investigators suggest that correction not be utilized, correction continue throughout childhood or further, or that it be applied in an incremental fashion (e.g. partial correction) depending on the infant's gestational age, age at time of measurement, and area of function being assessed [32]. Use of correction reflects a biological/maturational perspective, while adoption of chronological age represents an environmentally based orientation. Adjustment for prematurity is assumed to help differentiate more transient effects of preterm birth from more significant and persistent deficits. However, some investigators argue that correction simply obscures these deficits. Current arguments for incremental correction or total lack of correction are unconvincing. Imprecision in gestational age estimation, concomitant medical issues, and a lack of consensus regarding whether to correct to 37 or 40 weeks are additional confounds. Conclusions about the early outcome of premature infants will differ, depending on whether corrected or uncorrected scores are used [3].

Correction raises several other issues. If a child is followed longitudinally and correction is applied over the first 2 years but discontinued at the 3-year evaluation, decline in scores at that time could be partially attributable to cessation of age adjustment, even if the same test has been used throughout. Correction is more of an issue in those children who fall in the suspect range or who are very young at the time of assessment. If a child is functioning in the abnormal range despite utilizing adjustment for prematurity, the certainty of deficits is strong. If a child is performing at an above-average level with correction applied, there is a strong likelihood that at least average functioning will persist if correction is removed. Therefore, correction will primarily affect infants whose functioning is low average or marginal. Effects of correction will be restricted to studies focusing on early outcomes, raising duration of follow-up issues. This should have minimal impact on later high-prevalence/low-severity dysfunctions.

Consideration of biological risk issues

Prematurity is not a defined disease or syndrome, but rather is a condition with numerous aspects [2]. It is common knowledge that infants with the same birth weight or gestational age can differ markedly with respect to outcome. When one considers morbidity or mortality based on birth weight or gestational age, perinatal factors and physiological conditions of the individual infants must also be considered. How one views background risk variables, whether biomedical or environmental, will have an impact on our understanding of outcomes. Antecedents of prematurity, preterm labor, maternal infections, premature rupture of membranes, nutrition, exposure to tobacco, alcohol, or illicit drugs, maternal behaviors, stressful life events, maternal medical problems, and environmental toxicants will also affect outcome [2]. Ultimately, outcome is dependent on the cumulative effect of many environmental, biomedical, and genetic factors.

For example, with respect to consideration of background variables, Burchinal et al. [33] report intriguing differences in how the effects of social risk on early language and cognitive development can be represented. Individual risk variables were found to be appropriate to investigate the impact a social variable has on outcome at a particular age; however, this approach is not applicable for developmental patterns. Factor scores, derived from groups of risk variables subject to factor analysis, are useful with developmental trajectories in moderate to large samples. Risk indexes (tallying the number of risk factors) are useful with developmental patterns when a large number of risk variables are assessed in a small sample. The same may be true of biological risk issues. Quantifying risk conditions allows them to be used in statistical models to predict outcomes, and to be employed in risk adjustment comparisons across centers.

Various illness severity scores have been produced such as the Score for Neonatal Acute Physiology (SNAP; SNAP-II), the Revised Score for Neonatal Acute Physiology Perinatal Extension (SNAPPE-II), the Vermont-Oxford Network risk adjustment (VON-RA), the Neonatal Medical Index (NMI), and the Neurobiologic Risk Score [34,35]. These templates differ with respect to the number of items, time period the data are collected (e.g., 1 hour, 12 hours, 24 hours), the type of items (biochemical indicators, events [e.g., seizures], gender, non-physiological characteristics), and weighting of variables. Moreover, some recorded variables can be influenced by medical care decisions (e.g., fraction of inspired oxygen). Various schemes include baseline characteristics, others historical events, while still others involve more dynamic measurements. While all help to account for differences in patient populations, they often have different purposes (documenting illness severity, risk adjustment). Furthermore, several scoring schemes such as the clinical risk index for babies (CRIB) or SNAPPE were developed before the widespread use of surfactant or antenatal steroids. This underscores the need for such measures to be contemporary because differences in age cohorts often lead to medical improvements that can change relationships among measures. In addition, several risk indices are applicable to certain subgroups of infants (e.g., VLBW) but might not be useful in more heterogeneous samples [34,35]. Contributions of perinatal risk scores to neurodevelopmental outcome frequently are weak, this prediction being better suited to survival. This may be due to the nature of risk score measurements. More specifically, if these biomedical factors are not measured accurately, their importance can be erroneously underestimated or misinterpreted.

Measurement/outcome

Outcome measurements

Although global IQ or developmental scores have frequently been reported, these tend to obscure or mask individual components of IQ and preclude the opportunity to identify patterns of strengths and weaknesses.

Diffusing outcome to more global measures may also obscure more specific relationships among certain biomedical variables and particular areas of function. A full-scale IQ is an average of the child's performance on a variety of different subtests or areas of function. As such, it is subject to wide variations among those subtests or areas of function [3]. Conversely, if one were to adjust for global IQ, this would make a stronger case for selective sequelae if group differences are found [1,13]. However, many measures of specific cognitive functions or achievement are strongly associated with intelligence. Therefore, controlling for composite IQ measures may, in actuality, remove some of the variance of interest and obscure more subtle, specific problems [1].

Assessment

There are two ways to better document neurodevelopmental outcomes [36]. The first is to implement changes in interpretation of existing tests administered at early ages on the "front end," where critical items or groups of items are identified and used to predict outcomes. The second is to employ changes at a selected end point by refining outcome from a global score to specific subdomains. Inherent in the former is the assumption that continuity must exist in specific developmental functions over time. Parsing out functional subdomains during infancy, particularly verbal, cognitive, and motor, may enhance prediction [36], and it has been shown that robust developmental continuities exist in cognitive function, in the face of reorganization and change in behavior that make a new level of performance possible.

With respect to end-point measurement, assessment must extend beyond traditional IQ and achievement testing, because these measures provide a limited overview of functional abilities, and do not identify more circumscribed deficits. In the case of neurodevelopmental function, more specific tests or rating scales that measure the following areas should also be considered: (1) attention and executive functions (planning, organization, monitoring, inhibition, working memory); (2) language (phonological awareness, syntax, verbal fluency, comprehension of instructions, higher-order abstracting functions); (3) sensorimotor functions (visuomotor precision, fine motor speed); (4) visuospatial processes (design copying, visual closure, visuospatial planning); (5) memory and learning (list learning, delayed recall, assessment of semantic/strategic and rote/episodic verbal and visual functions);

and (6) behavioral adjustment (ADHD, internalizing and externalizing problems) [1]. The desired goal is to make the connection from early functional abilities to later outcome at school age and beyond. However, this approach may be difficult to fiscally justify, either in clinical or research settings. A compromise would be to employ representative tests measuring areas of function that have been identified in the literature as having an increased likelihood of problems in children born prematurely [1,3].

There is no true "gold standard" in developmental assessment, causing terms such as sensitivity and specificity to be misapplied. Instead, "co-positivity" and "co-negativity" are more appropriate in situations where scores on one test are compared to those obtained on a reference standard. The Bayley Scales of Infant Development (BSID), the BSID-II, and the most recent Bayley Scales of Infant and Toddler Development (BSID-III) [37,38] are traditionally considered the best criterion measures. However, analogous to changes in medical procedures having an effect on outcome studies over time, changes in outcome measures have a similar effect by limiting comparisons. Mean IQ/developmental quotient (DQ) scores on a given test are estimated to increase 3–5 points per decade, this phenomenon being referred to as the Flynn effect [39]. Therefore, the mean score of a test developed three decades ago conceivably could increase by as much as 15 points. Such adjustments must be considered when comparing scores in different age cohorts or longitudinally with different versions of the same test, because change could be due to real improvement or be an artifact of the different properties of the two instruments. To further complicate issues, the Flynn effect apparently has not been found with several new measurements such as the BSID-III [38]. Scores on these more contemporary tests actually are *higher* than their predecessors. Further compounding this problem is the recent difficulty in comparing results of the BSID-III to those of earlier versions of this test. Cognitive, language, and motor scores are produced in the most recent iteration. While motor scores and the previous Psychomotor Developmental Index (PDI) are grossly comparable, this is not the case with cognitive scores and the MDI because language and selected sensorimotor functions are not included in the cognitive score (as was the case in the BSID and BSID-II) [37,38].

Specific outcome measures should be folded into a basic outcome framework that could be compared across studies and centers. This basic framework should include a follow-up protocol with age at assessment, areas covered, and techniques used being uniform. However, more study-specific, narrow-band foci (e.g., the relationship between a specific condition such as hypothyroxinemia and a specific outcome such as cerebral palsy [CP]) could also be employed. This approach would allow for investigation of specific deficits pertinent to the purpose of the follow-up study in conjunction with more "standard" cognitive, behavioral/social, functional, and health-related outcomes that would be of interest across studies. The challenge is to accomplish this in a reasonable amount of time and at an acceptable cost [3].

There is a lack of consistency in terms of diagnostic criteria. Arguments are made both for and against viewing data as categorical or continuous. For example, in our meta-analysis of LBW studies, use of a binary "normal/not normal" categorization would have precluded identification of group differences [8]. However, viewing the data in a continuous fashion yielded a six point difference between LBW and control infants. It would appear that analyses of continuous data require decisions to include or delete severely involved infants and either option would alter results. Use of categorical methods allows inclusion of these babies, but masks more subtle findings. Floor effects and missing data are particularly problematic. "Outliers" whose raw scores cannot be converted into scaled scores (as in the case of a BSID-II score < 50) often are "censored" or excluded, and a high frequency of deletions may occur in populations with severely affected infants. As a solution, imputed values may be used (e.g., a score of 49 is recorded to indicate an unscalable score) and data analyzed using standard methods. Means, corrected for censoring, can be compared to means based on inclusion of imputed values to verify that imputation is appropriate. It is recommended that the mean IQ (and standard deviation [SD]), effect sizes and confidence intervals for each group, the proportion of mental retardation and borderline intelligence, and the proportion of major disorders (CP, blindness, deafness) be reported. Comparisons excluding children with major handicaps provide insight as to how children who survive without major handicap fare [3].

Age at time of evaluation

Early evaluation below 9 months of age often is negatively affected by recovery from medical issues, effects of infant state, higher variability in behaviors, and a more limited behavioral repertoire. Conversely, early involvement with a follow-up program will increase the likelihood of continued participation. These concerns are heightened if the evaluation occurs earlier than 6-months' corrected age. By 12 months environmental factors are less influential and biomedical issues such as oxygen supplementation may be less intrusive on testing procedures. Cognitive processes and emerging language are better assessed. At 18–24 months, environmental factors become more influential, cognitive and motor functions diverge, language becomes more elaborate, and there is improved prediction of later function. Developmental, versus intelligence tests, are typically employed because IQ tests have weak floors at this age and may lead to underestimation of disabilities. Correction for prematurity also is discontinued at 24 months and, as mentioned previously, this may have an impact on infants who were functioning in the low average or borderline range when gestational age adjustment was implemented [21].

By 3–4 years, "intelligence" can be assessed, as can pre-academic skills, early indicators of executive functions, and visuomotor integrative skills. Verbal and non-verbal functions are better differentiated, and prediction to later IQ is more reliable. More distal SES influences on outcome become stronger. At 6 years, a wider variety of tests can be employed and more precise assessment of attention and school achievement is possible. Previously existing problems, not apparent earlier, become evident when functions involving these deficits are now challenged. By age 8, IQ, neuropsychological functions, learning disabilities and behavioral adjustment can be adequately measured [21]. Assessment in adolescence and early adulthood provides the most complete representation of deficits.

Conversely, evaluation at older ages may be increasingly affected by environmental and genetic influences rather than early medical procedures and standards of care.

The trend of worsening outcome of children born prematurely as they reach school age is a significant concern [40–42]. Mild to moderate disabilities are identified later for a variety of reasons. Perhaps demands for higher-level skills cannot be met because of underlying cognitive or neuropsychological deficiencies. These previously existing deficiencies simply may not have been challenged earlier. As a result, these individuals are less likely to take advantage of educational opportunities because of deficits in basic skills, or increasing frustration and loss of motivation [43].

Children born prematurely more often have clusters of problems, versus a single issue in isolation. They also seem to have a greater tendency to be untestable (totally or partially) due to refusals. Whether this reflects the child's emerging sensitivity to areas of weakness, behavioral issues (ADHD, oppositional defiant disorder, executive dysfunction), the consequences of a vulnerable child status, or some combination of such is not clear. Nonetheless, further investigation of this issue is needed.

Conclusion

Long-term outcome studies are necessary for a host of reasons: for subsequent NICU decision-making, intervention strategies, and to enhance early identification of those at risk for later neurodevelopmental problems. Parents also need to be provided with a reasonable understanding about long-term problems that may subsequently develop in their high-risk newborn. Because of these ramifications and the tremendous investment of human and financial capital, it is imperative that follow-up data be obtained from scientifically rigorous studies which should be hypothesis-driven. As mentioned elsewhere [1] prediction of later outcome will most likely improve with the combined use of brain imaging techniques, functional activity of the brain (functional magnetic resonance imaging; diffusion-weighted imaging; and perfusion and blood-oxygenation-dependent imaging), magnetic resonance spectroscopy (to study brain metabolism), biochemical markers, serial neurodevelopmental assessments, and refinement of evaluation techniques employed at later ages.

References

1. Aylward GP. Neurodevelopmental outcomes of infants born prematurely. *J Dev Behav Pediatr* 2005; **26**: 427–40.

2. Institute of Medicine. *Preterm Birth: Causes, Consequences, and Prevention.* Washington, DC: The National Academies; 2007.

3. Aylward GP. Methodological issues in outcome studies of at-risk infants. *J Pediatr Psychol* 2002; **27**: 37–45.

4. O'Shea TM, Goldstein DJ. Follow-up data: their use in evidence-based decision-making. *Clin Perinatol* 2003; **30**: 217–50

5. Finer NN, Craft A, Vaucher YE, Clark RH, Sola A. Postnatal steroids: short-term gain, long-term pain? *J Pediatr* 2000; **137**: 9–13.

6. Aylward GP. Conceptual issues in developmental screening and assessment. *J Dev Behav Pediatr* 1997; **18**: 340–9.

7. Aylward GP. *Infant and Early Childhood Neuropsychology.* New York: Plenum; 1997.

8. Aylward GP, Pfeiffer SI, Wright A, Verhulst SJ. Outcome studies of low birth weight infants published in the last decade: a meta-analysis. *J Pediatr* 1989; **115**: 515–20.

9. McCormick MC. The outcome of very low birth weight infants: are we asking the right questions? *Pediatrics* 1997; **99**: 869–76.

10. Tyson JE, Broyles RS. Progress in assessing the long-term outcome of extremely low birth-weight infants. *JAMA* 1996; **276**: 492–3.

11. Aylward GP. Cognitive and neuropsychological outcomes: more than IQ scores. *Ment Retard Dev Disabil Res Rev* 2002; **8**: 234–40.

12. Rose BM, Holmbeck GN, Coakley RM, Franks EA. Mediator and moderator effects in developmental and behavioral research. *J Dev Behav Pediatr* 2004; **25**: 58–67.

13. Breslau N. Psychiatric sequelae of low birth weight. *Epidemiol Rev* 1995; **17**: 96–106.

14. Jacobson JL, Jacobson SW. Methodological considerations in behavioral toxicology in infants and children. *Dev Psychol* 1996; **32**: 390–403.

15. Baron R, Kenny DA. The moderator-mediator variable distinction in school psychological research: conceptual, strategic and statistical considerations. *J Pers Soc Psychol* 1986; **51**: 1173–82.

16. Liaw FB, Brooks-Gunn J. Patterns of low-birth-weight children's cognitive development. *Dev Psychol* 1993; **27**: 1024–35.

17. Koller H, Lawson K, Rose SA. Patterns of cognitive development in very low birth weight children during the first six years of life. *Pediatrics* 1997; **99**: 383–9.

18. Taylor HG, Burant CJ, Holding PA, *et al.* Sources of variability in sequelae of very low birth weight. *Child Neuropsychol* 2002; **8**: 163–78.

19. Lawrence FR, Blair C. Factorial invariance in preventive intervention: Modeling the development of intelligence in low birth weight, preterm infants. *Prev Sci* 2003; **4**: 249–61.

20. Hack M, Fanaroff AA. How small is too small? Considerations in evaluating the outcome of the tiny infant. *Clin Perinatol* 1988; **15**: 773–88.

21. Vohr B, Wright LL, Hack M, Aylward GP, Hirtz D. Follow-up care of high-risk infants. *Pediatrics* 2004; **114**: (Suppl) 1377–97.

22. Aylward GP, Hatcher RP, Stripp B, Gustafson NE, Leavitt LA. Who goes and who stays: subject loss in a multicenter, longitudinal follow-up study. *J Dev Behav Pediatr* 1988; **6**: 3–8.

23. Hollingshead AB. *Four-factor Index of Social Status.* Working paper. New Haven CT: Department of Sociology, Yale University; 1975.

24. Aylward GP. The relationship between environmental risk and developmental outcome. *J Dev Behav Pediatr* 1992; **13**: 222–9.

25. Bradley RH, Corwyn RF. Socioeconomic status and child development. *Annu Rev Psychol* 2002; **53**: 371–99.

26. Resnick MB, Gomatam SV, Carter RL, *et al*. Educational disabilities of neonatal intensive care graduates. *Pediatrics* 1998; **102**: 308–316.

27. Hunt JV, Cooper BA, Tooley WH. Very low birth weight infants at 8 and 11 years of age: role of neonatal illness and family status. *Pediatrics* 1988; **82**: 596–603.

28. Sameroff AJ, Chandler MJ. Reproductive risk and the continuum of caretaking casualty. In Horowitz FD, ed. *Review of Child Development Research,* Vol. 4. Chicago: University of Chicago Press. 1975; 187–244.

29. Aylward GP, Kenny TJ. Developmental follow-up: inherent problems and a conceptual model. *J Pediatr Psychol* 1979; **4**: 331–43.

30. Kato Klebanov P, Brooks-Gunn J, McCarton C, *et al*. The contribution of neighborhood and family income to developmental test scores over the first three years of life. *Child Dev* 1998; **69**: 1420–36.

31. Entwisle DR, Astone NM. Some practical guidelines for measuring youth's race/ethnicity and socioeconomic status. *Child Dev,* 1994; **65**: 1521–40.

32. Blasko PA. Preterm birth: to correct or not to correct. *Dev Med Child Neurol* 1989; **31**: 816–26.

33. Burchinal MR, Roberts JE, Hooper S, Zeisel SA. Cumulative risk and early cognitive development; a comparison of statistical risk models. *Dev Psychol* 2000; **36**: 793–807.

34. Gagliardi L, Cavazza A, Brunelli A, *et al*. Assessing mortality risk in very low birthweight infants: a comparison of CRIB, CRIB-II and SNAPPE-II. *Arch Dis Child Fetal Neonatal Ed* 2004; **89**: F419–22.

35. Zupancic JA, Richardson DK, Horbar JD, *et al*. Revalidation of the Score for Neonatal Acute Physiology in the Vermont Oxford Network. *Pediatrics* 2004; **119**: e156–63.

36. Aylward GP. Prediction of function from infancy to early childhood: implications for pediatric psychology. *J Pediatr Psychol* 2004; **29**: 555–64.

37. Bayley N. *The Bayley Scales of Infant Development,* 2nd edn. San Antonio, TX: The Psychological Corporation; 1993.

38. Bayley N. *The Bayley Scales of Infant and Toddler Development*, 3rd edn. San Antonio, TX: PsychCorp; 2006.

39. Flynn Jr. Searching for justice. The discovery of IQ gains over time. *Am Psychol* 1999; **54**: 5–20.

40. Taylor HG, Klein N, Hack M. School-age consequences of birth weight less than 750 g: a review and update. *Dev Neuropsychol* 2000; **17**: 289–321.

41. Marlow N, Wolke D, Bracewell MA, Samara M. Neurologic and developmental disability at six years of age after extremely preterm birth. *N Engl J Med* 2005; **352**: 9–19.

42. Szatmari P, Saigal S, Rosenbaum P, *et al*. Psychiatric disorders at five years among children with birthweights less than 1000g: a regional perspective. *Dev Med Child Neurol* 1990; **32**: 954–62.

43. O'Callaghan MJ, Burns YR, Gray PH, *et al*. School performance of ELBW children: a controlled study. *Dev Med Child Neurol* 1996; **38**: 917–26.

Chapter 13

Language function after preterm birth

Teresa M. Rushe

Introduction

Normal language development is a highly complex and protracted process. As such, it is not surprising that the brain damage often associated with very preterm birth may give rise to problems in this domain. To date, several studies have documented problems in multiple domains of language function at every stage of development in very preterm born individuals. Following a brief outline of normal language development, this chapter will proceed to review studies of language function in very preterm-born samples. Throughout the review a number of important questions are addressed. For example, do language difficulties in very preterm-born preschoolers represent a delay in the acquisition of language skills which over time recede? Or is it the case that early deficits in infants born very preterm hamper the ongoing acquisition of increasingly complex skills throughout the course of development? The factors which have been shown to predict good/bad language outcome for very preterm-born children will be also discussed.

Normal language development

Language is a complex cognitive process which typically emerges during the first 3 years of life, though the mastery and proficient use of language continues throughout the school years of the child and beyond. Prerequisites to language, such as the production of vowel sounds (e.g., cooing) and reduplicative babbling (e.g., dadada) typically occur in the first 8 months of life, with the first signs of word comprehension and true word production typically beginning between 11 and 13 months [1]. Word combinations emerge between 18 and 20 months, and grammatical development typically occurs between 20 and 36 months [1]. The acquisition of this preliterate speech involves the ability to discriminate speech sounds (phonetics), the

acquisition of grammatical rules (syntax), learning to associate objects and actions with their meanings (semantics), use of words for conversational purposes (pragmatics) and the ability to articulate intelligible words. Later spoken language developments in vocabulary, pragmatics, syntax, and meta-linguistic awareness all contribute to improvements in narrative discourse throughout the school years [2]. In normally developing children, verbal fluency increases from childhood to adolescence [3–5], and increases into young adulthood have also been documented [6]. Later language development also depends on the child's "cognitive readiness to advance" [2], so generalized cognitive problems are likely to affect the ongoing mastering of linguistic skills.

Literacy is a central component of later language development, which is associated with increased schooling and socialization of peers in the older child [2]. Improvements in writing, reading, and spelling occur throughout childhood, with children producing and recognising letter-like forms by age 3–4 years [7]. At the earliest stage, children make marks on paper randomly with little muscular control and by the end stage (age 7 years) the child writes with punctuation, and in the Roman alphabet words are organized in lines with spaces between words, moving from left to right, and from the top to the bottom of the page [7].

Very preterm birth and language development in preschool years

Many studies have documented problems in language acquisition in the early childhood period in survivors of very preterm birth. Foster-Cohen et al. [8] examined a variety of language outcomes in 2-year-old children born very preterm (VPT, < 33 weeks) and/or had a birth weight less than 1500 g (very low birth weight, VLBW). They found delays compared to term-born children on

Neurodevelopmental Outcomes of Preterm Birth, ed. Chiara Nosarti, Robin M. Murray, and Maureen Hack. Published by Cambridge University Press. © Cambridge University Press 2010.

a range of measures, including vocabulary size, quality of word use, syntax, and morphology.

By age 3.5 normally developing children can produce complete sentences, yet delays in expressive language are evident in children born very preterm [9–12]. Sansavini *et al.* [12] examined grammatical ability, such as mean length utterance, and total morphological errors (including omissions, substitutions, errors in bounded morphemes) in a sample of very preterm-born (from 25–33 weeks' gestation) children aged 3.5 years (corrected age). None of the children showed evidence of significant brain injury on ultrasound at birth, though as a group they had significantly lower scores across all outcomes compared to age-matched full-term-born children. Phonological working memory skills were also investigated (using repetition of sentences composed of nonsense and real words) and very preterm-born children performed significantly worse on the nonsense word repetition tasks than term controls. Repetition of real word sentences was not impaired, but performance on both tasks was related to mean length utterances. This is consistent with the reciprocal influence between phonological working memory and language acquisition [13], and suggests that very preterm-born children learn language in the same way as term peers. That is, before speech production and comprehension become automatic processes, phonological working memory may aid the learning, not only of new words, but also the syntactic structures important for grammatical competence.

Understanding the neuropsychological basis of language impairment in very preterm-born children is important if remediation programs aimed at improving social and academic function are to be successful. These studies show that problems already exist for very preterm children in their preschool years. The sooner such problems are identified, the more likely they are to be susceptible to remediation, as early deficits have the potential to interfere with ongoing development by reducing the child's capacity to acquire more complex skills later in development. This could lead to increasing cognitive gaps between very preterm-born children and term peers at school age.

Very preterm birth and language development in school years

The nature and significance of language problems in children born very preterm cannot be fully appreciated until the period for normal language acquisition has passed. More detailed assessment of language functions can be performed in the older child, and such studies permit the assessment of whether age-appropriate gains in language have been made. It remains unclear whether early problems reflect a delay in the acquisition of language skills which can, over time, recede, and/or whether later problems emerge when the child is faced with increasing cognitive challenges, such as the acquisition and mastery of literacy during school years. Later language development also depends on the child's cognitive readiness to advance to higher levels of thought [2], so also important is whether or not deficits in language function manifest as part of general cognitive difficulties, or whether they represent specific language impairments.

Luoma *et al* conducted a detailed assessment of speech and language production and comprehension in a sample of very preterm-born 5-year-olds born before 33 weeks' gestation. On the composite measure of speech and language function, the preterm children performed significantly worse than age-matched term controls. When very preterm children with major neurological disability were excluded from the analyses, global measures of language function failed to differentiate the two study groups, but very preterm children without major disability showed significant deficits on some aspects of language function, including rapid word retrieval and comprehension of relative concepts [14].

Many other studies of school-age (6 years plus) early birth survivors have found evidence of a variety of language impairments in this population [15–18]. Delays in expressive language and phonological processing skills at ages 6 and 7 years have been reported [15,16], though many of these were no longer evident after controlling for general cognitive ability [16]. The study by Wolke and Meyer [16] is notable because it included a large sample size of very preterm children (n = 264), the same number of sociodemographically matched term controls, as well as a detailed assessment of language function, including measures of sentence production, comprehension, and grammatical competence. They additionally tested for pre-reading skills using tasks of naming, rhyming, and sound to word matching. Six-year-old very preterm-born children performed significantly worse on all language measures compared to term peers, but they also performed worse on measures of general cognitive processing (the Kaufman Assessment Battery of sequential and simultaneous processing). After controlling for mental processing, the only language deficit to remain was on performance on a measure of speech articulation and quality of speech [16]. This suggests that many of the language deficits in very preterm-born children are part of a generalized reduction in cognitive capacity, rather than indicative of specific language impairment.

A number of other studies have also addressed the question of whether or not very preterm-born children showed evidence of specific language impairment (SLI) at school age [17,18]. Specific language impairment describes a developmental language disorder which occurs in the absence of known sensory, intellectual or neurological dysfunction or disease, and is typically diagnosed on the basis of a discrepancy between performance IQ and scores on standardized measures of expressive language [19]. Aram *et al.* studied speech and language development in 8-year-old children born very preterm and found that they scored significantly lower than normal birth weight controls on measures of speech and language [17]. They went on to assess the clinical significance of these group differences, using a discrepancy (between performance IQ and language scores) definition to identify those with SLI, and found that a higher percentage of the control group had SLI than did the very preterm-born children. However, the very preterm-born children had significantly lower performance IQ scores than the controls (hence the discrepancy between performance IQ and language scores was smaller in the preterm group), which may explain why there was a higher rate of SLI in controls. Aram *et al.* concluded that language problems of the very preterm children were more likely a result of general cognitive problems [17], which are in line with the results of Wolke and Meyer described earlier [16]. These findings are also consistent with those of Samuelsson *et al.* [18]. In their sample of 9-year-olds born with very low birth weight, 24% were classified as being poor readers (compared with 8% of normal birth weight children), but only 7% of the very low birth weight group compared with 13% of the normal birth weight children were classified as being dyslexic. They also used an IQ-language achievement discrepancy definition for dyslexia and argued that the reason why fewer of the very low birth weight group were identified as being dyslexic was because they tended to have worse IQ scores than reading scores [18].

These findings suggest that school-age language difficulties in very preterm subjects are in line with what would be expected in full-term children with low cognitive abilities, rather than evidence of SLI. As later language development also depends on the child's cognitive capacity, it would be expected that continuing general cognitive problems would impact on the achievement of age-appropriate language abilities in adolescence.

Very preterm birth and language development in adolescence

Knowledge and use of language develops throughout adolescence and beyond, with improvements in vocabulary size and quality, more sophisticated grammatical structures, increased meta-linguistic awareness, and extended discourse [2]. A number of studies have now reported results of language function in older survivors of preterm birth. In Rushe *et al.*, we reported evidence of differential impairment in language (verbal fluency) in very preterm-born (< 33 weeks) adolescents aged 14–15 years [20]. Performance on other measures of neuropsychological function, such as executive function, memory, and visuomotor function, was not impaired. However, because we did not include a measure of IQ, we were unable to ascertain the extent to which the language production deficits were due to general cognitive dysfunction.

We subsequently addressed this problem by including a measure of IQ (to test for the specificity of observed deficits), in our extended adolescent sample [21]. Additionally, we conducted a more detailed assessment of language function. Verbal fluency, phonological processing, and literacy were the particular focus of the study, given the ongoing development of these particular language functions throughout school age into adolescence. Compared to term controls, the adolescents born very preterm were found to have deficits in multiple measures of language function, including reading, spelling, verbal fluency, and phonological processing [21]. Intelligence quotient was found to be the best predictor of performance on all language tests, and the analyses suggested that with the exception of verbal fluency, these language deficits were best explained as part of generalized cognitive dysfunction.

Similarly, Breslau *et al.* reported that deficits in reading and mathematics in their large heterogeneous sample of low birth weight adolescents (< 2501 g) at age 17 were largely accounted for by IQ scores obtained at age 6 years [22]. On the basis of their findings, Breslau *et al.* suggested that interventions aimed at preventing persistent effects of low birth weight in the classroom should be targeted towards enhancing general intelligence [22]. There is, however, some evidence that primary deficits in phonological processing and working memory continue to account for some of the variance in reading and spelling in later childhood and adolescence, over and above that accounted for by generalized cognitive deficits [23]. Downie *et al.* found phonological processing and working memory ability to be a better predictor of reading and spelling than IQ in their sample of very preterm-born children at age 11 [23]. The results of this study argue for early targeted intervention of these skills, which are associated with the acquisition of literacy [13], in order to prevent accumulation of deficits and lags in cognitive development. As the need for special assistance has been estimated as being increased fourfold in this population [24] (please see Chapter 16 for a detailed account of academic performance and learning disabilities in very preterm and very low birth weight populations), the impact of language deficits in the classroom remains an areas of ongoing concern. More detailed neuropsychological studies of language function are required in order to fully understand the nature of language deficits, and how best to target educational remediation.

Methodological considerations

Although many studies have examined language function in very preterm-born children, particularly at school age, comparison across studies is limited by methodological inconsistencies. These include the heterogeneity of samples with respect to perinatal and social factors, age at which the assessment takes place, as well as the variability in language functions assessed. Furthermore, some studies include an age-matched control group, whereas others report performance in relation to normative standards. Prospective follow-up studies of the same population have the advantage over cross-sectional comparisons of very preterm populations in that biological and social factors remain constant. As such, they provide a better opportunity to address the question of whether deficits in language acquisition persist into school age and beyond, or whether very preterm-born children catch up with their peers.

Ment *et al.* [25] reported findings on their sample of very preterm subjects, nearly 300 of which had assessments at 36, 54, 72, and 96 months. At each age children were tested using the Peabody Picture Vocabulary Test (PPVT: a test of receptive vocabulary skills with

age-standardized normative data). They were also tested for IQ. The PPVT scores increased at each of the four assessment ages, and the change between the first and the last assessment (from age 3 to age 8) was statistically significant. During this time, nearly half of the children improved 10 points or more, whereas 17% of the sample deteriorated by at least 10 points. Those who deteriorated over time were those children who had evidence of brain injury at birth [25].

Saavalainen *et al.* also followed up their sample of 5-year-olds at age 9 and again at age 16 [26]. Deficits in naming skills at age 5 and 9 years were no longer evident at age 16. While taken together these studies suggest improvement of function with increasing age, it is worth highlighting that the language assessment in these studies was limited to the domain of vocabulary/naming tasks. In the study by Saavalainen *et al* [26], 16-year-olds were tested on color naming, and showed normal performance. Color naming is a skill that is expected to be complete by middle childhood, therefore, the deficit evidenced by the very preterm-born children at age 9 years likely reflects a delay in the acquisition of this skill. By age 16, however, the fact that the deficit was no longer evident probably reflected that very preterm individuals had ample time to catch up with their peers in this respect. On the contrary, studies which employed more age-appropriate language tasks have suggested that language deficits do persist in very preterm-born young people. For example, in a follow-up of the very preterm-born 14- to 15-year-old adolescents reported in Rushe *et al.* [20] very preterm-born subjects displayed verbal fluency deficits at age 19 years compared to age-matched term peers [6]. Furthermore, the very preterm group did not make the same age-related gains that were seen in the term group with respect to verbal fluency [6]. Further follow-up of a similar sample of very preterm individuals in adulthood (mean age 23 years) also showed lower scores compared to controls on a phonological verbal fluency task [27].

The above studies suggest that for at least some children born very preterm improvements in vocabulary throughout early school age is possible [25,26], but studies of adolescent/early adulthood samples suggest residual language impairments with respect to verbal fluency [6,27]. Absence of impairments and/or improvement in cognitive function has typically been interpreted as evidence of neural and functional plasticity in response to early brain damage [28]. When deficits in language production are shown to persist, however, it could be an indication that there are limits to the plasticity of the developing brain. Bishop, for example, suggested that a consequence of the brain's reorganization of structure–function relationships in response to early brain damage is that complex cognitive functions that are acquired later in development might suffer due to lack of synaptic sites [29]. Thus, the finding that 19- and 23-year-olds fail to make age-appropriate gains in verbal fluency in late adolescence and early adulthood might be interpreted within this framework. The extent and limits of the plasticity of the developing brain to injury is an area of ongoing research. Despite the widely held view that the young people's brains are more able to adapt to brain injury, more recent research suggests that age at injury interacts with multiple factors, including injury severity. Anderson *et al.* followed up 122 children (aged 3–13 years) with traumatic brain injury for 30 months after injury. They found that injury severity was the best predictor of cognitive outcome for all children, but that severe injury before age 3 years was associated with worse outcome than severe injury sustained after 3 years of age [30].

Brain injury and language outcome

Studies that investigate the relationship between extent of brain damage at birth (typically measured using ultrasound techniques in the days and weeks after birth) in very preterm-born samples tend to show a positive relationship between extent of perinatal brain injury and functional outcome. For example, Downie *et al.* [23] reported that reading and spelling in their very preterm-born 11-year-olds was present in those children with periventricular hemorrhage, but those children without evidence of periventricular brain injury performed as well as their term peers. The longitudinal study by Ment *et al.* further suggests that recovery of function may be related to the extent of brain damage sustained at birth. In their sample, very preterm-born children with evidence of periventricular brain injury at birth performed worse on the PPVT at all ages (3, 4.5, 6, and 8 years) than those children without evidence of brain injury. Furthermore, while language function in the "no brain injury" group improved with age, the performance of the "brain injury" group deteriorated over the follow-up period [25].

It is to be expected that those children with significant brain injury at birth fare less well than very preterm-born children without evidence of significant injury. Even in the absence of evidence of cerebral damage on neonatal ultrasound, brain development of the very preterm-born children must proceed outside the normal environment of the uterus, and additionally is frequently exposed to invasive medical interventions [24], the long-lasting effects of which are not fully understood. In a magnetic resonance imaging (MRI) study of adolescents born very preterm, MRI identified more brain lesions than had the neonatal ultrasound [31]. Fifty-five percent of very preterm adolescents had evidence of brain abnormality, as determined by two consultant neuroradiologists blind to subject status, compared with only one of the 21 age-matched full-term controls. The most common abnormality was ventricular enlargement, followed by thinning/atrophy of the corpus callosum [31]. However, those adolescents with evidence of brain abnormality did not perform worse on neuropsychological tests, including verbal fluency, than those adolescents without evidence of brain abnormality [20]. The relative preservation of function in the context of brain abnormality was interpreted as evidence of the brain's capacity to compensate for very early brain damage.

However, more recent studies which employ quantitative measures of brain volume are more consistent in showing that brain damage associated with very preterm birth is associated with functional outcome. In adolescents drawn from the same cohort, total corpus callosum area was found to be 7.5% smaller in very preterm-born adolescents, and furthermore, the extent of corpus callosum volume decrease was associated with reduced verbal IQ and reduced verbal fluency scores [32]. Lateral cerebellar volume decreases were also associated with reduced scores on language tasks [33]. More extensive analysis on a larger sample of the same cohort showed evidence of widespread gray and white matter increases and decreases in the very preterm sample [34]. Additionally, these brain abnormalities accounted for 28% of the variance of reading and spelling scores in the group of very preterm-born adolescents.

Environmental factors and language outcome

The above studies suggest that the brain damage associated with very preterm birth is an important determinant of language outcome. Recent studies from neuroscience have also shown that experience and learning can alter and determine brain structure [35,36]. As such, the developmental trajectory of cognitive function must be understood as a dynamic process where biological factors interact with environmental factors throughout the protracted stage of development. Social factors have also been shown to predict functional outcome in very preterm-born children, though the data are not always consistent. Maternal education was associated with language function at 3.5 years [12], but another study found that very preterm preschool children at risk for persistent language difficulties did not differ in terms of environmental support indices (lower social class, lower levels of maternal education, or lone parenthood) from very preterm subjects without language deficits [10]. Downie et al. also failed to find a relationship between social factors (household income, maternal education) and academic outcome in their sample of very preterm-born children at age 11 years [23]. They speculated that the direct impact of these factors may become attenuated as the children get older, but they also allow for the possibility that their findings may be an artifact of reduced variability in social factors in their sample of predominantly middle-class white families. A number of studies of adolescent samples have shown that social class remains a significant predictor of reading and spelling ability [22]. However, more specific measures of language function, such as verbal fluency and phonological processing, were not predicted by social class but were by perinatal factors, such as birth weight and gestational age [21]. It is perhaps not surprising that core linguistic skills are less susceptible to non-specialist intervention from parents than reading and spelling, but persist as a long-lasting consequence of premature birth. In their follow-up of children from age 3 to 8 years, Ment et al. found that higher maternal education was associated with improvement in scores with age, but only in those children without evidence of significant brain injury [25]. This suggests that while social factors can impact on subsequent recovery of function, such recovery is limited in those with significant brain injury.

Understanding the neural basis of language deficits after very preterm birth

During normal brain development, neural systems responsible for cognitive behaviors progress from diffuse, undifferentiated systems to specialized systems, and the bulk of development occurs during the last trimester of gestation and a few years postnatally [24],

but continues through childhood and adolescence and beyond [37,38]. Later gray matter changes in the brain are well documented with a non-linear pattern of cortical growth and loss that continues throughout adolescence [37]. Paus et al. showed age-related changes in white matter density in a sample of 111 normally developing children and adolescents aged 4–17 years [38]. Age-related changes in the left arcuate fasciculus (the white matter tract which connects frontal and temporal language centers) and in the internal capsule were suggested as supporting developmental improvements in speech and motor function, respectively [38].

As increasing specialization of neural systems is thought to underpin advances in cognitive function in typically developing children, atypical development is likely to have functional consequences throughout development. The brain damage associated with very preterm birth has been well documented, and it is likely that alternative structure and functional relationships have developed over time. Functional neuroimaging studies offer the potential to study the neural correlates of cognitive function in vivo and are of special significance in understanding the neural basis of language function after preterm birth. A small number of these have been conducted to date and are reviewed in Chapter 7 [39–41]. Using functional MRI (fMRI,) Peterson et al. and Ment et al. studied the neural basis of language function in 8-year-old and 12-year-old children, respectively [39,40]. Both studies drew children from the same birth cohort (all born at 33 weeks or less gestation), and employed the same cognitive paradigm to investigate the neural basis of phonological and semantic processing. Rushe et al. also examined the functional neuroanatomy of phonological processing in a group of young adults (aged 18–20 years) who were born very preterm and who additionally showed evidence of thinning of the corpus callosum [41]. Taken together, the results from these studies suggest alternative specialization of the neural systems for semantic and phonological processing after very preterm birth.

Conclusion

Delays in the acquisition of language have been reported in very preterm-born children in the preschool years, and studies of school-age children and adolescents suggest that these difficulties persist into adolescence and beyond. Given the importance of language skills in both the social and academic life of the child, early identification and remediation of such difficulties are necessary in order to prevent increasing cognitive gaps between the very preterm child and his/her peers. Biological factors such as lower birth weight, younger gestational age, and evidence of cerebral brain injury have been associated with worse cognitive outcome, whereas social advantage has been associated with better outcome. There remains considerable inconsistency in the available literature, however, most likely due to methodological inconsistencies across studies.

There are now a few longitudinal studies that have attempted to explore the stability of language function from early childhood onwards and these are important in that biological and social factors remain relatively constant in the samples investigated. Evidence from behavioral neuroscience shows that structural and functional brain development is a dynamic process, so it remains a challenge for researchers in this area to explore how biological and social factors interact with each other to affect the cognitive and behavioral outcome of individuals who were born very preterm. Long-term (into adolescence and adulthood) outcome studies are important because a detailed understanding of the persistent effects of very preterm birth cannot be appreciated until the stage of acquisition or mastery of certain functions has passed. This is especially true for studies of language ability, where improvements are seen up until adulthood in normally developing subjects. Research should also capitalize on recent developments in neuroimaging in order to further understand the neural basis of language difficulties in very preterm-born subjects. The few fMRI studies conducted to date suggest altered neural specialization for linguistic systems, which may explain the persistent language deficits in very preterm-born children. White matter is preferentially affected by very preterm birth, so it is of interest to measure the longer-lasting consequences of such early damage, and particularly how it might affect the ongoing development of cognitive function. White matter integrity is particularly important for complex functions such as language, which rely on the effective communication between multiple neural networks. Using diffusion tensor imaging (DTI) (a magnetic resonance technique that can be used to investigate white matter microstructure) Klingberg *et al.* compared poor adult readers with normal readers and reported that white matter of the poor readers had significantly lower diffusion anisotropy (i.e., less organization) in temporoparietal cortex bilaterally [42]. The combination of imaging techniques, such as DTI and fMRI, in very preterm samples will additionally show how white matter abnormalities are related to altered cortical activation patterns.

References

1. Tomasello M, Bates E. *Language Development: The Essential Readings*. Oxford: Blackwell; 2001.

2. Berman R. Developing linguistic knowledge and language use across adolescence. In: Hoff E, Shatz M, eds. *Blackwell Handbook of Language Development*. Oxford: Blackwell. 2004; 347–67.

3. Cohen MJ, Morgan AM, Vaughn M, Riccio CA, Hall J. Verbal fluency in children: developmental issues and differential validity in distinguishing children with attention-deficit hyperactivity disorder and two subtypes of dyslexia. *Arch Clin Neuropsychol* 1999; **14**(5): 433–43.

4. Tombaugh TN, Kozak J, Rees L. Normative data stratified by age and education for two measures of verbal fluency: FAS and animal naming. *Arch Clin Neuropsychol* 1999; **14**(2): 167–77.

5. Matute E, Rosselli M, Ardila A, Morales G. Verbal and nonverbal fluency in Spanish-speaking children. *Dev Neuropsychol* 2004; **26**(2): 647–60.

6. Allin M, Walshe M, Fern A, *et al.* Cognitive maturation in preterm and term born adolescents. *J Neurol Neurosurg Psychiatry* 2008; **79**(4): 381–6.

7. Garton A, Pratt C. *Learning to be Literate: The Development of Spoken and Written Language*, 2nd edn. New York: Blackwell; 1998.

8. Foster-Cohen S, Edgin JO, Champion PR, Woodward LJ. Early delayed language development in very preterm infants: evidence from the Mac Arthur-Bates CDI. *J Child Lang* 2007; **34**(3): 655–75.

9. Grunau RV, Kearney SM, Whitfield MF. Language development at 3 years in pre-term children of birth weight below 1000 g. *Br J Disord Commun* 1990; **25**(2): 173–82.

10. Briscoe J, Gathercole SE, Marlow N. Short-term memory and language outcomes after extreme prematurity at birth. *J Speech Lang Hear Res* 1998; **41**(3): 654–66.

11. Le Normand MT, Cohen H. The delayed emergence of lexical morphology in preterm children: the case of verbs. *J Neurolinguistics* 1999; **12**: 235–46.

12. Sansavini A, Guarini A, Alessandroni R, *et al.* Are early grammatical and phonological working memory abilities affected by preterm birth? *J Commun Disord* 2007; **40**(3): 239–56.

13. Archibald LM, Gathercole SE. Short-term and working memory in specific language impairment. *Int J Lang Commun Disord* 2006; **41**(6): 675–93.

14. Luoma L, Herrgard E, Martikainen A, Ahonen T. Speech and language development of children born at < or = 32 weeks' gestation: a 5-year prospective follow-up study. *Dev Med Child Neurol* 1998; **40**(6): 380–7.

15. Largo RH, Molinari L, Kundu S, Lipp A, Duc G. Intellectual outcome, speech and school performance in high risk preterm children with birth weight appropriate for gestational age. *Eur J Pediatr* 1990; **149**(12): 845–50.

16. Wolke D, Meyer R. Cognitive status, language attainment, and prereading skills of 6-year-old very preterm children and their peers: the Bavarian Longitudinal Study. *Dev Med Child Neurol* 1999; **41**(2): 94–109.

17. Aram DM, Hack M, Hawkins S, Weissman BM, Borawski-Clark E. Very-low-birthweight children and speech and language development. *J Speech Hear Res* 1991; **34**(5): 1169–79.

18. Samuelsson S, Bylund B, Cervin T, *et al*. The prevalence of reading disabilities among very-low-birth-weight children at 9 years of age. *Dyslexia* 1999; **5**: 94–112.

19. Leonard L. *Children with Specific Language Impairment*. Cambridge: The MIT Press; 2000.

20. Rushe TM, Rifkin L, Stewart AL, *et al*. Neuropsychological outcome at adolescence of very preterm birth and its relation to brain structure. *Dev Med Child Neurol* 2001; **43**(4): 226–33.

21. Frearson SJ. Academic and neural correlates of neuropsychological outcome of adolescents born very preterm. Unpublished PhD thesis, Institute of Psychiatry, King's College London; 2004.

22. Breslau N, Paneth NS, Lucia VC. The lingering academic deficits of low birth weight children. *Pediatrics* 2004; **114**(4): 1035–40.

23. Downie AL, Frisk V, Jakobson LS. The impact of periventricular brain injury on reading and spelling abilities in the late elementary and adolescent years. *Child Neuropsychol* 2005; **11**(6): 479–95.

24. Aylward GP. Neurodevelopmental outcomes of infants born prematurely. *J Dev Behav Pediatr* 2005; **26**(6): 427–40.

25. Ment LR, Vohr B, Allan W, *et al*. Change in cognitive function over time in very-low-birth-weight infants. *JAMA* 2003; **289**(6): 705–11.

26. Saavalainen P, Luoma L, Bowler D, *et al*. Naming skills of children born preterm in comparison with their term peers at the ages of 9 and 16 years. *Dev Med Child Neurol* 2006; **48**(1): 28–32.

27. Nosarti C, Giouroukou E, Micali N, *et al*. Impaired executive functioning in young adults born very preterm. *J Int Neuropsychol Soc* 2007; **13**(4): 571–81.

28. Aram DM, Eisele JA. Plasticity and recovery of higher function following early brain injury. In: Boller F, Grafman J, eds. *Handbook of Neuropsychology*. Amsterdam: Elsevier. 1992; 73–91.

29. Bishop DVM. Language development after focal brain damage. In: Bishop DVM, Mogford K, eds. *Language Development in Exceptional Circumstances*. Edinburgh: Churchill Livingstone. 1988; 203–19.

30. Anderson V, Catroppa C, Morse S, Haritou F, Rosenfeld J. Functional plasticity or vulnerability after early brain injury? *Pediatrics* 2005; **116**(6): 1374–82.

31. Stewart AL, Rifkin L, Amess PN, *et al*. Brain structure and neurocognitive and behavioural function in adolescents who were born very preterm. *Lancet* 1999; **353**(9165): 1653–7.

32. Nosarti C, Rushe TM, Woodruff PW, *et al*. Corpus callosum size and very preterm birth: relationship to neuropsychological outcome. *Brain* 2004; **127**(Pt 9): 2080–9.

33. Allin M, Matsumoto H, Santhouse AM, *et al*. Cognitive and motor function and the size of the cerebellum in adolescents born very pre-term. *Brain* 2001; **124**(Pt 1): 60–6.

34. Nosarti C, Giouroukou E, Healy E, *et al*. Grey and white matter distribution in very preterm adolescents mediates neurodevelopmental outcome. *Brain* 2008; **131**(Pt 1): 205–17.

35. Rubia K. The dynamic approach to neurodevelopmental psychiatric disorders: use of fMRI combined with neuropsychology to elucidate the dynamics of psychiatric disorders, exemplified in ADHD and schizophrenia. *Behav Brain Res* 2002; **130**(1–2): 47–56.

36. Maguire EA, Gadian DG, Johnsrude IS, *et al*. Navigation-related structural change in the hippocampi of taxi drivers. *Proc Natl Acad Sci U S A* 2000; **97**(8): 4398–403.

37. Giedd JN, Blumenthal J, Jeffries NO, *et al*. Brain development during childhood and adolescence: a longitudinal MRI study. *Nat Neurosci* 1999; **2**(10): 861–3.

38. Paus T, Zijdenbos A, Worsley K, *et al*. Structural maturation of neural pathways in children and adolescents: in vivo study. *Science* 1999; **283**(5409): 1908–11.

39. Peterson BS, Vohr B, Kane MJ, *et al*. A functional magnetic resonance imaging study of language processing and its cognitive correlates in prematurely born children. *Pediatrics* 2002; **110**(6): 1153–62.

40. Ment LR, Peterson BS, Vohr B, *et al.* Cortical recruitment patterns in children born prematurely compared with control subjects during a passive listening functional magnetic resonance imaging task. *J Pediatr.* 2006; **149**(4):490–8.

41. Rushe TM, Temple CM, Rifkin L, *et al.* Lateralisation of language function in young adults born very preterm. *Arch Dis Child Fetal Neonatal Ed* 2004; **89**(2): F112–18.

42. Klingberg T, Vaidya CJ, Gabrieli JD, Moseley ME, Hedehus M. Myelination and organization of the frontal white matter in children: a diffusion tensor MRI study. *Neuroreport* 1999; **10**(13): 2817–21.

A cognitive neuroscience perspective on the development of memory in children born preterm

Michelle de Haan

Introduction

Memory is an important component of cognitive function, allowing individuals to build a stable knowledge base and to remember the details of everyday life. Abnormalities in the brain regions involved in memory, including the prefrontal cortex, caudate nucleus, and hippocampus, as well as the connections between them, have been documented in children who were born preterm and may result in compromised memory. The aim of this chapter is to briefly review what studies in cognitive neuroscience have revealed about the normal development and neural bases of different types of memory and to consider whether and how these skills are affected by premature birth.

Types of memory

Memory is not a unitary skill, but instead consists of a number of different components relying on different neural systems. One fundamental distinction is between implicit and explicit memory. Implicit memory is typically described as non-conscious, automatic, or not amenable to verbal recall, and examples include procedural skills such as knowledge of how to ride a bicycle. Explicit memory is typically described as knowledge that can be consciously brought to mind, and examples include knowledge of the definitions of words or memory for the "what, where, and when" of specific events such as a summer holiday. Explicit memory itself can be further divided into short-term or working memory, and long-term memory. Working memory refers to the type of memory used to hold information in mind for short periods until it is used to solve a problem or carry out a task, such as remembering a phone number until it is dialed. Long-term memory refers to memory systems used to store information once it is no longer in immediate attention. Long-term memory itself can be divided into two subcomponents,

memory for facts that is relatively independent of context (semantic memory), and memory for events linked to their spatial and temporal context (episodic memory). For example, remembering a fact such as "Paris is the capital of France" is considered semantic memory, whereas recalling the details of your last visit to France is considered episodic memory. Below, the neural bases and development of these different types of memory will be described in typical development and following preterm birth.

Working memory

Working memory is the "moment to moment monitoring, processing and maintenance of information" [1, p. 28]. It "allows humans … to maintain a limited amount of information in an active state for a brief period of time and to manipulate that information [2, p. 12 061]. For adults, the number of items is estimated at 1–10 over a time span of 0–60 seconds [2].

Working memory is often divided into three components: the central executive that controls and regulates the working memory system, and two domain-specific slave systems responsible for processing information in the phonological (phonological loop) or visuospatial (visuospatial sketchpad) form [3,4]. More recently an "episodic buffer" component has been added to this model that is involved in binding information from different sources [5], but it will not be discussed further here as there is little work on its development.

Visuospatial working memory

Studies with adults show that a fronto-parietal network plays an important role in visuospatial working memory (possibly especially on the right and possibly with a dorsal-ventral distinction in frontal areas for visual vs. spatial [6,7]). This has been studied mainly for visuospatial working memory but there is some evidence

Neurodevelopmental Outcomes of Preterm Birth, ed. Chiara Nosarti, Robin M. Murray, and Maureen Hack. Published by Cambridge University Press. © Cambridge University Press 2010.

for activation of similar pathways during audio-spatial working memory tasks [8] (though single-cell studies suggest different but parallel populations of neurons are involved [9]). The inferior posterior parietal and anterior occipital cortices appear to mediate short-term storage (whose contents decay rapidly; [2]), while the visual superior posterior parietal, premotor areas and dorsolateral prefrontal areas appear to be involved in rehearsal (allowing reactivation of the rapidly decaying contents of the storage component).

A fronto-parietal network also appears to be involved in children [10–16]. Activation in the superior frontal and intraparietal cortex is greater in older than younger children and working memory capacity is significantly correlated with brain activity in the same regions [12,17]. Interestingly, studies with adults also show increased activity in the fronto-parietal network with improvements in working memory following training [18]. In children, regions thought to underlie the phonological loop are additionally activated during spatial tasks [12]. Together, these results thus suggest that increases in working memory are associated with increases in activation in the fronto-parietal network and with an increased localization and specialization of activity [15]. Diffusion tensor imaging studies suggest that developmental increases in gray matter activation in frontal and parietal cortices could be due to maturation of white matter connections [19].

The developmental increases in working memory coincide with the timing of several neurodevelopmental processes including a decrease in synaptic density [20], axonal elimination [21], changes in global cerebral metabolism [22], and myelination [23]. The inferior parietal cortex is one of the last areas to myelinate, a change which would increase transmission locally within parietal cortex and also its communication with frontal cortex which could result in more stable fronto-parietal activity [17]. Synaptic pruning and axonal pruning could also result in less competition with input from other areas leaving the fronto-parietal network more stable. A more stable network would be less susceptible to interference and thus perform better. Neural network models support the idea that stronger fronto-parietal synaptic connectivity between cells coding for similar stimuli contributes to development of working memory [24].

Several studies have reported that visuospatial working memory is impaired in children born preterm. This includes children as young as 2–5 years of age [25–28] (but see [29]) to children aged 8–16

[30–33] (but see [34]). The deficits have been observed both in children selected for low risk (normal neonatal ultrasound; no global developmental delay) [26,27,33] and in unselected groups [28,32]. Working memory impairment is related to behavioral problems (inattentive behavior) in preterm individuals [35].

These impairments in working memory may not be surprising given that structural abnormalities in both gray and white matter have been reported in the fronto-parietal regions in children born preterm (e.g., [36–38]). However, few studies have directly examined links between brain structure or function and working memory performance in this population. In one study [28], both qualitative and quantitative assessment of magnetic resonance imaging (MRI) scans taken at term equivalent related to spatial working memory performance at 2 years of age (corrected). Qualitative assessment of white matter injury, and quantitative measures of total cerebral spinal fluid volume and total cerebral volume in dorsal regions predicted performance, while quantitative measures of cortical gray matter, myelinated or unmyelinated white matter, and deep nuclear gray matter did not. A secondary analysis examining subregions within cortical gray matter did show that tissue volumes in fronto-parietal subregions bilaterally predicted performance on the working memory task. In another study, adolescents who were born preterm showed atypical activation in the caudate nucleus, but not the hippocampus, during a spatial working memory task [39]. In a third study, adolescents born preterm scored lower than those born full term on spatial working memory and also had lowered hippocampal volumes bilaterally [31].

Phonological working memory

Phonological working memory is typically described as including two subcomponents, a phonological short-term store, within which memory traces fade after a few seconds, and a controlled articulatory rehearsal process, which is capable of refreshing the trace and thereby preventing its decay. As for visuospatial working memory, a fronto-parietal network is implicated in these abilities. Both studies of patients with brain injury [40] and neuroimaging studies of healthy individuals [41] suggest that the supramarginal gyrus of the inferior parietal lobe mediates the short-term store whereas premotor regions (Brodmann's areas 44 and 46) mediate the rehearsal process.

The development of neural networks underlying phonological working memory has been studied less frequently than the development of those involved in visuospatial working memory. As discussed above, there is evidence that the neural processes involved in visuospatial working memory and phonological working memory may be less distinct and more overlapping in young children, and become more differentiated with age. It is important to note however that behavioral studies do show that verbal and visuospatial working memory are separable even in children as young as 4–6 years of age [42–43].

Several studies have reported that children who were born very preterm ranging in age from 3 to 15 years tend to have impaired digit spans [25,44–47], though word span can be normal [25,44]. Such studies have also reported impairments in more complex working memory tasks such as mental arithmetic [25], phrase and sentence repetition [44], Behavior Rating Inventory Executing Function (BRIEF) working memory scales [45], and non-word repetition [47]. One study estimated that about one third of preterm preschoolers show very poor phonological working memory that puts them at risk for persisting language difficulties [48]. While some studies have examined the neural correlates of phonological processing in the context of language perception and comprehension in children born preterm (e.g., [49]), there has been little attention to the relationship between phonological working memory abilities and brain structure or function in this population.

Central executive

The central executive component of working memory acts as a supervisory system and controls attention and flow of information to and from the phonological loop and visuospatial sketchpad. It is closely related to a range of skills known more generally as "executive functions," which includes abilities such as planning ahead and organizing goal-directed behavior.

Studies in adults suggest that the dorsolateral prefrontal cortex and parietal association areas are an important part of the neural substrate of the central executive [50,51]. The central executive component of working memory is believed to be in place by at least 6 years of age, though it, together with the other components of working memory, expands considerably in its functional capacity throughout childhood into adolescence [43].

Few studies have specifically examined the central executive component of working memory in children born preterm, though several studies have examined the development of executive functions. Such studies have generally found that executive functions are impaired in children born preterm compared to children born full term, even when controlling for IQ [25,34]. There is evidence that white matter abnormalities, including those in the anterior corpus callosum [52], are related to impairments in executive functioning in children born preterm .

Summary

Working memory relies on a fronto-parietal network that normally shows greater activation and greater anatomical localization with increasing age during childhood. Studies with preterm individuals suggest that working memory is impaired in this population, though the extent to which such deficits are due to problems with the slave systems or with the central executive has not been studied in detail. A small number of studies have examined links between altered brain structure or function and working memory performance in preterm individuals. These studies suggest that there may be links between alterations in gray and white matter and working memory performance, however, more studies are needed to look in greater detail at the link between fronto-parietal networks and working memory in such populations.

Explicit long-term memory

Explicit long-term memory includes memory both for facts (semantic memory) and personal experiences (episodic memory) that can be brought to mind. Recall of items from episodic memory is by definition associated with retrieval of contextual details related to the encoding, whereas recall of items from semantic memory is not [53]. A similar distinction applies to recognition, whereby it can occur with retrieval of contextual details related to encoding ("recollection-based recognition") or without these additional details ("familiarity-based recognition" [54,55]).

There is consensus that the medial temporal lobe-cortical (MTL) circuit, involving the hippocampus and the perirhinal, entorhinal, and parahippocampal cortices, supports cognitive memory in human adults. According to one view [56] (see also [57]), these structures function in a hierarchy, wherein perceptual information first enters the parahippocampal regions mediating semantic memory (and familiarity-based recognition) and only then passes to hippocampal regions necessary for episodic memory (and recollection-based recognition). Others acknowledge the possibility of a division of labor within the MTL memory system, but argue that the hippocampus itself is involved in both semantic and episodic memory [58]. In addition to the MTL, the prefrontal cortex is known to play a role in explicit long-term memory, particularly recall memory.

Infancy

Visual recognition memory in infants born preterm has been examined using the visual paired comparison procedure. This task is believed to rely on the medial temporal lobe. Adult humans [59] and monkeys [60,61] with bilateral MTL lesions, including those restricted to the hippocampus [62] show the normal pattern of longer looking to novel than familiar stimuli when there is little or no delay between familiarization and test, but are impaired if a delay is imposed. Unlike these adults with lesions, full-term human infants show evidence of delayed memory: 3- to 4-day-olds look longer at a novel face than a familiar one even when a 2-minute delay is imposed [63], and 3-month-olds can do the same over a 24-hour delay [64]. Studies have shown that infants born preterm show reduced novelty preferences at 5–12 months' corrected age compared to full terms (e.g., [65,66]). Novelty preference scores are particularly affected in preterm infants who suffer respiratory distress syndrome postnatally, especially if they also required prolonged mechanical ventilation [66]. Event-related potential (ERP) studies of auditory recognition memory also suggest impairments: ERPs recorded at term show that preterm infants fail to recognize the mother's voice [67], and ERPs at 4 months of age show that novelty detection is present but smaller in size [68] (but see [69] for evidence of intact auditory recognition in a behavioral task). However, none of the studies imposed a delay between familiarization and memory test. Since novelty preferences are thought to require the hippocampus only if a delay is involved, the impairments observed in immediate tests might be due to damage in surrounding cortices or other brain regions. The finding of impaired novelty preference at immediate test also suggests a more general impairment in information processing, as such impairments have been linked to impaired speed of processing and to later IQ [70].

The earliest signs of recall memory seem to emerge in normally developing infants by approximately 6–9 months of age (e.g., [71,72]). This has been shown using a task called deferred imitation, where recall is inferred from better production of single actions or action sequences after observation of an experimenter

modeling actions compared to a pre-modeling baseline. Two studies demonstrate that memory in this task involves the MTL, one showing impairments in amnesic adults with MTL damage (but not in adults with frontal lobe damage [73]) and the other in individuals who sustained selective bilateral hippocampal lesions during infancy or early childhood [74].

Two studies have found that children born preterm are impaired on recall in deferred imitation tasks. In one study, toddlers tested at 19 months' corrected age showed poorer recall of 3-step sequences at immediate recall and after a 15-minute delay compared with their full-term counterparts [75]. Memory performance was related to gestational age at birth in this low-risk sample. Another study using a similar procedure found that deficits are present by 12 months' corrected age and persist until at least 36 months [76]. Although performance improves considerably from 12 to 36 months for both children born full term and those born preterm, there was no evidence of preterm "catch-up": the deficits detected at 12 months did not diminish with age. This study also found links between performance and medical risk factors: lower birth weight and lengthier postnatal hospitalization were associated with poorer performance in preterm children at 24 and 36 months. It is important to note that in neither study was the specificity of the memory impairment assessed, so it is not clear whether it reflects a particular difficulty with memory or whether it is part of a more widespread impairment of cognitive abilities.

Preschool and School Age

There is agreement that long-term memory skills improve over the preschool and school-age period, but few studies have examined the neural basis of these changes in typical development. Existing studies have provided some evidence for the role of the MTL, but very little is known about the role of the prefrontal cortex in the normal development of explicit memory.

Some studies have used ERPs to examine the development of recollection-based recognition. In adults, recollection-based recognition has a neural signature distinct from familiarity-based recognition. The studies with children indicate that the ERPs associated with recollection are present in children's ERPs by 10 years of age, suggesting that the medial temporal lobe memory systems believed to underlie recollection-based recognition are functioning by this age [77,78].

There is evidence that the hippocampus is important specifically for the normal development of the episodic component of long-term memory, as individuals who sustain selective, bilateral hippocampal damage in infancy or childhood show impairments in episodic memory with relative preservation of semantic memory and general intellectual abilities [79]. This type of memory impairment has been labeled "developmental amnesia" [80] and is thought to be related to hypoxic-ischemic injury. A hippocampal volume reduction of 20–30% bilaterally appears to be necessary to result in developmental amnesia [81].

Difficulties with explicit long-term memory might be expected in children born preterm, since neuroimaging studies suggest that structures in the medial temporal lobe, including the hippocampus, are abnormal in this population (e.g., [82]). Studies with preschool and school-age children who have been born preterm have primarily used standardized neuropsychological assessments of memory abilities. Generally, these studies have suggested that there are either no impairments in long-term memory [46,83–85] or that any impairments observed are in line with the level of general intellectual function and do not reflect specific memory deficits [83,85].

Some studies have attempted to link brain and memory in children born preterm. One line of study examined whether neonatal hydrocortisone treatment for bronchopulmonary dysplasia affects memory or the hippocampus, since corticosteroids are known to influence this brain structure. These studies have found no difference in memory or hippocampal structure in these children, and no relation between the development of the hippocampus to memory ability [86,87]. Other studies have more directly compared preterm individuals with term controls. One such study found that the hippocampus was reduced in size in adolescents who were born preterm who were selected for having spent a long period on ventilation postnatally [31]. Some aspects of memory were also impaired in these children, including working memory. However, long-term episodic memory did not appear to be particularly affected. Since the hippocampus was the only structure measured in this study, it is difficult to know whether other brain structures may have contributed to the memory difficulties that were observed.

Summary

The medial temporal lobe and surrounding cortices play an important role in explicit long-term memory. There is limited information about the normal development of brain systems underlying this type of memory,

existing studies implicate the medial temporal lobes and it is likely that development of prefrontal areas also contributes to development of explicit long-term memory. Overall, studies with children born preterm suggest that long-term memory is not affected, at least not disproportionately relative to their level of general intellectual functioning. So far, studies have not typically compared episodic and semantic memory to examine whether both are equally affected or unaffected.

Implicit long-term memory

Implicit long-term memory encompasses a variety of abilities, which share the distinction from cognitive memory in being skills that are not easily verbalized and typically measured instead as changes in performance, such as decreased reaction times. Three commonly studied examples of implicit memory are priming, conditioning, and procedural learning [88]. This chapter will focus on procedural learning, since the literature on the neural bases of development in humans is greatest for this type of implicit memory.

Procedural learning is long-term memory for skills or procedures, often described as the slow acquisition over time of "how to do things," such as riding a bicycle or playing a piano. Although the individual may be intentionally trying to learn such skills, he/she is typically unaware of what exactly is being learned. Procedural learning is mediated by regions including a fronto-striatal circuit. This aspect of implicit long-term memory may be especially at risk following preterm birth since it relies on motor abilities which can often be affected in this population (reviewed in [89]).

Development of procedural learning has been studied using the serial reaction time task [90]. In this task, individuals are asked to map a set of spatial or object stimuli onto an equal number of response buttons. Without the knowledge of the individual, the stimuli are presented in a predictable and repeating sequence. Implicit learning is said to occur when individuals show faster reaction times during the repeating sequences than during comparison intervals when stimuli are presented randomly, even though they have no conscious awareness of the regularities. There is some controversy regarding the development of procedural learning as measured by the serial reaction time task, with some studies finding that performance is similar in young children and adults [91], but others finding that abilities improve with age [92]. Regardless, neuroimaging evidence does suggest that a fronto-striatal circuit is also involved in procedural learning in typically developing children [93]. However, children and adults differ in that children show more subcortical activity and adults show more cortical activity.

There is limited information about the development of procedural memory in children born preterm. One study examined implicit sequence learning in children who had been born preterm and who had sustained intraventricular hemorrhage [94], as severe intraventricular hemorrhage is associated with basal ganglia injury [95]. Results showed that children who had sustained unilateral grade 2 hemorrhage or less severe insults performed similarly to age- and gender-matched full-term children, whereas those who had sustained bilateral grade 2 hemorrhage or more severe insults performed more poorly. Another study used a simpler motor learning task suitable for infants and compared performance in preterm and full-term infants at 5, 7, and 12 months of age [96]. In this visual expectancy task, infants are shown a repeating pattern of visual stimuli, and eye movements are measures to determine if infants learn to anticipate the location of the upcoming stimulus over time. The authors reported similar findings for both preterm and full-term infants, with both groups showing decreased reaction times and increase anticipation with age.

Conclusion

Delays in perceptual and cognitive development have often been reported in children born preterm, and memory appears to be no exception. Overall, the evidence suggests that working memory is impaired in children born preterm, whereas explicit long-term memory is less likely to be affected. There is much more limited data with respect to implicit long-term memory, with studies of procedural learning suggesting that it may only be impaired in cases of frank basal ganglia damage.

Impairments in both visuospatial and phonological working memory have been reported in children born preterm. It is not entirely clear whether these deficits reflect primary deficits in these slave systems or whether they are a consequence of damage to the central executive components. It is important to note also that children born preterm can often experience perceptual deficits that could affect their performance on working memory tasks, though there is evidence that limitations in visual perception do not necessarily affect complex cognitive skills [97]. Understanding the neural bases, developmental course, and cognitive source of impairments in working memory may

provide insight into the poor school achievement that has been reported in children born preterm, because working memory ability has been shown to be a predictor of academic achievement in this population (e.g., [98]). Existing evidence suggests that development of a fronto-parietal network is important for improvements in working memory with age. In particular, increasing stability of this network and localization and specialization of its activation has been associated with increases in working memory capacity. Future studies can illuminate whether the impairments observed in preterm individuals are associated with disruption of these typical developmental processes.

Specific impairment in explicit long-term memory does not seem to be a general feature of children born preterm. This is perhaps surprising given that neuroimaging studies have shown that structures considered critical for this ability, such as the hippocampus, are abnormal in preterm groups. It is possible that, in the case of the hippocampus, the degree of volume reduction observed in children born preterm is not typically sufficient to make a full-blown impairment in episodic long-term memory, a common feature in this group of children [81]. Another possibility is that additional damage that co-occurs with hippocampal injury results in a more general lowering of cognitive abilities rather than a selective memory impairment. Future studies which examine in more detail the semantic and episodic components of explicit long-term memory may help to clarify the nature and extent of any deficits in this skill.

Relatively few studies have focused on long-term implicit memory development and its neural correlates in children born preterm. The procedural type of implicit learning relies on a fronto-striatal circuit, and thus might be anticipated to be affected in children born preterm, particularly those experiencing hypoxic-ischemic injury or intraventricular hemorrhage, since both can affect the basal ganglia. Existing studies suggest that impairments in procedural learning are not a general characteristic of preterm individuals, but that they can be found in those children in whom basal ganglia injury is suspected. There is little information about other types of implicit learning in children born preterm such as priming and conditioning. Given that implicit memory is believed to play a role in functions such as language acquisition (e.g., [99]), a more detailed understanding of its development in preterm individuals would be useful.

Understanding of the prevalence and neural bases of specific memory impairments in children born preterm is clearly still limited. Future studies should try to dissociate a possible memory deficit from other impairments seen in this group, for example language deficits, which might overshadow everyday memory problems. In addition, investigating the relationships between different cognitive abilities can illuminate how a deficit in one affects the development of others, or possibly how recovery of function may occur at the expense of other skills. It would be valuable to apply knowledge gained from developmental cognitive neuroscience to preterm research in terms of the cognitive organization and neural bases of memory systems in typical development and the tasks best used to assess these specific abilities. In addition, more investigations into the brain lesions of these children in relation to their cognitive profiles might further elucidate the common structural and functional deficits in this group. Structural and functional neuroimaging will play an important role in these goals, particularly as these techniques develop to allow more precise characterization of the extent of brain injuries and how these may impact brain development more generally (see Chapters 4–8). Longitudinal studies are also important, to understand how brain plasticity may allow functional recovery or how deficits may become more apparent as the brain matures. These types of studies may help to provide a better support for the cognitive development and educational outcome of children born preterm.

References

1. Baddeley A, Logie RH. Working memory: the multiple component model. In: Miyake A, Shah P, eds. *Models of Working Memory*. New York: Cambridge University Press. 1999; 28–61.

2. Smith EE, Jonides J. Neuroimaging analyses of human working memory. *Proc Natl Acad Sci U S A*, 1998; **95**: 12061–8.

3. Baddeley A, Hitch GJ. Working memory. In: Bower G, ed. *The Psychology of Learning and Motivation,* Vol. 8. San Diego: Academic Press. 1974; 47–90.

4. Baddeley A. *Working Memory*. Oxford: Clarendon Press; 1986.

5. Baddeley A. The episodic buffer: a new component of working memory? *Trends Cogn Sci* 2000; **4**: 417–23.

6. Ruchkin DS, Johnson R, Jr., Grafman J, Canoune H, Ritter W. Multiple visuospatial working memory buffers: evidence from spatiotemporal patterns of brain activity. *Neuropsychologia* 1997; **35**: 195–209.

7. Sala JB, Rama P, Courtney SM. Functional topography of a distributed neural system for spatial and nonspatial information maintenance in working memory. *Neuropsychologia* 2003; **41**: 341–56.

8. Martinkauppi S, Rama P, Aronen HJ, Korvenoja A, Carlson S. Working memory of auditory localization. *Cereb Cortex* 2000; **10**: 889–98.

9. Kikuchi-Yorioka Y, Sawaguchi T. Parallel visuospatial and audiospatial working memory processes in the monkey dorsolateral prefrontal cortex. *Nat Neurosci* 2000; **3**: 1075–6.

10. Casey BJ, Cohen JD, Jezzard P, *et al.* Activation of prefrontal cortex in children during a nonspatial working memory task with functional MRI. *Neuroimage* 1995; **2**: 221–9.

11. Crone EA, Wendelken C, Donohue S, van Leijenhorst L, Bunge SA. Neurocognitive development of the ability to manipulate information in working memory. *Proc Natl Acad Sci U S A* 2006; **103**: 9315–20.

12. Kwon H, Reiss AL, Menon V. Neural basis of protracted developmental changes in visuo-spatial working memory. *Proc Natl Acad Sci U S A* 2002; **99**: 13336–41.

13. Nelson CA, Monk CS, Lin J, *et al.* Functional neuroanatomy of spatial working memory in children. *Dev Psychol* 2000; **36**: 109–16.

14. Olesen PJ, Macoveanu J, Tegner J, Klingberg T. Brain activity related to working memory and distraction in children and adults. *Cereb Cortex* 2007; **17**: 1047–54.

15. Scherf KS, Sweeney JA, Luna B. Brain basis of developmental change in visuospatial working memory. *J Cogn Neurosci* 2006; **18**: 1045–58.

16. Thomas KM, King SW, Franzen PL, *et al.* A developmental functional MRI study of spatial working memory. *Neuroimage* 1999; **10**: 327–38.

17. Klingberg T, Forssberg H, Westerberg H. Increased brain activity in frontal and parietal cortex underlies the development of visuospatial working memory capacity during childhood. *J Cogn Neurosci* 2002; **14**: 1–10.

18. Olesen PJ, Westerberg H, Klingberg T. Increased prefrontal and parietal activity after training of working memory. *Nat Neurosci* 2004; **7**: 75–9.

19. Olesen PJ, Nagy Z, Westerberg H, Klingberg T. Combined analysis of DTI and fMRI data reveals a joint maturation of white and grey matter in a fronto-parietal network. *Brain Res Cogn Brain Res* 2003; **18**: 48–57.

20. Bourgeois JP, Rakic P. Changes of synaptic density in the primary visual cortex of the macaque monkey from fetal to adult stage. *J Neurosci* 1993; **13**: 2801–20.

21. LaMantia AS, Rakic P. Axon overproduction and elimination in the corpus callosum of the developing rhesus monkey. *J Neurosci* 1990; **10**: 2156–75.

22. Chugani HT, Phelps, ME. Maturational changes in cerebral function in infants determined by 18FDG positron emission tomography. *Science* 1986; **231**: 840–3.

23. Paus T, Zijdenbos A, Worsley K, *et al.* Structural maturation of neural pathways in children and adolescents: in vivo study. *Science* 1999; **283**: 1908–11.

24. Edin F, Macoveanu J, Olesen P, Tegner J, Klingberg T. Stronger synaptic connectivity as a mechanism behind development of working memory-related brain activity during childhood. *J Cogn Neurosci* 2007; **19**: 750–60.

25. Bohm B, Smedler AC, Forssberg H. Impluse control, working memory and other executive functions in preterm children when starting school. *Acta Paediatr* 2004; **93**: 1363–71.

26. Caravale B, Tozzi C, Albino G, Vicari S. Cognitive development in low risk preterm infants at 3–4 years of life. *Arch Dis Child Fetal Neonatal Ed* 2005; **90**: F474–9.

27. Vicari S, Caravale B, Carlesimo GA, Casadei AM, Allemand F. Spatial working memory deficits in children ages 3–4 who were low birth weight, preterm infants. *Neuropsychology* 2004; **18**: 673–78.

28. Woodward LJ, Edgin JO, Thompson D, Inder TE. Object working memory deficits predicted by early brain injury and development in the preterm infant. *Brain* 2005; **128**: 2578–87.

29. Matthews A, Ellis AE, Nelson CA. Development of preterm and full-term infant ability on AB, recall memory, transparent barrier and means-ends tasks. *Child Dev* 1996; **67**: 2658–76.

30. Curtis WJ, Lindeke LL, Georgieff MK, Nelson CA. Neurobehavioural functioning in neonatal intensive care unit graduates in late childhood and early adolescence. *Brain* 2002; **125**: 1646–59.

31. Isaacs EB, Lucas A, Chong W, *et al*. Hippocampal volume and everyday memory in children of very low birth weight. *Pediatrics* 2000; **47**: 713–20.

32. Luciana M, Lindeke L, Georgieff M, Mills M, Nelson CA. Neurobehavioural evidence for working-memory deficits in school-aged children with histories of prematurity. *Dev Med Child Neurol* 1999; **41**: 521–33.

33. Saavalainen PM, Luoma L, Bowler D, *et al*. Spatial span in very prematurely born adolescents. *Dev Neuropsychol* 2007; **32**: 769–85.

34. Bayless S, Stevenson J. Executive functions in school-age children born very prematurely. *Early Hum Dev* 2007; **83**: 247–54.

35. Nadeau L, Boivin M, Tessier R, Lefebvre F, Robaey P. Mediators of behavioral problems in 7-year-old children born after 24–28 weeks of gestation. *J Dev Behav Pediatr* 2001; **22**: 1–10.

36. Anjari M, Srinivasan L, Allsop JM, *et al*. Diffusion tensor imaging with tract-based spatial statistics reveals local white matter abnormalities in preterm and infants. *Neuroimage* 2007; **35**: 1012–27.

37. Kesler SR, Ment LR, Vohr B, *et al*. Volumetric analysis of regional cerebral development in preterm children. *Pediatr Neurol* 2004; **31**: 318–25.

38. Nosarti C, Giouroukou E, Healy E, *et al*. Gray and white matter distribution in very preterm adolescents mediates neurodevelopmental outcome. *Brain* 2008; **131**: 205–17.

39. Curtis WJ, Zhuang J, Townsend EL, Hu X, Nelson CA. Memory in early adolescents born prematurely: a functional magnetic resonance imaging investigation. *Dev Neuropsychol* 2006; **29**: 341–77.

40. Vallar G, DiBetta AM, Silveri MC. The phonological store-rehearsal system: patterns of impairment and neural correlates. *Neuropsychologia* 1997; **35**: 795–812.

41. Henson RN, Burgess N, Frith CD. Recoding, storage, rehearsal and grouping in verbal short-term memory: an fMRI study. *Neuropsychologia* 2000; **38**: 426–40.

42. Alloway TP, Gathercole SE, Pickering SJ. Verbal and visuospatial short-term and working memory in children: are they separable? *Child Dev* 2006; **77**: 1698–716.

43. Gathercole SE, Pickering SJ, Ambridge B, Wearing H. The structure of working memory from 4 to 15 years of age. *Dev Psychol* 2004; **40**: 177–90.

44. Sansavini A, Guarini, A, Alessandroni R, *et al*. Are early grammatical and phonological working memory abilities affected by preterm birth? *J Commun Disord* 2006; **40**: 239–56.

45. Anderson PJ, Doyle LW; the Victorian Infant Collaborative Study Group. Executive functioning in school-aged children who were born very preterm or with extremely low birth weight in the 1990s. *Pediatrics* 2004; **114**: 50–7.

46. Rushe TM, Rifkin L, Stewart AL, *et al*. Neuropsychological outcome at adolescence of very preterm birth and its relation to brain structure. *Dev Med Child Neurol* 2001; **43**: 226–33.

47. Pasman JW, Rotteveel JJ, Massen, B. Neurodevelopmental profile in low-risk preterm infants at 5 years of age. *Eur J Pediatr Neurol* 1998; **2**: 7–17.

48. Briscoe J, Gathercole, SE, Marlow N. Short-term memory and language outcomes after extreme prematurity at birth. *J Speech, Lang Hear Res* 1998; **41**: 654–66.

49. Peterson BS, Vohr B, Kane MJ, *et al*. A functional magnetic resonance imaging study of language processing and its cognitive correlates in prematurely born children. *Pediatrics* 2002; **110**: 1153–62.

50. D'Esposito M, Detre JA, Aslop DC, *et al*. The neural basis of the central executive system of working memory. *Nature* 1995; **378**: 279–81.

51. Salmon E, Van der Linden M, Collette, F, *et al*. Regional brain activity during working memory tasks. *Brain* 1996; **119**: 1617–25.

52. Narberhaus A, Segarra D, Caldu X, *et al*. Corpus callosum and prefrontal functions in adolescents with history of very preterm birth. *Neuropsychologia* 2008; **46**: 111–16.

53. Tulving E. Episodic and semantic memory. In Tulving E, Donaldson W, eds. *Organisation of Memory*. London: Academic Press. 1972; 381–403.

54. Tulving E. How many memory systems are there? *Am Psycholo* 1985; **40**: 395–8.

55. Yonelinas AP. Receiver-operating characteristics in recognition memory: evidence for a dual-process model. *J Exp Psychol Learn Mem Cogn* 1994; **20**: 1341–54.

56. Mishkin M, Suzuki WA, Gadian DG, Vargha-Khadem F. Hierarchical organization of cognitive memory. *Philos Trans R Soc Lond B Biol Sci* 1997; **352**: 1451–67.

57. Aggleton JP, Brown MW. Episodic memory, amnesia, and the hippocampal-anterior thalami axis. *Behav Brain Sci* 1999; **22**: 424–44.

58. Squire LR, Stark CE, Clark RE. The medial temporal lobe. *Annu Rev Neurosci* 2004; **27**: 279–306.

59. McKee RD, Squire LR. On the development of declarative memory. *J Exp Psychol Learn Mem Cogn* 1993; **19**: 397–404;

60. Bachevalier J, Brickson M, Hagger C. Limbic-dependent recognition memory in monkeys develops early in infancy. *Neuroreport* 1993; **4**: 77–80.

61. Pascalis O, Bachevalier J. Neonatal aspirations of the hippocampal formation impair visual recognition memory when assessed by paired-comparison task but not by delayed nonmatching to sample task. *Hippocampus* 1999; **9**: 609–16.

62. Pascalis O, Hunkin NM, Holdstock JS, Isaac CL, Mayes AR. Visual paired comparison performance is impaired in a patient with selective hippocampal lesions and relatively intact item recognition. *Neuropsychologia* 2004; **42**: 1293–300.

63. Pascalis O, de Schonen S. Recognition memory in 3- to 4-day-old infants. *Neuroreport* 1994; **5**: 1721–4.

64. Pascalis O, de Haan M, Nelson CA, de Schonen S. Long-term recognition memory for faces assessed by visual paired comparison in 3- and 6-month-olds. *J Exp Psychol Learn Mem Cogn* 1998; **24**: 249–60.

65. Rose SA, Feldman JF, Jankowski J. Attention and recognition memory in the 1st year of life: a longitudinal study of preterm and full-term infants. *Dev Psychol* 2001; **37**: 135–51.

66. Rose SA, Feldman JF, McCarton CM, Wolfson J. Information processing in seven-month-old infants as a function of risk status. *Child Dev* 1988; **59**: 589–603.

67. Therien JM, Worwa CT, Mattia FR, deRegnier RA. Altered pathways for auditory discrimination and recognition memory in preterm infants. *Dev Med Child Neurol* 2004; **46**: 816–24.

68. Tokioka AB, Pearce JW, Crowell DH. Endogenous event-related potentials in term and preterm infants. *J Clin Neurophysiol* 1995; **12**: 468–75.

69. O'Connor MJ. A comparison of preterm and fullterm infants on an auditory discrimination at four months and on Bayley Scales of Infant Development at 18 months. *Child Dev* 1980; **51**: 81–8.

70. Rose SA, Feldman JF. Memory and speed: their role in the relation of infant information processing to later IQ. *Child Dev* 1997; **68**: 630–41.

71. Carver LJ, Bauer PJ. The dawning of a past: The emergence of long-term explicit memory in infancy. *J Exp Psychol Gen* 2001; **130**: 726–45.

72. Herbert J, Gross J, Hayne H. Age-related changes in deferred imitation between 6 and 9 months of age. *Infant Behav Dev* 2006; **29**: 136–9.

73. McDonough L, Mandler JM, McKee RD, Squire, LR. The deferred imitation task as a nonverbal measure of declarative memory. *Proc Natl Acad Sci U S A* 1995; **92**: 7580–4.

74. Adlam AL, Vargha-Khadem F, Mishkin M de Haan M. Deferred imitation of action sequences in developmental amnesia. *J Cogn Neurosci 2005;* **17**: 240–8.

75. de Haan M, Bauer PJ, Georgieff MK, Nelson CA. Explicit memory in low-risk infants aged 19 months born between 27 and 42 months of gestation. *Dev Med Child Neurol* 2000; **42**: 304–12.

76. Rose SA, Feldman JF, Jankowski J. Recall memory in the first three years of life : a longitudinal study of preterm and term children. *Dev Med Child Neurol* 2005; **47**: 653–9.

77. Czernochowski D, Mecklinger A, Johansson M, Brinkmann, M. Age-related differences in familiarity and recollection: ERP evidence from a recognition memory study in children and young adults. *Cogn Affect Behav Neurosci* 2005; **5**: 417–33.

78. de Chastelaine M, Friedman D, Cycowicz YM. The development of control processes supporting source memory discrimination as revealed by event-related potentials. *J Cogn Neurosci* 2007; **19**: 1286–301.

79. Vargha-Khadem F, Gadian DG, Watkins KE, *et al.* Differential effects of early hippocampal pathology on episodic and semantic memory. *Science* 1997; **277**: 376–80.

80. Gadian DG, Aicardi J, Watkins KE, *et al.* Developmental amnesia associated with early hypoxic-ischemic injury. *Brain* 2000; **123**: 499–507.

81. Isaacs EB, Vargha-Khadem F, Watkins KE, *et al.* Developmental amnesia and its relationship to degree of hippocampal atrophy. *Proc Natl Acad Sci U S A* 2003; **100**: 13060–3.

82. Nosarti C, Al Asady MH, Frangou S, *et al.* Adolescents who were born very preterm have decreased brain volumes. *Brain* 2002; **125**: 1616–23.

83. Hoff Esbjorn B, Hansen BM, Greisen G, Mortensen EL. Intellectual development in a Danish cohort

of prematurely born preschool children: specific or general difficulties? *J Dev Behav Pediatr* 2006; **27**: 477–84.

84. Briscoe J, Gathercole SE, Marlow N. Everday memory and cognitive ability in children born very prematurely. *J Child Psychol Psychiatry* 2001; **42**: 749–54.

85. Narberhaus A, Segarra D, Gimenez M, *et al.* Memory performance in a sample of very low birth weight adolescents. *Dev Neuropsychol* 2007; **31**: 129–35.

86. Rademaker KJ, Rijpert M, Uiterwaal CS, *et al.* Neonatal hydrocortisone treatment related to 1H-MRS of the hippocampus and short-term memory at school age in preterm born children. *Pediatr Res* 2006; **59**: 309–13.

87. Rademaker KJ, Uiterwaal CS, Groenendaal F, *et al.* Neonatal hydrocortisone treatment: neurodevelopmental outcome and MRI at school age in preterm-born children. *J Pediatr* 2007; **150**: 351–7.

88. Squire LR, Knowlton B, Musen G. Structure and organization of memory. *Annu Rev Psychol* 1993; **44**: 453–99.

89. Bracewell M, Marlow, N. Patterns of motor disability in very preterm children. *Men Retard Dev Disabil Res Rev* 2002; **8**: 241–8.

90. Nissen M, Bullemer P. Attentional requirements of learning. Evidence from performance measures. *Cogn Psychol* 1987; **19**: 1–32.

91. Meulmans T, van der Linden M, Perrucher P. Implicit sequence learning in children. *J Exp Child Psychol* 1998; **69**: 199–221.

92. Thomas KM, Nelson CA. Serial reaction time learning in preschool- and school-aged children. *J Exp Child Psychol* 2001; **79**: 364–87.

93. Thomas KM, Hunt R, Vizueta N, *et al.* Evidence of developmental differences in implicit sequence learning: an fMRI study of children and adults. *J Cogn Neurosci* 2004; **16**: 1339–51.

94. Thomas KM, Vizueta N, Teylan M, Eccard C, Casey BJ. Implicit learning in patients with presumed basal ganglia insults: Evidence from a serial reaction time task. Paper presented at the annual meeting of the Cognitive Neuroscience Society, New York; 2003.

95. Soghier LM, Vega M, Aref K, *et al.* Diffuse basal ganglia or thalamus hyperechogenicity in preterm infants. *J Perinatol* 2006; **26**: 230–6.

96. Rose SA, Feldman JF, Jankowski J, Caro DM. A longitudinal study of visual expectation and reaction time in the first year of life. *Child Dev* 2002; **73**: 47–61.

97. Stiers P, Vandenbuscche, E. The dissociation of perception and cognition in children with early brain damage. *Brain Dev* 2004; **26**: 81–92.

98. Gathercole SE, Pickering SJ. Working memory deficits in children with low achievements in the national curriculum at 7 years of age. *Br J Educ Psychol* 2000; **70**: 177–84.

99. Ullman MT. The declarative/procedural model of lexicon and grammar. *J Psycholinguist Res* 2001; **30**: 37–69.

Chapter 15

Executive function development in preterm children

Peter J. Anderson, Kelly Howard, and Lex W. Doyle

Introduction

Prematurity is a major public health issue given the increasing rate of preterm births, the improved survival rate for children born extremely preterm, and the substantial costs associated with caring for these children in the neonatal period and beyond [1]. For the families of preterm children, the most common concern is the long-term intellectual, educational, and behavioral outcome for their child, as these issues greatly affect social and adaptive functioning and vocational opportunities. The concerns of parents are warranted, as many preterm children will develop an impairment in at least one of these areas, with the rate of impairment increasing with decreasing weight and gestational age at birth [2–4].

In the past 20 years a number of outcome studies have focused on children born very preterm (VPT; born prior to 32 completed weeks' gestation) or very low birth weight (VLBW; birth weight <1500 g). Research indicates that VPT/VLBW children frequently display cognitive impairment [3], with the rate of intellectual impairment being approximately three times greater in VPT/VLBW children compared with full-term-born peers [2]. An array of cognitive deficits have been reported in this population including visuomotor problems [5], attentional difficulties [6], impaired memory [7], delayed language skills [8], and executive dysfunction [9]. Consistent with this profile of cognitive impairment, relatively high rates of learning disabilities are cited (see also Chapter 16) [2,4]. Very preterm/very low birth weight children also tend to have higher rates of social and emotional difficulties, such as poorer social skills, social withdrawal, anxiety, and depression [10]. In addition, an increased prevalence of developmental disorders (i.e., attention deficit hyperactivity disorder [ADHD], autism) has been described in the preterm population [11,12].

One area of cognitive functioning that has attracted recent interest in VPT/VLBW children is executive functioning. Executive function is an umbrella term that refers to a collection of cognitive processes, which are responsible for goal-directed or future-oriented behavior [13]. The key elements of executive function include (a) anticipation and deployment of attention; (b) impulse control and self-regulation; (c) initiation of activity; (d) working memory; (e) mental flexibility and utilization of feedback; (f) planning ability and organization; and (g) selection of efficient problem-solving strategies [14]. Given the broad nature of this construct, impaired executive functioning can be inferred from a variety of presentations including an inability to focus or maintain attention, impulsivity, disinhibition, reduced working memory, difficulties monitoring or regulating performance, inability to plan actions in advance, disorganization, poor reasoning ability, difficulties generating and/or implementing strategies, perseverative behavior, a resistance to change activities, difficulties shifting between conflicting demands, and a failure to learn from mistakes [14]. Executive dysfunction is also often associated with maladaptive affect, energy level, initiative, and moral and social behavior.

Executive dysfunction may lead to secondary problems such as academic, social, communication, and adaptive difficulties, and thus can have considerable ramifications to a child's quality of life. In VPT/VLBW children, a number of studies have examined specific elements of executive function, and this chapter will review this research. A conceptual model of executive function will be presented to provide a framework for examining different aspects of executive functioning across development. We will discuss risk factors that may be associated with executive dysfunction in this population, and also propose possible neural mechanisms underpinning executive dysfunction in VPT/VLBW children.

Neurodevelopmental Outcomes of Preterm Birth, ed. Chiara Nosarti, Robin M. Murray, and Maureen Hack. Published by Cambridge University Press. © Cambridge University Press 2010.

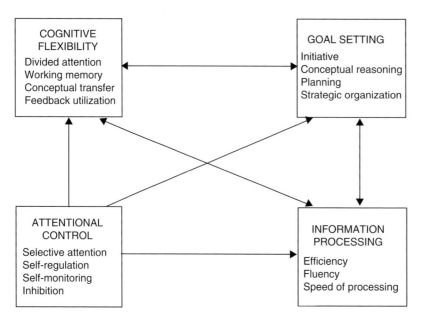

Fig. 15.1. The executive control system. Adapted from "Assessment and development of executive function (EF) during childhood," by P. Anderson, *Child Neuropsychol* 2002; **8**(2), p. 73.

Conceptual model of executive function

Operational frameworks for psychological constructs are important, as they provide the basis for interpreting behavior and studying development. Various theoretical models of executive function have been proposed, although no model has been uniformly accepted. For the purposes of this review, we will adopt the executive control system [13,14]. This framework conceptualizes executive function as an overall control system which comprises four distinct domains: attentional control, cognitive flexibility, goal setting, and information processing (Fig. 15.1). While these domains are independent and comprise discrete functions, in order to operate in a functional manner they interact and have bidirectional relationships. Task requirements determine the level of input from each domain, and thus the operation of the executive control system is task dependent.

The *attentional control* domain includes the capacity to selectively attend to specific stimuli and the ability to focus attention for a prolonged period. This domain also involves the regulation and monitoring of actions, so that plans are executed in the correct order, errors are identified, and goals are achieved. Impulse control is also an integral component of attentional control, such as the capacity to delay gratification and inhibit prepotent responses. The *cognitive flexibility* domain includes the ability to shift between

response sets, learn from mistakes, devise alternative strategies, divide attention, and process multiple sources of information concurrently. The manipulation component of working memory is also an aspect of this domain. The *goal setting* domain includes the ability to initiate, or the capacity to start an activity and devise a plan to complete a task/activity. It also comprises the ability to plan. Planning ability involves anticipating future events, formulating a goal or end point, and devising a sequence of steps or actions that will achieve the goal or end state. Related to planning ability is organization. Organization in this model refers to the ability to arrange complex information, or a sequence of steps, in a logical, systematic, and strategic manner. Organization has important consequences as to how efficiently and effectively goals are attained, and is associated with how well information or plans are remembered and retrieved. The fourth domain in this model is *information processing*, as executive functioning cannot be assessed without taking into account issues of fluency, efficiency, and speed of output.

Methodological considerations

Given the above conceptualization of executive function, it is possible for individuals to display global executive dysfunction (i.e., deficits across all executive domains) or specific executive dysfunction (i.e., deficits restricted to selective executive processes), although clinical research suggests that global executive dysfunction is rare [15]. Most studies examining executive function in VPT/VLBW children have focused either on a specific executive process or set of processes, and as a consequence, from individual studies it has been difficult to ascertain whether VPT/VLBW children exhibit a global or specific impairment in executive functioning.

Furthermore, some studies have employed a narrow assessment protocol, focusing on executive processes and ignoring other cognitive domains such as perceptual, language, visuospatial, and memory processes. Executive processes are considered higher-order processes, and, as such, are dependent on lower-order processes such as sensory processing, perception, and memory. Given that deficits in lower-order processes have been reported [5,7], it is reasonable to hypothesize that executive impairments exhibited by VPT/VLBW children reflect deficient functioning in "ingredient" processes, or in other words, those that are necessary for higher-order processing. Some authors have attempted to deal with the issue by controlling for IQ [16–20], but this approach does not adequately account for the contributions of lower-order processes. When broader assessment protocols are adopted that include measures of executive and non-executive processes, a differential analysis may be useful for identifying the presence and severity of deficits across different cognitive domains [21]. Usually, a differential analysis involves a qualitative assessment of the pattern of deficits, in order to identify those cognitive processes that are more frequently and/or severely affected within a clinical population. While this approach has merit, it does not adequately account for the integrative and hierarchical features of general information processing. For example, higher-order processes such as executive function have a far greater reliance and dependency on other processes than more basic processes, such as sensation and perception. Another approach is to assess those non-executive, or "ingredient," functions that may contribute to performance on specific executive measures, and adjust for those in analyses [22,23]. This approach allows one to determine if specific executive deficits are secondary to other cognitive deficits.

An examination of studies that have investigated executive functioning in VPT/VLBW cohorts reveals marked differences in sample selection. For example, studies often differ in terms of (1) the birth weight and/or gestational age criteria used to define groups, (2) the inclusion and exclusion of children at high or low biological and/or social risk, and (3) the representativeness of groups, such as whether the sample is recruited from a single hospital or from a geographic region. Another important difference between studies is the era in which the cohorts were born. Over the past 20 years the treatment for VPT/VLBW infants has improved greatly, resulting in significant reductions in mortality. As a consequence, the VPT/VLBW population born today is quite different from that born in the 1970s and 1980s in terms of the infants who survive, as well as in terms of the treatment received, which may have positive and negative long-term implications. Furthermore, many studies report on relatively small samples, compromising the power of the study to identify true deficits. In addition, small samples are unlikely to be representative given the significant heterogeneity of the VPT/VLBW population, and are more likely to have an over- or underrepresentation of rare but clinically important neonatal complications, such as high-grade intraventricular hemorrhage (IVH) and periventricular leukomalacia (PVL) (see also Chapter 12 on methodological considerations).

Executive functioning in VPT/VLBW children

With these limitations in mind, we have reviewed previous research to determine the nature of executive deficits in VPT/VLBW children in early childhood (< 5 years), middle childhood (5–12 years), and adolescence (> 12 years). The review has been divided into these developmental stages in order to highlight the evolution of the executive dysfunction across childhood. Some studies that include more mature or heavier infants are also cited if they are pertinent and have a significant proportion of VPT/VLBW children.

Early childhood (0–4 years)

It is now well established that certain executive processes emerge in infancy [13], and a small number of studies have examined elements of executive functioning in VPT/VLBW preschoolers. However, the assessment of executive processes during early childhood is difficult, due to the limited attentional and memory capacity, and verbal comprehension of children in this age range. Furthermore, there are few validated measures available for this age group, and as a consequence, studies have generally used experimental paradigms. Studies have tended to focus on the attentional control (inhibition, encoding, and maintenance of information) and cognitive flexibility (shifting response patterns) domains, which is appropriate given that these domains emerge in infancy and early childhood. A limitation of much of the early childhood research is the reliance on small non-representative low-risk samples [16,22,24,25], making it difficult to generalize these findings to the VPT/VLBW population.

Studies that have assessed multiple aspects of executive functioning in VPT/VLBW preschoolers tend to report variable findings [24]. Espy and colleagues [24] examined working memory and cognitive flexibility in a small sample of 29 low-risk preterm infants (28–36 weeks' gestation) and matched full-term controls at a mean age of 3.25 years. Delayed alternation (DA) was used to assess working memory, and involves searching for a reward in one of two locations that alternates after each correct search. Spatial reversal (SR) was used to assess shifting and flexibility, and requires the child to learn a specific response pattern (i.e., search under cup A) and after a period of time inhibit that established behavior and shift to a new response pattern (i.e., search under cup B). While the preterm group made significantly more errors than the control group on the working memory task (DA), the two groups performed similarly on the cognitive flexibility task (SR). This pattern of performance was considered to be indicative of a selective deficit in maintaining information on-line in order to guide future action.

Caravale, Vicari, and associates [16,22] also reported working memory deficits in a small sample of 30 low-risk preterm children (30–34 weeks' gestation) when compared with a matched full-term control group. This ex-preterm sample did not exhibit neurodevelopmental deficits on routine clinical examination, but performed significantly more poorly than controls on a spatial working memory task. Children born preterm also exhibited attentional deficits, as demonstrated by their poorer performance on a measure of selective and sustained attention [16]. Significant group differences on these working memory and attention tasks remained after adjusting for IQ [16]. Further analysis of these data revealed that the magnitude of the group difference on the working memory task increased with longer delays [22], indicating that the preterm preschoolers had problems maintaining information on-line (i.e., working memory) and encountered no problems encoding information. Interestingly, the spatial working memory deficits in the preterm group also remained after controlling for attention and perceptual difficulties [22], which provides strong evidence that in this group working memory was a primary deficit and not secondary to deficits in related cognitive domains (see also Chapter 14).

While these studies indicate that preterm children are at risk for working memory and attention deficits, both report on small low-risk selected samples. However, a recent New Zealand study assessed executive functioning in a reasonably large and representative cohort of 92 VPT/VLBW and 103 full-term children [17,26]. Other advantages of this New Zealand study are that it is longitudinal, with assessments conducted at 2 and 4 years of age, and that neonatal brain scans were conducted on the VPT/VLBW sample using magnetic resonance imaging (MRI). At 2 years of age, Woodward et al. [26] assessed object working memory using a three-step multi-search multi-location (MSML) task. The MSML task is similar to SR in that it requires the child to shift his/her established response pattern to an alternative response; however, the MSML task includes three search locations while SR involves only two search locations. In this task the VPT/VLBW group was slower to learn the demands of the task, and was less likely to correctly switch to the new location of the reward. The VPT/VLBW group made more non-perseverative errors, which was interpreted to reflect a difficulty encoding and maintaining information associated with the location of the reward, probably reflecting a deficit in working memory. While the MSML task also involves cognitive flexibility, the VPT/VLBW group made slightly fewer perseverative errors than the control group suggesting that their difficulty on this task was not associated with inflexibility, which is consistent with the findings of Espy et al. [24]. Interestingly, Woodward et al. [26] found a relationship between task performance and brain pathology, with increasing degree of white matter abnormality associated with lower rates of task completion and higher rates of atypical search behavior. Furthermore, task performance was associated with neonatal brain volumes, specifically the dorsolateral prefrontal, premotor, sensorimotor and parieto-occipital regions.

At the 4-year follow-up, the impact of neonatal white matter injury on cognitive flexibility was evaluated [17]. This time a version of the Detour Reaching Box (DRB) task was used to examine the capacity to switch from a previously reinforced rule and alternate between multiple rules. Somewhat surprisingly, severity of white matter pathology was not associated with the capacity to inhibit a previously established behavior; however, it was associated with the capacity to switch between different response patterns with the children with moderate to severe white matter pathology exhibiting the most difficulty. An important finding was that VPT/VLBW children with no detectable white matter abnormality exhibited no deficits in relation to cognitive flexibility and performed similarly to the full-term controls. Edgin *et al.* [17] also examined continuity of performance at 2 and 4 years of age and reported that while task failure decreased with age, failure rates were consistently higher for children with brain pathology. For example, only 10% of VPT/VLBW children without white matter pathology failed the tasks at both time points, in contrast to 39% of those with mild pathology and 69% of those with moderate to severe pathology. From this finding it may be postulated that executive dysfunction in VPT/VLBW preschoolers may be largely related to diffuse white matter pathology.

An earlier study by Ross *et al.* [27] provides additional support that executive deficits in VPT/VLBW preschoolers may be associated with brain pathology. Using measures of visual attention, cognitive flexibility, and working memory at 2 years of age, Ross *et al.* [27] reported selective executive deficits in a small sample of VPT children (28–32 weeks' gestation) with grade 1/2 IVH when compared with VPT children with no detectable abnormalities on neonatal ultrasound and full-term children. Intraventricular hemorrhages refer to bleeds that originate in the germinal matrix (transient embryonic structure located along the lining of the lateral ventricles), and this study was interested in the consequences of mild hemorrhages that are confined to the germinal matrix (grade 1) or lateral ventricles (grade 2). The VPT group without IVH performed similarly to full-term controls on most measures, including general cognitive development, visual attention, cognitive flexibility, and working memory, although they displayed a less systematic search strategy. The VPT group with IVH exhibited more significant deficits, performing less well than the VPT group without IVH and full-term controls on tests of working memory and cognitive flexibility, but did not differ on a test of visual attention.

In summary, based on the research reported to date, VPT/VLBW preschoolers are at increased risk for executive dysfunction, in particular reduced working memory capacity and cognitive inflexibility. An inability to hold or maintain information on-line in order to guide future action was evident even in low-risk preterm children, while cognitive inflexibility at this age seems to be strongly associated with brain pathology.

Middle childhood (5–12 years)

More research has been conducted examining executive functioning in VPT/VLBW in middle childhood; however, quality studies are still lacking. In this age group there have been a mix of studies conducted with large representative samples [4,9,18,28] and studies conducted with small [19,29] or low-risk [30–33] samples.

Attentional control (e.g., selective and sustained attention, impulse control, self-monitoring) is the most investigated executive domain in VPT/VLBW children in middle childhood. The research published to date demonstrates that this population is at significant risk for exhibiting selective attention deficits in contrast to full-term peers [4,18,28], which means these children are more likely to have lapses in attention or be distracted by non-relevant stimuli. Selective attention deficits have also been reported in low-risk LBW samples [33], however, the magnitude of the deficit is likely to increase with decreasing birth weight [4,33]. Very preterm/very low birth weight school-age children also appear to have more difficulty sustaining attention for a prolonged period, especially on monotonous tasks such as the continuous performance tasks (CPT) [30,34]. Sustained attention seems to be particularly related to brain pathology, with children with mild and severe lesions identified on neonatal cranial ultrasound committing significantly more commission errors (reflecting impulsivity) than children without lesions [34]. Research confirms that the capacity to inhibit a natural or reinforced behavior is another concern for VPT/VLBW school-age children when compared with full-term children [18,19,28,30], Thus, these children tend to have difficulty restraining themselves when they have a natural urge to respond in a particular fashion. For example, VPT/VLBW school-age children are likely to perform more slowly and less accurately when asked to say "night" when shown a card of a sun and "day" when shown a card of a moon. Working memory deficits have also been consistently reported in VPT/VLBW school-age children [9,18,31,32], in particular verbal and spatial maintenance tasks which involve the retention of information for a short period of time. Parents of VPT/VLBW school-age children also report concerns regarding working memory, with 20% of a VPT/VLBW sample scoring more than 1.5 standard deviations (SD) above the normative mean on a working memory scale [9]. One aspect of attentional control that has been neglected in this age group is self-monitoring,

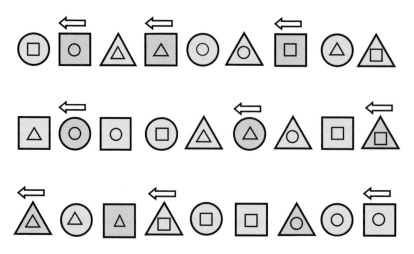

Fig. 15.2. The Contingency Naming Test. In trial 1 children are requested to name the colors of the shape, and in trial 2 the outside shape. In trial 3, the color of the shape is named if the internal and external shapes match, and otherwise the outside shape is named. The same contingency applies for trial 4, except in this trial the rule is reversed for those shapes with a backward arrow. See plate section for color version.

that is, the ability to regulate and monitor the accuracy of behavior and make changes if needed. While this element of attentional control is difficult to evaluate using traditional cognitive paradigms, behavioral questionnaires such as the Behavior Rating Inventory of Executive Function (BRIEF) [35] are often helpful. Using the parent form of the BRIEF, Anderson and Doyle [9] found subtle deficits in monitoring behaviors in a large representative cohort of VPT/VLBW school-age children.

Impaired cognitive flexibility has also been reported in VPT/VLBW school-age children. For example, a number of studies have demonstrated VPT/VLBW children to be either slower, less accurate, or both when required to shift response patterns [4,18,19]. An example of a shifting task for this age group is the Contingency Naming Test (CNT; Fig. 15.2) [36], which involves the naming of different colored shapes according to specific rules and contingencies. Using the CNT, Taylor *et al.* [4] found the children with birth weights < 750 g to be significantly slower to complete the task than children with birth weights between 750 and 1499 g and full-term controls. In addition to slower completion times, Bohm *et al.* [18] found VLBW school-age children made more errors than matched term controls on a similar but less demanding shifting task. Consistent with these findings, parents of VPT/VLBW children tend to note increased levels of inflexibility in contrast to parents of full-term children, with twice the rate of clinically significant problems [9]. However, shifting deficits are not a universal finding [31,32]. On a set-shifting task from the Cambridge Neuropsychological Test Automated Battery (CANTAB) [37] a low-risk

sample of predominantly preterm neonatal intensive care unit (NICU) survivors performed similarly to that of controls at 7 years and 11 years of age. This contrasting result may reflect differences in sample characteristics, a lack of power, or differences in the measures as the set-shifting task on the CANTAB also taps inhibition and conceptual reasoning abilities. An important aspect of cognitive flexibility that has not been investigated is the manipulation aspect of working memory, which is referred to as the central executive component of working memory [38] and involves the maintenance and manipulation of that information in some form. This aspect of working memory is clearly important for shifting and dividing attention, as well as planning and organization.

With regards to the goal setting domain, planning ability has been assessed in a number of VPT/VLBW school-aged outcome studies. Planning ability refers to the capacity to devise a plan to successfully attain a specific goal, and generally involves formulating a sequence of steps or actions in advance. To assess planning ability, versions of the Tower of London (TOL; Fig. 15.3) and Tower of Hanoi (TOH) have been administered to VPT/VLBW cohorts. Harvey *et al.* [29] reported significant planning deficits in a sample of extremely low birth weight (ELBW) school-age children in comparison to controls on the TOH, while Anderson and Doyle [9] found that VPT/ELBW correctly solved fewer items on the TOL than matched full-term peers. On complex five-move problems in the TOL, planning difficulties were found in a low-risk sample of preterm children at 7 years of age [32], however, no planning problems were identified when this cohort was followed up at a mean age of 11 years

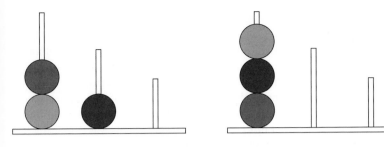

Fig. 15.3. The Tower of London (TOL). The object of the TOL is to move the balls on the pegs from a starting position (left diagram) to achieve a specific configuration (right diagram) following certain rules. In this item the child is allowed five moves. See plate section for color version

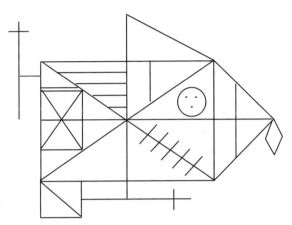

Fig. 15.4. The Rey-Osterrieth Complex Figure (RCF). Children are asked to copy this geometric figure as accurately as possible.

[31]. In a more ecologically valid measure of planning ability, Taylor *et al.* also reported deficits in VPT/VLBW school-age children, in particular those with birth weights < 750 g, who also tend to perform more poorly on the Rey-Osterrieth Complex Figure (RCF; Fig. 15.4), [4,9] especially those high-risk children (birthweights < 750 g) [4]. The RCF involves copying a complex geometric figure as accurately as possible and is sensitive to planning and organizational difficulties. Not surprisingly, in real-life situations parents are also reporting planning and organizational problems in this population [9]. Another element of the goal setting domain is conceptual reasoning, which is the capacity to identify the concept linking words, themes, objects or figures. A study by Anderson and Doyle [9] suggests that VPT/VLBW children also exhibit subtle deficits in this aspect of executive functioning.

While research has not explicitly investigated higher-order information processing, VPT/VLBW school-age children have been reported to require more time to complete cognitive flexibility tasks and are less fluent in generating words [4]. Thus, one may presume from these findings that this population also exhibits less efficient information processing.

In summary, in middle childhood, the VPT/VLBW population exhibits at least subtle deficits across all executive domains (attentional control, cognitive flexibility, goal setting, and information processing), which is characteristic of global executive dysfunction. However, it is important to note that only a minority of school-age VPT/VLBW children display signs of significant impairment, although the study by Taylor *et al.* [4] indicates that the incidence and severity of executive deficits increase in the higher-risk children, such as those born at the limits of viability. Also, from a clinical perspective, marked interindividual differences are observed. None of the studies reported above utilized advanced neuroimaging techniques so it is not clear how structural brain abnormalities are contributing to these executive deficits. However, the study by Katz *et al.* [34] found a significant relationship between cranial ultrasound abnormalities and inattention, and another study reported a reduction in scores on the RCF in 8-year-old VPT/VLBW infants who had grades 3 and 4 IVH diagnosed by ultrasound in the newborn period [39]. These studies suggest there is likely to be a strong association between brain pathology and executive dysfunction in VPT/VLBW school-age children.

Adolescence and early adulthood (13+ years)

Relatively few studies have studied VPT/VLBW adolescents and young adults; however, some of the studies that have been reported have assessed a broad range of executive processes [20,40] or included structural or functional neuroimaging [41,42].

At a mean age of 16 years, Taylor *et al.* [40] found executive deficits in a group of adolescents born with birth weights < 750 g. These adolescents performed below full-term peers on the RCF (planning and organization), a version of the TOL (planning ability), the CNT (cognitive flexibility), the CANTAB Spatial Working Memory task, as well as verbal fluency which assesses efficient lexical organization, in addition to working memory and self-monitoring. Quite large rates of impairment were reported, with 63% of this group exhibiting a deficit on the RCF, 67% on the CANTAB Spatial Working Memory task, 64% on the CNT, and 52% on the TOL. In contrast, children with birth weights between 750 and 1499 g did not differ significantly from the full-term controls in any of the executive measures, although there was clearly a gradient effect, with this group performing between the < 750 g and full-term groups. Approximately a third of the 750–1499 g group exhibited deficits on the various executive measures, compared with 12–20% of full-term controls. In terms of neonatal predictors, Taylor et al. [40] found that birth weight and respiratory problems (length of oxygen dependency) significantly predicted performance on most of these executive measures. It is also worth noting that although significant executive deficits were identified in this cohort of VLBW adolescents, language, perceptual-motor, and memory deficits were also reported.

A recent study by Saavalainen et al. [23] suggest that the working memory deficits observed in VPT children may improve with age. When compared with full-term controls, the group of very preterm adolescents assessed in this study had a specific deficit in a spatial working memory task (Spatial Span Backwards) that involved both the maintenance and manipulation of spatial information. For example, in the Spatial Span Backwards task the examinee observes the examiner tap a configuration of blocks in a certain order and then is required to tap the blocks in the *reverse* order. No deficits were found on spatial memory tasks that involved only the maintenance of information (i.e., tapping the blocks in the same order as the examiner), or on verbal working memory tasks, regardless of whether they involved maintenance of information only or maintenance and manipulation. Taylor et al. [40] also reported spatial working memory deficits in their < 750 g group; however, their task did not require the manipulation of information, but did require elements of strategic organization and self-monitoring. Thus, based on these findings it may be hypothesized that working memory deficits in VPT adolescents are restricted to the visuospatial modality and to tasks where attentional control and flexibility elements are also critical.

In a sample of VPT adolescents Rushe et al. [41] also found deficits in a verbal fluency task in comparison to full-term controls; however, somewhat surprisingly this was not associated with the presence of brain pathology on MRI. This sample of VPT adolescents also performed below peers on tests of cognitive flexibility (Trails B) and verbal working memory, although these group differences failed to reach statistical significance. This VPT sample also performed similarly to controls on the RCF and tests of visuomotor speed, memory, and learning, and object naming, indicating that this group of VPT adolescents was exhibiting few deficits. In relation to brain pathology on MRI, abnormalities were not associated with performance on any of the measures reported. While Rushe et al. [41] failed to find a relationship between qualitative abnormalities on brain MRI and cognitive functioning, other studies have found an association between regional volumes and cognitive functioning, and reported differences in functional activation. For example, verbal fluency has been found to be associated with corpus callosum volumes in VPT adolescents [43], and despite performing similarly to controls in a response inhibition task, VPT adolescent boys tended to activate different functional networks, which may reflect alternative cognitive strategies or functional plasticity [42].

Research examining executive function in adulthood is even rarer. However, Nosarti and colleagues [20] have recently reported deficits in a sample of VPT adults aged between 20 and 24 years. This study included measures of response inhibition, verbal fluency, cognitive flexibility, and divided attention. Deficits in verbal fluency and response inhibition were observed, as well as lapses in attention. Three inhibition tasks were administered involving inhibition of verbal response or motor response, and only the difference on the verbal inhibition task reached significance. Thus, it would appear that these VPT young adults were exhibiting verbal inhibition and organizational difficulties, as well as attentional control and cognitive flexibility deficits. Unfortunately this important study did not include goal setting measures, in particular measures of planning and organization.

In summary, it seems that VPT/VLBW survivors are still at risk for executive deficits in adolescence and young adulthood, although the results are mixed with inconsistencies across studies. While deficits are observed in all executive domains, the deficits do not appear to be as severe as those observed in middle childhood, although the findings from Taylor et al. [40] suggest that high rates of problems are still present in adolescence for high-risk survivors such as those with birth weights < 750 g, and those who suffer significant respiratory problems in the neonatal period.

Table 15.1 Summary of executive deficits in very preterm/very low birth weight survivors across childhood

	Attentional control	Cognitive flexibility	Goal setting
Early childhood	Deficits in: Maintenance of information on-line ? Attention	Deficits in : Shifting to new response pattern Switching between response patterns	NA
Middle childhood	Deficits in: Selective attention Sustained attention Inhibition Maintenance of information on-line ? Self-monitoring	Deficits in: Switching response patterns Set-shifting	Deficits in: Planning ability Spatial organization Reasoning ability
Adolescence +	Deficits in: Verbal response inhibition Attention lapses	Deficits in: Working memory Switching response patterns	Deficits in: Planning ability Spatial organization Verbal fluency

NA = not assessed.

Based on research conducted to date, the evolution of executive impairments in VPT/VLBW children is summarized in Table 15.1. The capacity to hold information on-line for a short period of time tended to be reduced in VPT/VLBW survivors in early and middle childhood, but by adolescence this deficit has not been reported. With regards to more complex working memory that also involves strategic organization and/or manipulation, deficits with spatially presented information are observed in middle childhood and adolescence. Selective and sustained attentional deficits are reported across childhood. The ability to inhibit behavior also appears to be a concern for VPT/VLBW children across development, although by early adulthood this deficit seems to be restricted to the inhibition of verbal responses and not visuomotor responses. In early childhood high-risk VPT/VLBW children can experience some difficulties with the transition to a new task or response pattern within the same activity, and across development VPT/VLBW children tend to have problems switching fluently and accurately between different response patterns. Finally, planning and organizational deficits are commonly reported in this population in middle childhood and adolescence. While we are in a reasonable position to speculate which executive processes are impaired in VPT/VLBW children, longitudinal research with large representative samples and a specific focus on executive functioning is clearly required.

Neuroanatomical factors

Brain injury and alterations to normal brain development are likely to be associated with executive deficits in VPT/VLBW children [9]. Neuroimaging studies in both healthy and clinical populations clearly demonstrate that executive processes are subserved by complex and interrelated neural systems [44,45], and damage to any link in these systems may result in deficits. Differentiating the neural correlates of executive deficits is a difficult task, as it may be the result of damage to the prefrontal cortex, white matter tracts, or subcortical and posterior brain regions [13].

Diffuse white matter abnormalities are common in infants born VPT [46]. This type of diffuse injury is thought to be caused by hypoxia-ischemia and/or cytokine attack, both of which injure immature oligodendrocytes, can lead to axonal damage, and have negative consequences for neural development [47]. For example, a recent series of studies has found that diffuse white matter injury affects subsequent myelination, maturation of gray matter structures [48], cerebellar growth [49], and development of subcortical structures such as the basal ganglia and thalamus [50]. Diffusion tensor imaging (DTI) has also been applied to investigate the effects of preterm birth on the integrity and connectivity of white matter tracks [51,52]. Using this imaging technique, Hüppi et al. [53] demonstrated that neonatal white matter injury in preterm infants had "major deleterious effects on subsequent development of fiber tracts" (p.455). For further discussion on DTI studies see also Chapter 8.

While these diffuse white matter abnormalities may be related to the high incidence of cognitive and behavioral problems observed in VPT/VLBW children [54], the functional significance of this pathology is not well understood. To date, there have been only a few studies that have examined the relationship between diffuse white matter abnormalities and later outcomes [26,41,55]. The two studies that utilized neonatal neuroimaging report strong associations between diffuse white matter injury on MRI at term equivalent and adverse neurodevelopmental outcomes [55] and working memory difficulties [26] at 2 years of age. White matter integrity is an essential component of the prefrontal neural networks associated with executive processes [56], and damage to periventricular white matter tracts as seen in many VPT/VLBW infants may compromise these prefrontal systems, in particular the fronto-striatal pathways. In addition to a direct impact on prefrontal networks, diffuse white matter abnormalities are also likely to reduce information processing and response speed [56].

Volumetric studies have also demonstrated structural brain changes as a result of being born VPT. At term-equivalent age (40 weeks' gestation), VPT/VLBW infants have significantly less cortical and subcortical gray matter relative to term infants [54], as well as regional reductions in the parieto-occipital area [57]. Volumetric studies with school-age children reveal enlarged lateral ventricles, thinning of the corpus callosum, and smaller hippocampi, basal ganglia, thalamus, amygdala, and cerebellum structures [43,58–60]. Overall, these findings demonstrate that prematurity, in particular extreme prematurity, alters neural development in the neonatal period and has ramifications for subsequent brain development. Factors that are likely to influence brain development in the neonatal period in the VPT/VLBW include (a) white matter injury, (b) inadequate provision of nutritional substrates and hormones essential for brain growth and development, (c) medical complications (e.g., bronchopulmonary dysplasia, sepsis, patent ductus arterosis), (d) medical interventions (e.g., surgery, corticosteroids, caffeine, ventilation), and (e) environmental stresses (e.g., high noise levels, bright lights, prolonged separation from parents, invasive medical procedures) [60]. While the evidence linking volumetric discrepancies and executive deficits are lacking, a few studies have reported significant associations. For example, Nosarti et al. [43,61] found reductions in the corpus callosum and left caudate nucleus were related to poor verbal fluency and higher ratings of hyperactivity respectively in VPT/VLBW adolescents, while Woodward et al. [26] found significant associations between reduced cerebral tissue volumes in the dorsolateral prefrontal cortex, sensorimotor, parieto-occipital, and premotor regions at term equivalent and working memory difficulties at 2 years of age.

The pervasiveness of executive deficits in VPT/VLBW children, together with evidence that these deficits are present even in young children, implies damage to white matter tracts or subcortical and posterior brain regions, rather than direct injury to the prefrontal cortex [62]. Animal models of brain injury indicate that early damage to late maturing areas of the brain, such as the prefrontal cortex, may not be evident in infancy and may take several years to emerge [63,64]. In contrast, the functional consequences of early white matter injury or damage to early maturing areas are present from a young age and persist throughout development [65]. Furthermore, neuroimaging studies demonstrate that children display a greater reliance on subcortical systems than adults when performing executive tasks [66].

In summary, while structural brain abnormalities are well documented in VPT/VLBW children, the impact of these abnormalities on executive functioning is not fully understood. Longitudinal research incorporating serial neuroimaging and neuropsychological evaluations at critical developmental stages are needed to clarify the neural basis of deficits in these skills at different ages.

Social and environmental factors

Social and environmental risk factors account for variability in outcomes independent of biological risks [67]. Factors such as family functioning, parenting characteristics, quality of the home environment, and socioeconomic status have the potential to moderate the effects of prematurity on cognitive and behavioral development. Few studies have systematically investigated the contribution of these factors to executive dysfunction in VPT/VLBW samples. However, Robson and Pederson [68] found that a LBW child's exposure to structured and developmentally appropriate activities in the home environment was predictive of vigilance and impulsivity. Similarly, Landry et al. [69] documented the importance of early parenting for the development of executive skills in VPT and full-term children. These investigators found that mothers' early use and quality of verbal support to foster their children's learning (scaffolding) directly supported early language and non-verbal problem-solving skills, and indirectly influenced later mental flexibility and problem-solving skills.

Other researchers have examined the effects of social risk or disadvantage on behavioral development of preterm children, although the findings are inconsistent. Levy-Shiff et al. [70] and Taylor et al. [6] found that behavior problems, such as inattention and hyperactivity, were more pronounced in VPT children at greatest social disadvantage. Conversely, studies of cognitive outcomes have reported that the effects of prematurity are reduced for children from more disadvantaged backgrounds[71,72]. To explain the latter pattern of results, Hack *et al.* [72] suggests the negative consequences of birth risk on cognition may be overwhelmed by the adverse effects of the environment. These contrasting results nevertheless point to the importance of considering different moderating effects, depending on the type of outcome measured and age at assessment [73,74].

Issues for clinical practice

When assessing a VPT/VLBW child it is important to remember that outcomes in this population are highly variable, and in many cases infants with similar neonatal characteristics have quite different outcomes. Furthermore, in addition to problems in executive function, difficulties in other cognitive and behavioral domains are frequently observed, including sensory, perceptual, and motor problems, slowed information processing, and memory and learning difficulties. At present it is not clear whether deficits in executive function are more severe than deficits in other cognitive domains, or whether deficits in other cognitive domains are secondary to deficits in executive function. Thus, for standard follow-up programs a broad-based assessment is warranted for VPT/VLBW children. Also, the nature of executive dysfunction in this population has been shown to change during development, and some problems may not emerge until later in life. Thus, ongoing surveillance of these children is recommended.

The effectiveness of early interventions with this population has been poorly investigated, although at some institutions early developmental programs in the NICU, or shortly after discharge, are standard practice. Research to date suggests that early developmental interventions tend to be associated with enhanced cognitive development in early childhood, but by middle childhood these benefits have diminished (see also Chapter 18). The impact these early interventions have on the development of executive functioning has not been examined.

Conclusion

Current research indicates that VPT/VLBW survivors are at risk for executive dysfunction across childhood and into early adulthood; however, further research is required to determine the differential nature of these deficits. It appears that the features of executive dysfunction evolve across development, but more specific longitudinal studies are needed to investigate this issue. While executive dysfunction has been reported in even low-risk children, it seems that it is more frequent and severe in high-risk preterm infants, such as those with birth weights < 750 g. It is also important to acknowledge that a considerable proportion of VPT/VLBW children show no executive impairment and outcomes are variable. Certain risk factors have been associated with executive dysfunction such as IVH, diffuse white matter injury, and volumetric differences, but at this stage the mechanisms underlying this impairment are not well understood, and further research is required to enhance our understanding of these brain–behavior relationships.

References

1. Institute of Medicine of the National Academies. *Preterm birth: Causes, Consequences, and Prevention.* Washington, DC: The National Academies Press; 2007.

2. Anderson PJ, Doyle LW; Victorian Infant Collaborative Study Group (VICS). Neurobehavioral outcomes of school-age children born extremely low birth weight or very preterm in the 1990s. *JAMA* 2003; **289**(24): 3264–72.

3. Bhutta AT, Cleves MA, Casey PH, Cradock MM, Anand K. Cognitive and behavioral outcomes of school-aged children who were born preterm: a meta-analysis. *JAMA* 2002; **288**(6): 728–37.

4. Taylor HG, Klein N, Minich NM, Hack M. Middle-school-age outcomes in children with very low birthweight. *Child Dev* 2000; **71**(6): 1495–511.

5. Goyen TA, Lui K, Woods R. Visual-motor, visual-perceptual, and fine motor outcomes in very-low-birthweight children at 5 years. *Dev Med Child Neurol* 1998; **40**(2): 76–81.

6. Taylor HG, Hack M, Klein NK. Attention deficits in children with < 750 gm birth weight. *Child Neuropsychol* 1998; **4**(1): 21–34.

7. Rose SA, Feldman JF. Memory and processing speed in preterm children at eleven years: a comparison with full-terms. *Child Dev* 1996; **67**(5): 2005–21.

8. Luoma L, Herrgard E, Martikainen A, Ahonen T. Speech and language development of children born at < = 32 weeks' gestation: a 5-year prospective follow-up study. *Dev Med Child Neurol* 1998; **40**(6): 380–7.

9. Anderson PJ, Doyle LW. Executive functioning in school-aged children who were born very preterm or with extremely low birth weight in the 1990s. *Pediatrics* 2004; **114**(1): 50–7.

10. Zelkowitz P, Papageorgiou A, Zelazo PR, Salomon Weiss MJ. Behavioral adjustment in very low and normal birth weight children. *J Clin Child Psychol* 1995; **24**(1): 21–30.

11. Wilkerson DS, Volpe AG, Dean RS, Titus JB. Perinatal complications as predictors of infantile autism. *Int J Neurosci* 2002; **112**(9): 1085–98.

12. Botting N, Powls A, Cooke RW, Marlow N. Attention deficit hyperactivity disorders and other psychiatric outcomes in very low birthweight children at 12 years. *J Child Psychol Psychiatry* 1997; **38**(8):931–41.

13. Anderson P. Assessment and development of executive function (EF) during childhood. *Child Neuropsychol* 2002; **8**(2): 71–82.

14. Anderson P. Towards a developmental model of executive function. In: Anderson V, Jacobs R, Anderson P, eds. *Executive Functions and the Frontal Lobes: A Lifespan Perspective.* London: Psychology Press. 2008; 3–21.

15. Grattan L, Eslinger P. Frontal lobe damage in children and adults: a comparative review. *Dev Neuropsychol* 1991; **7**(3): 283–326.

16. Caravale B, Tozzi C, Albino G, Vicari S. Cognitive development in low risk preterm infants at 3–4 years of life. *Arch Dis Child Fetal Neonatal Ed* 2005; **90**(6): F474–9.

17. Edgin J, Inder T, Anderson P, *et al.* Executive functioning in preschool children born very preterm: relationship with early white matter pathology. *J Int Neuropsychol Soc* 2008; **14**(1): 90–101.

18. Bohm B, Smedler AC, Forssberg H. Impulse control, working memory and other executive functions in preterm children when starting school. *Acta Paediatr* 2004; **93**(10): 1363–71.

19. Bayless S, Stevenson J. Executive functions in school-age children born very prematurely. *Early Hum Dev.* 2006; **83**(4): 247–54.

20. Nosarti C, Giouroukou E, Micali N, *et al.* Impaired executive functioning in young adults born very preterm. *J Int Neuropsychol Soc* 2007; **13**(4): 571–81.

21. Taylor H. Children born preterm or with very low birth weight can have both global and selective cognitive deficits. *J Dev Behav Pediatr* 2006; **27**(6): 485–6.

22. Vicari S, Caravale B, Carlesimo GA, Casadei AM, Allemand F. Spatial working memory deficits in children at ages 3–4 who were low birth weight, preterm infants. *Neuropsychology* 2004; **18**(4): 673–8.

23. Saavalainen P, Luoma L, Bowler D, *et al.* Spatial span in very prematurely born adolescents. *Dev Neuropsychol* 2007; **32**(3): 769–85.

24. Espy KA, Stalets MM, McDiarmid MM, *et al.* Executive functions in preschool children born preterm: application of cognitive neuroscience paradigms. *Child Neuropsychol* 2002; **8**(2): 83–92.

25. Matthews A, Ellis A, Nelson C. Development of preterm and full-term infant ability on AB, recall memory, transparent barrier detour, and means-end tasks. *Child Dev* 1996; **67**(6): 2658–76.

26. Woodward LJ, Edgin JO, Thompson D, Inder TE. Object working memory deficits predicted by early brain injury and development in the preterm infant. *Brain* 2005; **128**(Pt II): 2578–87.

27. Ross G, Boatright S, Auld PAM, Nass R. Specific cognitive abilities in 2-year-old children with subependymal and mild intraventricular hemorrhage. *Brain Cogn* 1996; **32**(1): 1–13.

28. Marlow N, Hennessy E, Bracewell M, Wolke D; EPICure Study Group. Motor and executive function at 6 years of age after extremely preterm birth. *Pediatrics* 2007; **120**(4): 793–804.

29. Harvey JM, O'Callaghan MJ, Mohay H. Executive function of children with extremely low birthweight: a case control study. *Dev Med Child Neurol* 1999; **41**(5): 292–7.

30. Elgen I, Lundervold AJ, Sommerfelt K. Aspects of inattention in low birth weight children. *Pediatr Neurol* 2004; **30**(2): 92–8.

31. Curtis WJ, Lindeke LL, Georgieff MK, Nelson CA. Neurobehavioural functioning in neonatal intensive care unit graduates in late childhood and early adolescence. *Brain* 2002; **125**(Pt 7): 1646–59.

32. Luciana M, Lindeke L, Georgieff M, Mills M, Nelson CA. Neurobehavioral evidence for working memory deficits in school-aged children with histories of prematurity. *Dev Med Child Neurol* 1999; **41**(8): 521–33.

33. Breslau N, Chilcoat H, DelDotto J, Andreski P, Brown G. Low birth weight and neurocognitive status at six years of age. *Biol Psychiatry* 1996; **40**(5): 389–97.

34. Katz KS, Dubowitz LMS, Henderson S, *et al.* Effect of cerebral lesions on continuous performance test responses of school age children born prematurely. *J Pediatr Psychol* 1996; **21**(6): 841–55.

35. Gioia GA, Isquith PK, Guy SC, Kenworthy L. *Behavior Rating Inventory of Executive Function. Professional Manual.* Lutz, FL: Psychological Assessment Resources, Inc; 2000.

36. Anderson P, Anderson V, Northam E, Taylor HG. Standardization of the Contingency Naming Test for school-aged children: a new measure of reactive flexibility. *Clin Neuropsychol Assess* 2000; **1**: 247–73.

37. CeNeS Cognition. *Cambridge Neuropsychological Test Automated Battery (CANTAB).* Cambridge, UK: CeNeS Limited; 1996.

38. Baddeley A. Exploring the central executive. *Q J Exp Psychol* 1996; **49A**: 5–28.

39. Sherlock R, Anderson P, Doyle L; Victorian Infant Collaborative Study Group. Neurodevelopmental sequelae of intraventricular haemorrhage at 8

years of age in a regional cohort of ELBW/very preterm infants. *Early Hum Dev* 2005; **81**(11): 909–16.

40. Taylor H, Minich N, Banget B, Filipek P, Hack M. Long-term neuropsychological outcomes of very low birth weight: associations with early risks for periventricular brain insults. *J Int Neuropsychol Soc* 2004; **10**(7): 987–1004.

41. Rushe T, Rifkin L, Stewart A, *et al.* Neuropsychological outcome at adolescence of very preterm birth and its relation to brain structure. *Dev Med Child Neurol* 2001; **43**: 226–33.

42. Nosarti C, Rubia K, Smith A, *et al.* Altered functional neuroantanomy of response inhibition in adolescent males who were born very preterm. *Dev Med Child Neurol* 2006; **48**(4): 265–71.

43. Nosarti C, Rushe T, Woodruff P, *et al.* Corpus callosum size and very preterm birth: relationship to neuropsychological outcome. *Brain* 2004; **127**(Pt 9): 2080–9.

44. Collette F, Van der Linden M, Laureys S, *et al.* Exploring the unity and diversity of the neural substrates of executive functioning. *Hum Brain Mapp* 2005; **25**(4): 409–23.

45. Fan J, McCandliss BD, Fossella J, Flombaum JI, Posner MI. The activation of attentional networks. *Neuroimage* 2005; **26**(2): 471–9.

46. Inder TE, Wells SJ, Mogridge NB, Spencer C, Volpe JJ. Defining the nature of the cerebral abnormalities in the premature infant: a qualitative magnetic resonance imaging study. *J Pediatr* 2003; **143**(2): 171–9.

47. Volpe JJ. Brain injury in the premature infant – neuropathology, clinical aspects, pathogenesis, and prevention. *Clin Perinatol* 1997; **24**(3): 567–87.

48. Inder TE, Huppi PS, Warfield S, *et al.* Periventricular white matter injury in the premature infant is followed by reduced cerebral cortical gray matter volume at term. *Ann Neurol* 1999; **46**(5): 755–60.

49. Shah DK, Anderson PJ, Carlin JB, *et al.* Reduction in cerebeller volumes in preterm infants: relationships to white matter injury and neurodevelopment at two years of age. *Pediatr Res* 2006; **60**(1): 97–102.

50. Inder TE, Wang H, Volpe JJ, Warfield S. Premature infants with PVL have altered deep nuclear structures – a volumetric MR study. *Pediatr Res* 2003; **53**(4): 538A.

51. Nagy Z, Westerberg H, Skare S, *et al.* Preterm children have disturbances of white matter at 11 years of age as shown by diffusion tensor imaging. *Pediatr Res* 2003; **54**(5): 672–9.

52. Partridge SC, Mukherjee P, Henry RG, *et al.* Diffusion tensor imaging: serial quantitation of white matter tract maturity in premature newborns. *Neuroimage* 2004; **22**(3): 1302–14.

53. Hüppi PS, Murphy B, Maier SE, *et al.* Microstructural brain development after perinatal cerebral white matter injury assessed by diffusion tensor magnetic resonance imaging. *Pediatrics* 2001; **107**(3): 455–60.

54. Inder TE, Warfield SK, Wang H, Hüppi PS, Volpe JJ. Abnormal cerebral structure is present at term in premature infants. *Pediatrics* 2005; **115**(2): 286–94.

55. Woodward LJ, Anderson PJ, Austin NC, Howard K, Inder TE. Neonatal MRI to predict neurodevelopmental outcomes in preterm infants. *N Engl J Med* 2006; **355**(7): 685–94.

56. Filley CM. *The Behavioural Neurology of White Matter.* New York: Oxford University Press; 2001.

57. Peterson BS, Anderson AW, Ehrenkranz R, *et al.* Regional brain volumes and their later neurodevelopmental correlates in term and preterm infants. *Pediatrics* 2003; **111**(5): 939–48.

58. Allin M, Matsumoto H, Santhouse A, *et al.* Cognitive and motor function and the size of the cerebellum in adolescents born very pre-term. *Brain* 2001; **124**(Pt I): 60–6.

59. Isaacs EB, Lucas A, Chong WK, *et al.* Hippocampal volume and everyday memory in children of very low birth weight. *Pediatr Res* 2000; **47**(6): 713–20.

60. Peterson BS, Vohr B, Staib LH, *et al.* Regional brain volume abnormalities and long-term cognitive outcome in preterm infants. *JAMA* 2000; **284**(15): 1939–47.

61. Nosarti C, Allin M, Frangou S, Rifkin L, Murray R. Hyperactivity in adolescents born very preterm is associated with decreased caudate volume. *Biol Psychiatry* 2005; **57**(6): 661–6.

62. Luciana M. Cognitive development in children born preterm: implications for theories of brain plasticity following early injury. *Dev Psychopathol* 2003; **15**(4): 1017–47.

63. Goldman P, Rosvold H, Mishkin M. Selective sparing of function following prefrontal lobectomy in infant monkeys. *Exp Neurol* 1970; **29**(2): 221–6.

64. Goldman P. Functional developmental of the prefrontal cortex in early life and the problem of neuronal plasticity. *Exp Neurol* 1971; **32**(3): 366–87.

65. Goldman P, Rosvold H. The effects of selective caudate lesions in infant and juvenile Rhesus monkeys. *Brain Res* 1972; **43**(1): 53–66.

66. Casey B, Galvan A, Hare T. Changes in cerebral functional organization during cognitive development. *Curr Opin Neurobiol* 2005; **15**(2): 239–44.

67. Taylor HG, Burant CJ, Holding PA, Klein N, Hack M. Sources of variability in sequelae of very low birth weight. *Child Neuropsychol* 2002; **8**(3): 163–78.

68. Robson AL, Pederson DR. Predictors of individual differences in attention among low birth weight

children. *J Dev Behav Pediatr* 1997; **18**(1): 13–21.

69. Landry SH, Miller-Loncar CL, Smith KE, Swank PR. The role of early parenting in children's development of executive processes. *Dev Neuropsychol* 2002; **21**(1): 15–41.

70. Levy-Shiff R, Einat G, Mogilner MB, *et al.* Biological and environmental correlates of developmental outcome of prematurely born infants in early adolescence. *J Pediatr Psychol* 1994; **19**(1): 63–78.

71. Bendersky M, Lewis M. Effects of intraventricular hemorrhage and other medical and environmental risks on multiple outcomes at age three years. *J Dev Behav Pediatr* 1995; **16**(2): 89–95.

72. Hack M, Breslau N, Aram D, *et al.* The effect of very low birth weight and social risk on neurocognitive abilities at school age. *J Dev Behav Pediatr* 1992; **13**(6): 412–20.

73. Aylward GP. The relationship between environmental risk and developmental outcome. *J Dev Behav Pediatr* Jun 1992; **13**(3): 222–9.

74. Taylor HG, Klein N, Hack M. School-age consequences of birth weight less than 750 g: a review and update. *Dev Neuropsychol* 2000; **17**(3): 289–321.

Applied research
Academic performance and learning disabilities

H. Gerry Taylor

Introduction

Recent advances in neonatal intensive care have resulted in survival of increasing numbers of children with very low birth weight (VLBW, < 1500 g) or very preterm birth (VPTB, < 32 weeks' gestational age [GA]) [1]. Because many of these survivors have neurological abnormalities and other neonatal complications, they are at high risk for an array of neurodevelopmental problems. Studies following children with VLBW or VPTB (i.e., VLBW/VPTB) into early childhood show that they have higher rates of neurosensory and other health disorders, more problems in behavior and socialization, and lower scores on tests of mental, language, and motor skills than control groups of children born at term with normal birth weight (NBW, ≥ 2500 g) [2]. These problems are more common and severe for children born at the limits of viability, such as those with extremely low birth weight (ELBW, < 1000 g) or extremely preterm birth (EPTB, GA < 28 weeks).

Problems in academic achievement and school performance are apparent soon after school entry [3–8]. Learning difficulties are manifest in failure to meet classroom expectations as indexed by grade repetition or the need for special education assistance, parent and teacher reports of poor school performance, and low scores on tests of academic skills, such as those assessing reading, spelling, mathematics, and writing. These problems are more common than persisting health disorders or global developmental impairments, with many survivors experiencing relatively selective impairments in academic achievement. The reason for the high prevalence of scholastic problems relative to other disorders is unclear, but may reflect the substantial numbers of children with mild generalized cognitive deficiency and specific neuropsychological weaknesses [9].

The adverse educational outcomes of VLBW/VPTB have consequences for both the child and society. Children who fail grades or require special education services in primary school are at greater risk than other children for long-term learning and behavior problems and even school dropout [10,11]. Children with VLBW/VPTB also require high levels of educational resources. Chaikind and Corman [12] estimated that the greater rates of special education provided to children with low birth weight (LBW, < 2500 g) in the USA in 1989–90 were accompanied by incremental educational costs of US$370.8 million. In a more recent study of children who entered kindergarten in the State of Florida from 1996 through 1999, Roth et al. [13] estimated incremental kindergarten costs of US$3150, US$2150, and US$950 per child for children with respective birth weights of < 1000 g, 1000–1499 g, and 1500–2499 g.

The primary aim of this chapter is to describe the educational consequences of VLBW/VPTB and the factors associated with these outcomes. The rationale for focusing on this subset of the LBW and/or preterm (< 37 weeks' GA) population is that most studies of educational outcomes have followed higher-risk survivors who meet criteria for VLBW/VPTB. Although GA cut-offs provide a more meaningful basis for classifying the degree of prematurity, information on GA can be unreliable and birth weight markers are thus frequently used in place of GA to identify samples. Specific sample criteria are given below for studies that recruited children based on birth weight or GA cut-offs other than VLBW/VPTB. This chapter first reviews the manifestations of adverse educational outcomes in the classroom and on formal tests of academic achievement, as well as evidence for developmental changes in these outcomes. Because educational outcomes vary dramatically even within subsets of VLBW/VPTB

Neurodevelopmental Outcomes of Preterm Birth, ed. Chiara Nosarti, Robin M. Murray, and Maureen Hack. Published by Cambridge University Press. © Cambridge University Press 2010.

cohorts with more extreme LBW or low GA, the biological and social predictors of these outcomes are then considered, along with associated cognitive and behavior problems. Research limitations and needs are listed in the subsequent section followed by a summary of the existing literature and of potentially fruitful directions for future research.

Evidence of adverse educational outcomes

Educational modifications and teacher ratings of school performance

Compared with NBW control groups, samples of children with VLBW/VPTB have higher rates of grade repetition and special learning assistance and are rated by their teachers as having weaknesses in school performance [11, 14–17]. These adverse educational outcomes are evident in follow-up studies of VLBW/VPTB or ELBW/EPTB cohorts born both before and after the advent of surfactant therapy [9,18–21]. Representative contemporary outcomes are reported by Saigal et al. [22]. These researchers recruited a large multinational sample of 5- to 11-year-old children with birth weight 500–1000 g. The children were born during the presurfactant era (1970s and 1980s) at sites in New Jersey, Ontario, Bavaria, and Holland. Despite between-site variations in educational policy, educational outcomes were similar. Respective rates of grade retention and/or special education assistance at the four sites were 63%, 57%, 68%, and 51%.

Similar results are reported in studies of children born in the post-surfactant era. Our research team found that 38% of a regional 1992–5 ELBW birth cohort followed to mean age 8 years formally qualified for a special education program, compared with significantly fewer (11%) of a NBW control group [9]. Anderson et al. also reported poor educational outcomes in an Australian ELBW/EPTB cohort compared with NBW controls [18]. Rates were higher at 8 years for the ELBW/EPTB group for both grade repetition (20% vs. 7%) and special education (39% vs. 22%). In this and other studies, children with VLBW/VPTB or ELBW/EPTB were rated by their teachers as performing less well than their NBW peers in the basic skills areas of reading, spelling, writing, and mathematics [14,20,23–25].

Findings from studies of educational outcomes reveal a "gradient" relation between the degree of

LBW/low GA and educational outcomes. Klebanov et al. [11] assembled a large multisite pre-surfactant sample comprised of three subgroups with LBW (≤ 1000 g, 1001–1500 g, and 1501–2500 g) and a NBW group. Rates of grade failure and/or special education placements at 9 years were higher for each of the LBW groups compared with the NBW group, with a clear gradient relation between the degree of LBW and educational modifications. Respective rates of grade failure for < 1000 g, 1001–1500 g, and 1501–2500 g groups were 37%, 26%, and 27% compared with 14% for the NBW group; and respective rates of special education for the three LBW groups were 12%, 6%, and 6% compared with 4% for the NBW group.

Several other studies provide further evidence for a gradient effect. Pinto-Martin et al. [26] examined the prevalence of special education placement at 9 years in a 1984–7 birth cohort of children weighing 500–2000 g. They found that grade retention was significantly more common in children with < 1000 g birth weight (18%) than in those with birth weight 1001–1500 g (10%) or 1501–2000 g (7%). Nearly half of the children with < 1000 g birth weight were in special education placements compared with about a third of the 1000–1500 g subgroup and slightly fewer (29%) of the 1501–2000 g subgroup. Higher rates of these placements were predicted by birth weight ≤ 1500 g or GA < 28 weeks. In following their ELBW cohort to adolescence, Saigal et al. [27] also documented a higher rate of grade repetition and/or special education in survivors with < 750 g birth weight compared with 750–1000 g birth weight (72% vs. 53%). An epidemiological survey of children born from 1982 to 1986 and attending public schools in the state of Florida during the 1996–7 school year suggests that risks for special education placement may increase incrementally with decreases in birth weight below 3500 g [28].

Our research team investigated educational consequences at age 11 years in a 1982–6 cohort with < 750 g birth weight compared with a higher birth weight VLBW group (750–1499 g) and term controls [25]. Compared with the term group, the < 750 g cohort had a significantly higher rate of grade repetition than the term group, and both VLBW groups had higher rates of special education. The rates of these outcomes varied along a gradient for both outcomes. Thirty percent of the < 750 g group had repeated a grade compared with 13% of the 750–1499 g group and 8% of the controls, and 50% of the < 750 g group compared with 27% of the 750–1499 g group and 8% of the controls had received special education.

The nature and intensity of special education assistance for children with VLBW/VPTB varies widely for school-age children in the USA. Pinto-Martin et al. found that 50% of the special education services received by the 9-year-old children in their 500–2000 g birth weight cohort were delivered within the regular classroom, 37% in a separate room within the regular school (part- or full-time), and 13% in a special school [26]. In their population study of factors related to special education placements in kindergarten in the state of Florida, Resnick et al. [5] found that children with VLBW had higher rates of remedial educational services and of placements in nearly all special education programs than children with 3000–4749 g birth weight. The only exception was the lack of an effect of VLBW on rates of placement in programs for the "emotionally handicapped." These researchers found that elevated rates of special education were especially pronounced for more severe handicapping conditions, including the physically impaired, sensory impaired, and trainable or profound mentally handicapped. The effects of VLBW were less marked for programs targeted to milder disabilities, including educable mentally handicapped and learning disabled. Findings from Avchen et al. [28] indicated that 12- to 15-year-old children with VLBW, and even those with birth weight 1500–2500 g, had higher rates of enrollment in all types of special education programs compared with NBW children. These and other findings suggest that children with VLBW/VPTB receive a broad range of academic supports during the school-age years [11,19,25–27].

Scores of tests of academic achievement

Learning problems in children with VLBW/VPTB are further documented by their poor performance on tests of academic achievement. Numerous studies indicate that these children score more poorly than NBW controls on tests of reading, spelling, writing, mathematics, and even handwriting [9,24,29–31]. Gradient effects are reported in several studies, with children born at the lower limits of birth weight or GA scoring less well than heavier children with VLBW/VPTB [7,11,18,22,25,26]. The effect sizes corresponding to group differences in achievement scores range from moderate to large. To illustrate, our study of outcomes at mean age 11 years revealed effect sizes of 1.0–1.9 in comparing the <750 g birth weight group with term controls, and of 0.3–0.4 in comparing the 750–1499 g birth weight group with controls [25]. Effect sizes represent differences between group means in units of standard deviation, referred

to as Cohen's d. In a more recent study by our research group comparing a post-surfactant ELBW cohort with NBW controls at mean age 8 years, effect sizes for group differences in achievement testing ranged from 0.5 to 0.7.[9] Anderson et al. [18] demonstrated similar group differences in achievement in comparing an ELBW/EPTB cohort with NBW controls on achievement tests at 8 years. Rates of low achievement scores provide an alternative gauge of the clinical significance of group differences. Substandard scores on achievement testing, defined as standard scores < 85, were twice as common in our ELBW sample than in NBW controls [9]. Similarly, O'Callaghan et al. found teacher reports of academic delays were three times more common in an ELBW group than in controls [24].

Deficiencies in academic skills are demonstrated even in analyses that exclude children with global intellectual deficits or neurosensory impairments [11,27,30,31,32,]. Problems in mathematics are especially prominent. Children with VLBW/VPTB score more poorly than NBW children in this academic domain even when controlling for IQ [14,18,33,34]. Analysis of data from our study of outcomes in two VLBW groups (<750 g and 750–1499 g) revealed significantly greater deficits in these children relative to term controls at mean age 11 years on tests of mathematics than on reading tests [34].

Rates and types of learning disabilities (LDs)

Learning disabilities are generally identified by first excluding children with neurosensory disorders and generalized mental deficiency and then determining if children's scores on tests of academic achievement meet criteria for either low achievement or for achievement that is below expected levels relative to IQ [32]. Using the "low-achievement" method, an LD is identified based on a standardized score that is below age or grade expectation (e.g., a standard score on an achievement test that is more than 1 standard deviation below the normative mean for age). The second or "IQ discrepancy" definition requires that the child's standard score fall below that predicted by IQ. To identify scores that satisfy this definition, regression analysis is conducted to estimate an "expected" score based on IQ. Data from the NBW controls are typically used for this purpose. Regression analysis also provides information on the variability of the predicted scores, or standard error of the estimate. The difference between the children's actual scores and the scores predicted by their IQs is then computed and divided by the standard error, yielding discrepancies between the observed and predicted scores in standard units. An LD on a given test is defined in terms of standard scores that fall a specified amount (e.g., 1 standard unit) below predicted scores.

Using one or both of these two definitions, several studies have demonstrated higher rates of LDs in children with VLBW/VPTB than in NBW controls. In our study of developmental outcomes of < 750 g birth weight, we investigated LDs in participants without neurosensory disorders and with at least low average composite (≥ 80) scores on the Kaufman Assessment Battery for Children [35]. Achievement testing included subtests of the Woodcock–Johnson Tests of Achievement measuring word reading (Letter/Word Identification), spelling (Dictation), mathematics reasoning (Applied Problems), and arithmetic computations (Calculation). The rates of these LDs in the < 750 g group and our two comparison groups (750–1499 g and term-born) are graphed in Figs 16.1 and 16.2. Group differences in rates of low-achievement LDs were observed on tests of mathematics reasoning, arithmetic computations, and word reading. Rates of any low-achievement LDs, as well as IQ-discrepant LD in mathematics reasoning, were significantly higher in the < 750 g group compared with term controls. Rates of low-achievement LD in mathematics reasoning were also significantly higher in the < 750 g group compared with the 750–1499 g group.

In a subsequent follow-up study of LDs in this sample at mean age 11 years, we again examined scores on reading and mathematics tests after excluding children from our sample with neurosensory disorders or with low global cognitive ability [36]. The < 750 g group continued to have higher rates of low-achievement LDs in both skill areas. At this visit, 60% of the < 750 g group had a low-achievement LD compared with 34% of the 750–1499 g group and 24% of the term controls. The majority (80%) of the children with a low-achievement LD at this assessment had a low-achievement LD at the previous visit at mean age 7 years, suggesting cross-age stability of LDs. Furthermore, the VLBW groups had higher rates of low-achievement LDs in both reading and mathematics (29% of the < 750 g group compared with 17% of the 750–1499 g group and 10% of the controls).

Two other studies offer additional evidence for higher rates of LDs in children with VLBW/VPTB compared with their NBW peers. Grunau et al.[30] examined low-achievement LDs in reading, written output, and arithmetic in a cohort of children with ≤ 800 g birth weight at ages 8–9 years. Learning disabilities on at least one of these test domains were identified in 65% of the ≤ 800 g group compared with 13% of the control group. Group differences in rates of LDs were greatest in the domains of written output and arithmetic, and rates of concurrent LDs in multiple achievement domains were ten times more frequent in the ELBW group than in controls (30% versus 3%). In another study, Johnson and Breslau[32] found higher rates of low-achievement LDs in reading and mathematics in a LBW sample at age 11 years, but only in boys. Higher rates of LDs were identified across the full range of LBW, with the rate of LD in mathematics increasing linearly with decreasing birth weight. Rates of LDs in LBW males were three times greater in reading and six times greater in mathematics than the corresponding rates in NBW males.

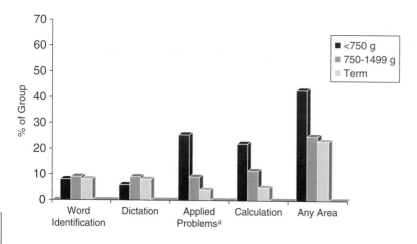

Fig. 16.1. Rates of IQ-discrepancy LDs on tests of word recognition, spelling to dictation, mathematics reasoning, and arithmetic computation in groups with < 750 g birth weight, 750–1499 g birth weight, and term birth. Discrepancies were defined as scores on the achievement tests that were greater than one standard error of the estimate from scores predicted by an IQ estimate obtained using the Kaufman Assessment Battery for Children. aRates significantly higher in < 750 g group compared with term group. Reproduced by permission of the publisher (Oxford University Press) from: Taylor HG, Hack M, Klein N, et al. Achievement in children with birth weights less than 750 grams with normal cognitive abilities: evidence for specific learning disabilities. J Pediatr Psychol, 1995; **20**: 703–19.

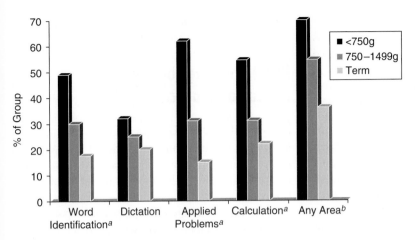

Fig. 16.2. Rates of low-achievement LDs on tests of word recognition, spelling to dictation, mathematics reasoning, and arithmetic computation in groups with < 750 g birth weight, 750–1499 g birth weight, and term birth. Low achievement was defined by standard scores for age on the tests of < 85. [a] Rates significantly higher in < 750 g group compared with term group. [b] Rates significantly higher in <750 g group compared with the 750–1499 g group. Reproduced by permission of publisher (Oxford University Press) from: Taylor HG, Hack M, Klein N, *et al.* Achievement in children with birth weights less than 750 grams with normal cognitive abilities: evidence for specific learning disabilities. *J Pediatr Psychol,* 1995; **20:** 703–19.

The finding of increased rates of LDs in males only is contrary to most of the literature on educational outcomes but is consistent with a greater male vulnerability to VLBW/VPTB [31,37]. This discrepancy between these findings and those of other investigations may reflect the study's sensitivity to this sex difference, but may also relate in part to the strategy of sampling children across the full spectrum of LBW.

Children with VLBW/VPTB also appear to have different types of reading problems than NBW children. Samuelsson *et al.* [38] classified children with VLBW at 9 years who scored poorly on a reading comprehension test into two subgroups. One subgroup had low scores in both reading and non-verbal reasoning skills, and the other subgroup had low scores in reading only. The two subgroups were referred to, respectively, as poor readers and dyslexics. The major finding was that the proportions of children in these two subgroups differed according to birth weight. Whereas there were more poor readers than dyslexics in the VLBW group (24% versus 7%), dyslexia was more common than poor reading in the NBW group (13% versus 8%). Another study of this same sample suggested group differences in the nature of children's reading problems [39]. Weaknesses in orthographic (spelling-based) reading skills were more prominent relative to phonological (sound-based) skills in the VLBW group than in the NBW controls. The VLBW group also scored more poorly on tests of other reading skills than the NBW group.

Developmental changes in educational outcomes

Learning difficulties in children with VLBW/VPTB emerge early in development. In addition to the increased rates of special education and grade repetition in kindergarten [5], delays in learning readiness skills are observed even in survivors without neurosensory deficits or mental deficiency. These delays include early childhood deficits in attention and task orientation, perceptual motor function, letter and number knowledge, and phonological processing and other speech and language competencies [3,6,8,21,40–42]. Saigal *et al.* [6] found that nearly half of their 501–1000 g birth weight cohort was at risk for future learning problems based on poor performance on kindergarten screening tests administered at age 5.5 years.

Longer-term follow-up studies indicate that children with VLBW/VPTB continue to have lower scores on achievement tests and on teacher ratings of academic performance and more need for special school interventions as they progress through the grades [23,32,43,44]. Botting *et al.* [14] found that educational difficulties identified in a cohort of children with < 1250 g birth weight at age 12 years were similar to those identified at age 8. Breslau *et al.* [45] also observed stable deficits in achievement testing between 11 and 17 years in a LBW sample. Other studies suggest educational outcomes may change with advancing age. Following children from age 8 to 12–16 years, Saigal *et al.* [27] observed more negative changes in achievement scores in an ELBW cohort compared with NBW controls. These differences were significant in comparisons between their subsample of children with < 750 g birth weight and NBW controls. Additional support for worsening outcomes is provided by Cohen *et al.* [46], who observed a tendency for increasing rates of learning problems from 8 to 12 years in a LBW sample with normal IQ. Consistent with this trend, O'Brien *et al.* [43] documented a significant increase in provision of extra education assistance between ages 8 and 14–15 years in following a sample of children from the UK with GA < 33 weeks.

In contrast, D'Angio *et al.* [19] documented a decline from 7–14 years in the proportion of a cohort of children with < 29 weeks' GA from New York State who received extra school services. The potential for positive change in educational outcomes is further supported by recent findings from Samuelsson *et al.* [47]. These investigators found more differences between a VLBW group and NBW controls in reading performance at 9 years than at 15 years. They also demonstrated that the VLBW group made significantly greater gains in reading comprehension across this age span than the NBW group. Similarly, Tideman [48] found lower school grades at age 16 years but not at 19 years in a Swedish sample of preterm children with < 35 weeks' GA. The inconsistency of these findings may reflect study differences in sample make-up, attrition, or the responsiveness of educational systems to children's learning needs.

Young adult educational outcomes are positive for many survivors. Saigal *et al.* [49] followed a regional cohort of ELBW survivors to mean age 23 years. Their NBW controls were selected randomly from lists provided by school boards at an earlier follow-up. Although the rate of self-reported LDs was higher in the ELBW group, results failed to reveal group differences in educational levels achieved. However, other findings confirm adverse effects on educational attainments. Hack *et al.* [50] reported lower high school graduation rates in a 1977–9 VLBW birth cohort examined at mean age 20 years than in a NBW control group selected from the same region using population-sampling methods (74% versus 83%). The VLBW cohort also scored lower on tests of word recognition and mathematics reasoning, and less of the VLBW men compared with NBW men were enrolled in post-secondary studies (30% versus 53%). Differences in educational attainment in this study were significant even when excluding survivors with neurosensory deficits or IQ < 70. Similar results were obtained by Cooke [51] from a postal questionnaire sent to a 1980–3 VLBW cohort and to term classmate controls at 19–22 years of age. According to survey findings, a smaller proportion of the VLBW group earned higher educational qualifications, including university degrees, and fewer were full-time students. Lower levels of educational attainment relative to NBW controls or population expectations are also reported in two other studies that

assessed pre-surfactant ELBW or VLBW cohorts in young adulthood [52,53].

Predictors and correlates of educational outcomes

Social and biological risk factors

Variability in educational outcomes of VLBW/VPTB is accounted for in part by social factors. These factors comprise measures of both family socioeconomic status (SES) and the home environment. Socioeconomic status is typically defined in terms of level of parent education, maternal marital status, and parent occupation and income, whereas the home environment is defined by more proximal measures of family functioning, parent psychiatric distress, and parent resources and stressors [54]. Higher rates of special education placement and lower scores on tests of academic achievement have been linked to single marital status, lower maternal education level, or lower family income [5,9,55–58]. In their follow-up study of a large sample of children with LBW and NBW controls drawn from urban and suburban settings, Breslau *et al.* [59] demonstrated slower growth in academic skills across the first 5 years in children from disadvantaged backgrounds. These negative environmental effects were independent of the effects of LBW. Investigations that have examined the home environment suggest that educational outcomes are additionally related to proximal family factors, such as the regularity of contact with both parents in single-parent households and maternal stimulation of children's early development [55,60].

Educational outcomes are also negatively associated with neonatal and postnatal medical risk factors, and these associations are independent of environmental risk factors [5,9,11,19,54,58]. The separate effects of biological risks are further supported by evidence of negative effects in ELBW cohorts at relative social advantage. For example, Halsey *et al.* [61] found that about half of the children with ELBW from their higher SES sample were receiving special education at 7 years. Individual neonatal factors associated with educational interventions or weaker academic skills at school age include intraventricular hemorrhage and other brain abnormalities on neonatal cranial ultrasound, chronic lung disease, necrotizing enterocolitis, meningitis, postnatal corticosteroid treatment, length of neonatal hospitalization, and numbers of neonatal complications [9,19,54,58,62,63]. Our research team found that early school-age children with VLBW with high numbers of these complications had three times the rate of special education placements than survivors with fewer complications [54].

Postnatal medical factors related to poorer educational outcomes include subnormal head circumference and neurosensory abnormalities, such as cerebral palsy and retinopathy of prematurity [4,16,64–66]. In analysis of data from our study of outcomes in two VLBW groups (< 750 g and 750–1499 g), Peterson *et al.* [67] observed that smaller head circumference at age 8 years was associated with lower scores on reading, spelling, and mathematics tests, even when controlling for the effects of neurosensory abnormality, SES, sex, weight for GA at birth, and neonatal medical complications. In a study of a < 29 weeks' GA sample, children with more severe physical impairments had more intensive special education services at age 4–10 years [19]. Other studies indicate that rates of special education are higher in VLBW survivors with early childhood neurological impairments than in those without these impairments [16,66], and that children with neurodevelopmental impairments so severe as to preclude standardized testing are likely to be placed in special schools [68].

Few studies have examined educational outcomes in relation to measures of brain volume or brain abnormalities as measured by postnatal magnetic resonance imaging (MRI). Stewart *et al.* [69] failed to find a link between abnormalities on MRI and school performance in a sample of children with < 33 weeks' GA. On the other hand, Allin *et al.* [70] reported that smaller cerebellar volume predicted poorer reading skills in a similarly defined preterm sample, and Isaacs *et al.* [71]

documented an association between smaller gray matter volume in the left parietal lobe and calculation ability in children with < 30 weeks' GA.

Behavior and neuropsychological correlates of educational problems

Scholastic deficits in VLBW/VPTB cohorts are frequently accompanied by concurrent weaknesses in cognitive functioning and behavior problems. With regard to cognitive skills, Downie *et al.* [72] reported that scores on a test of non-word reading were correlated with measures of IQ, phonological awareness, verbal working memory, and temporal order perception in a sample of children with ELBW and full-term controls at mean age 11–12 years. Other studies of samples with VLBW or ELBW have documented correlations of low achievement in reading, spelling, mathematics, and written output with weaknesses in IQ, perceptual motor abilities, memory, and executive functions (e.g., attention, verbal work memory, planning skills) [30,46,73]. Associations of achievement with some cognitive skills, such as perceptual motor and spatial abilities, phonological processing, and executive function, remain even when controlling for IQ [4,36,62,74]. Thus, the associations of neuropsychological impairments with poor achievement cannot be explained solely in terms of global mental deficiency.

Causal modeling analysis of data from our study of academic achievement in < 750 g and 750–1499 g groups supported the role of neuropsychological skills as mediators of the effects of biological risk on school-age achievement [34]. Figure 16.3 summarizes

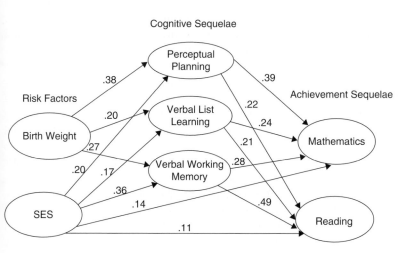

Fig. 16.3. Structural equation model of relationships between birth weight, socioeconomic status (SES), and cognitive and achievement outcomes at mean age 11. Cognitive outcomes were measured by neuropsychological abilities composites, and achievement outcomes by composites of reading and mathematics skills. The model provided a good fit to the data. Standardized path coefficients listed above the arrows indicate the strengths of the casual connections. Paths between birth weight and achievement were not significant and hence were excluded from the model. Reproduced by permission of the publisher (Taylor & Francis, Ltd.) from: Taylor HG, Burant CJ, Holding PA, *et al.* Sources of variability in sequelae of very low birth weight. *Child Neuropsychol,* 2002; **8:** 163–78.

the model that we successfully fit to our data. The model confirms associations of VLBW with specific cognitive skills which, in turn, were associated with achievement in reading and mathematics. These associations were independent of the effects of SES. Consistent with evidence that reading and mathematics skills have different neuropsychological correlates, the model shows that verbal working memory was more strongly related to reading and mathematics to perceptual planning. In view of the vulnerability of children with VLBW/VPTB to deficits on perceptual tasks, the strong association of perceptual planning skills with mathematics achievement helps explain survivors' pronounced deficits in this area [30,36].

Cognitive, motor, and language abilities in early childhood help account for variability in later educational modifications and academic achievement among children with VLBW/VPTB [16,75]. The Bavarian Longitudinal Study followed children with VLBW/VPTB to ages 6, 8, and 13 years [7]. Findings from this project revealed that phonological skills at 6 years predicted reading and spelling at 8 years, and that IQ at 6 years predicted mathematics at 8 years. Academic skills at 8 years, in turn, predicted academic success at 13 years as measured by the child's educational track and performance within the track.

Research with other LBW samples provides additional evidence for associations of early developmental problems with later educational outcomes. In a study of a normally intelligent LBW cohort, participants who had learning problems at 8 years had more neonatal sleep abnormalities and scored more poorly on early childhood assessments of cognitive ability than participants without learning problems [76]. In following a sample of children born at ≤ 37 weeks' GA from ages 4 to 8 years, Sullivan and McGrath [77] demonstrated that early weaknesses in motor skills presaged later school interventions and low achievement scores. Other follow-up studies of LBW samples documented associations of general cognitive deficiencies in early childhood with adverse educational outcomes at the end of compulsory schooling, including low achievement scores, low school grades, and the need for special services or early dropout from school [45,75].

Several studies suggest that symptoms of attention deficit hyperactivity disorder (ADHD) are also associated with grade failure, special education placement, and teacher ratings of poor school performance with VLBW/VPTB or ELBW samples [16,17,78,79].

Difficulties following directions, formulating questions, expressing thoughts, and remaining task oriented may underlie some of these children's scholastic difficulties [3,31,80]. In light of evidence of negative effects of VLBW/VPTB on academic self-esteem, motivational problems may additionally contribute to educational difficulties [7,30].

Research limitations and needs

Research on the educational consequences of VLBW/VPTB has been subject to several general methodological limitations [10]. To begin with, VLBW/VPTB cohorts are frequently not population based and the consequences of VLBW/VPTB may be affected by development of new medical technologies [26]. Differences between neonatal centers in efforts to save the highest-risk neonates and in methods of medical management may introduce cross-site differences in outcome. Likewise, newer methods of medical management raise questions about the applicability of findings from studies of earlier birth cohorts to more recent survivors [30]. Consideration of sample recruitment strategies and of variations in findings related to birth cohort is thus important in evaluating research findings. Follow-up studies of later-born children are needed to determine if changes in neonatal care have altered educational outcomes.

Secondly, past studies often fail to recruit NBW children who are matched to the index cases on background factors or to control for these factors in making group comparisons. In studies conducted by our research group, recruitment of comparison groups based on demographic factors (e.g., same hospital of birth or classroom) yielded index and control groups similar in background characteristics [9,25]. Selection of NBW matches from the same schools as the index children was especially critical given between-school variations in instructional approaches and education policy. However, we recognize that we failed to match on factors such as genetic influences on development, prenatal alcohol and drug exposure, and parenting characteristics, and that these factors may have contributed to group differences in educational outcomes. Even more critically, the ultimate effects of VLBW/VPTB on educational progress are likely moderated by a host of factors, such as genetic susceptibilities, early parenting and family circumstances, developmental and educational interventions, and the child's behavioral adjustment and motivation [7,10,14,31,81]. These factors can obscure and may even override the effects of VLBW/VPTB [82]. The educational consequences of VLBW/VPTB will be best appreciated in research that takes these other influences into account.

Thirdly, studies in this area have frequently employed inadequate measures of educational outcome. Reliance on parent reports is problematic, given that some parents are unaware of their child's school performance or of special educational interventions [15]. Although teachers are in a better position to assess educational progress, teacher ratings are also subjective and may be influenced by their expectations and teaching methods. While objective tests of academic achievement avoid these limitations, these tests may also be criticized as assessing too limited a range of learning skills. For example, tests of reading often have been restricted to word recognition and have not tapped more advanced text processing skills. Similarly, assessments of mathematics have been confined in large part to tests of basic arithmetic computations and have not examined diverse aspects of mathematical reasoning or problem-solving. More comprehensive assessments of academic skills, objective observations of children's classroom learning behaviors, and concurrent assessment of cognitive and behavioral outcomes would shed light on the nature of their scholastic deficiencies. These more extensive assessments may also be useful in identifying subtle learning problems that would otherwise go undetected, or in discovering the ways in which these problems differ from those present in NBW children [36,62].

Fourthly, educational outcomes are typically described only for total VLBW/VPTB samples, rather than in relation to the degree of biological or neurological risk. Evidence that outcomes are worse for children with more extreme low birth weight or low GA and for those with neonatal medical complications implies a need to consider variations in outcome in relation to the extent and type of biological risk. For example, it would be useful to know if the nature or severity of educational deficits relate to the type of neonatal medical complications or to characteristics of brain insult as evident on neonatal MRI. More information on residual neuropathology would also illuminate the neural mechanisms contributing to difficulties in school performance and academic achievement. Although neural abnormalities due to perinatal hypoxic-ischemic and pro-inflammatory brain insult are presumed to underlie these difficulties [10], we know little about relationships between

insults to specific neural structures and educational sequelae. Further investigation of education outcomes is also warranted in lower-risk children with birth weight 1500–2500 g. Despite the less pronounced effects on academic achievement in these children [59], they are more numerous than survivors with VLBW/VPTB and more information is needed on the nature and predictors of their educational outcomes.

Fifthly, it will be important to investigate developmental issues, including the precursors of adverse educational outcomes and longer-term effects of VLBW/VPTB on academic progress through the school-age years and into adulthood. In view of associations of scholastic problems with assessments of cognitive, motor, and language skills conducted prior to or shortly after school entry, it may be feasible to identify children with special learning needs early in childhood [7,31,59]. However, more research is needed to specify risks for poor early school progress and identify family and schooling factors that may facilitate learning [11,21,81]. Longer-term follow-up studies are required to chart scholastic development during the school-age years and assess the effects of VLBW/VPTB on adult educational attainment. For example, it would be useful to know if some children progress less rapidly than others, and if so to explore the reasons for such differences. Academic competencies in young adulthood and their implications for higher educational attainments and employment are also poorly understood, and no study has as yet described these attainments for a cohort of infants born in the post-surfactant era.

Sixthly, we need to better understand why many children with more extreme degrees of VLBW/VPTB function well academically despite high-risk birth [18,81]. It is unclear if these positive outcomes reflect an absence of severe neonatal brain insult, greater brain plasticity, provision of effective academic instruction or support systems, or some combination of these factors. The possibility of compensatory neural development is supported by a functional MRI (fMRI) study carried out by Ment et al. [83]. These researchers found that children with 600–1250 g birth weight had different patterns of brain activation during language and phonological processing tasks than a matched term-born group. Another fMRI study by Noble et al. [84] revealed effects of SES on brain activation patterns during a pseudoword reading task. While this study did not focus on effects of

VLBW/VPTB, the results support the possibility of environmental influences on brain development. Further investigations of the relation of educational outcomes to neonatal brain status, brain functioning in childhood, and family and school influences may help illuminate the mechanisms responsible for positive educational outcomes.

Finally, we know little of how to optimize academic progress in the VLBW/VPTB population. There is some evidence that intensive early developmental interventions improve long-term educational outcomes [85]. Early interventions to enhance parent–child interactions also have potential to facilitate early learning readiness [86]. But few if any instructional approaches have been designed to promote school performance and academic achievement in school-age children with VLBW/VPTB. Relevant methods to consider in intervention research would be application of phonics-based programs to prevent early reading failure [7]. Because deficiencies exist in multiple academic domains and in view of weaknesses in attention, executive function, and other non-verbal skills [30,72], intervention research might also examine other academic interventions, including structured approaches that break down learning tasks, teach explicit strategies for task completion and problem-solving, and allow for extended time and practice [36]. In view of the variability in academic outcomes in the VLBW/VPTB and changes in needs that may occur with advancing age, effective interventions are likely to require accommodation to individual learning characteristics.

Conclusion

As a result of recent increases in survival of children with VLBW/VPTB, more children are born with chronic medical conditions, such as cerebral palsy and severe cognitive impairment [87]. These survivors will require intensive educational programing from an early age. Survival has also increased for children without major forms of disability who have "high-prevalence/low-severity" problems, including subtle forms of learning, cognitive, and behavioral disturbances [81]. The manifestations of learning problems in this subset of survivors are elevated rates of grade failure, special educational placement, and LDs, lower teacher ratings of school performance, and lower scores on tests of academic achievement compared with NBW children. Although academic deficits are most pronounced in the area of mathematics, reading, spelling, and writing are also adversely affected.

Academic deficits cannot be fully attributed to mental retardation or neurosensory disorders. Scores on achievement tests remain lower for VLBW/VPTB samples than for NBW controls even when children with these conditions are excluded or when comparisons are made controlling for IQ. Findings showing that academic achievement is associated with deficits in attention, executive function, and other specific neuropsychological weaknesses, even when controlling for IQ, provides additional support for selective academic deficits. Consistent with selective effects on achievement, rates of LDs in reading, written output, and mathematics are higher in VLBW/VPTB cohorts than in NBW control groups. Children with VLBW/VPTB also display distinct patterns of LDs. Learning disabilities are frequently present in multiple academic domains. Furthermore, a high rate of "non-verbal" LD is suggested by the combination of deficiencies in both mathematics and visual-perceptual skills [30,36]. Although children with VLBW/VPTB score less well than their NBW peers on tests of phonological processing and other speech and language skills, they are less likely to have isolated forms of language-based LDs [7,8,38,39,72].

Children with more severe learning and other developmental impairments are placed in special schools or in full-time special education classrooms. Less severely affected survivors receive special assistance for a portion of the day within their regular classrooms or in resource rooms. Still other survivors appear to make academic progress within the educational mainstream. The numbers of academically "unaffected" children is a matter of some debate. Anderson et al. [18] found educational problems in only a minority of their Australian ELBW/EPTB cohort at 8 years of age. Similar findings are reported in studies of school outcomes in low GA cohorts in the UK, the Netherlands, and New Zealand [23,32]. In contrast, other studies documented grade failure or special education in the majority of their cohorts [25,27]. Differences in sample composition, procedures for assessing educational outcome, school policies for retaining students or providing special education assistance, or even in the quality of instructional support given by regular classroom teachers may help account for the discrepant findings. It is clear, however, that many children with VLBW/VPTB meet standard criteria for academic success.

The wide variability in educational outcomes within and between study samples can be attributed to several factors. Biological risks for poorer outcomes include lower birth weight or GA, neonatal medical complications such as abnormalities on cranial ultrasounds and chronic lung disease, postnatal neurosensory impairments, and subnormal head circumference. Adverse outcomes are especially pronounced in children with more extreme degrees of VLBW/VPTB. Social factors, such as low SES and disadvantaged family environments, also predict adverse educational outcomes. Because social factors contribute to outcomes independent of biological risks, children at both social and biological risk are especially prone to learning problems. A better understanding of the specific contribution of VLBW/VPTB to children's academic problems requires that we take social risks and other experiential and biological-genetic factors into account. These other factors include early developmental interventions, family and teacher supports for learning, prenatal exposure to drugs or alcohol, and family histories of learning problems. Consideration of these multiple influences on children's learning will also enhance prediction of individual outcomes.

Learning difficulties are evident in many children with VLBW/VPTB by the time of school entry and persist throughout the school-age years and into young adulthood. The persistence of these difficulties is confirmed by findings that adolescents with VLBW/VPTB have higher rates of special education and lower academic achievement than their NBW peers. Further confirmation comes from studies indicating that young adult survivors have more self-reported learning difficulties, lower rates of secondary school graduation, and lower post-secondary educational attainments compared with NBW controls or population expectations. While most longitudinal studies have found that educational problems remain constant relative to age-matched NBW controls or even worsen with advancing age, one study observed a reduction in special education from early school age to adolescence and another reported improved reading skills from ages 9–15 years [19,47]. The positive educational attainments observed in some studies of young adult survivors also suggest that later academic functioning is better than expected based on earlier outcomes [81]. The conflicting findings may reflect differences between studies in sample composition, the educational policies and learning supports of the schools

attended by study participants, and the measures used to assess outcome. The results imply a need for further longitudinal investigation of factors related to positive or negative changes over time.

Other topics for future research include:

1. description of educational outcomes in recent VLBW/VPTB birth cohorts and in children with birth weight 1500–2500 g;
2. evaluation of the specific nature of educational problems using comprehensive measures of academic skills (e.g., accuracy, fluency, higher-level comprehension and problem-solving) and observations of classroom behavior;
3. examination of an expanded range of influences on achievement to improve prediction and better delineate the role of VLBW/VPTB;
4. investigation of outcomes in relation to brain volumes and brain activation as measured by structural MRI and fMRI, to determine the neural basis of individual differences in scholastic performance and to investigate neural plasticity;
5. examine factors related to positive outcomes to explore protective or compensatory mechanisms;
6. study of the manifestations of educational problems at school entry or sooner to enhance early identification of children;
7. design and test instructional interventions geared to the particular problems of children with VLBW/VPTB to help optimize academic progress.

In conducting this research, it will be important to recruit representative samples of children with VLBW/VPTB, select NBW comparison groups with similar background characteristics, and make statistical adjustments for any measurable confounds. A final requirement is to be aware of the complexity of learning problems [81]. As outcomes that reflect "real-world" functioning [21,42], these problems reflect not only neuropsychological weaknesses but also children's behavioral dispositions, motivation, and contextual factors, such as the academic demands made of the child and the supports available to meet these demands. Finding ways to avoid or minimize learning problems will yield substantial savings for the child and society.

Acknowledgments

Work on this chapter was supported in part by grants HD50309 and HD39756 from the National Institutes of Health (NIH). Past studies by our research team cited in the chapter were funded by NIH grants HD39756, HD26554, and HD34177. The author is indebted to Maureen Hack, MB ChB for her collaboration and leadership.

References

1. Hintz SR, Kendrick DE, Vohr BR, *et al*. Changes in neurodevelopmental outcomes at 18 and 22 months' corrected age among infants of less than 25 weeks' gestational age born in 1993–1999. *Pediatrics* 2005; **115**: 1645–51.

2. Taylor HG, Klein N, Hack M. School-age consequences of < 750 g birth weight: a review and update. *Dev Neuropsychol* 2000; **17**: 289–321.

3. Klein N. Children who were very low birthweight: cognitive abilities and classroom behavior at 5 years of age. *J Spec Educ* 1988; **22**: 41–54.

4. Marlow N, Hennessy EM, Bracewell MA, *et al*. Motor and executive function at 6 years of age after extremely preterm birth. *Pediatrics* 2007; **120**: 793–804.

5. Resnick MB, Gueorguieva RV, Carter RL, *et al*. The impact of low birth weight, prenatal conditions, and sociodemographic factors on educational outcome in kindergarten. *Pediatrics* 1999; **104**: e74.

6. Saigal S, Szatmari P, Rosenbaum P, *et al*. Intellectual and functional status at school entry of children who weighed 1000 grams or less at birth: a regional perspective of births in the 1980s. *J Pediatr* 1990; **116**: 409–16.

7. Schneider W, Wolke D, Schlagmuller M, *et al*. Pathways to school achievement in very preterm and full term children. *Eur J Psychol Educ* 2004; **19**: 385–406.

8. Wolke D, Meyer R. Cognitive status, language attainment, and prereading skills of 6-year-old very preterm children and their peers: The Bavarian Longitudinal Study. *Dev Med Child Neurol* 1999; **41**: 94–109.

9. Taylor HG, Klein N, Drotar D, *et al*. Consequences and risks for < 1000-g birth weight for neuropsychological skills, achievement, and adaptive functioning. *Dev Behav Pediatr* 2006; **27**: 459–69.

10. Aylward GP. Neurodevelopmental outcomes of infants born prematurely. *Dev Behav Pediatr* 2005; **26**: 427–40.

11. Klebanov PK, Brooks-Gunn J, McCormick MC. School achievement and failure in very low birthweight children. *Dev Behav Pediatr* 1994; **15**: 248–56.

12. Chaikind S, Corman H. The impact of low birthweight on special education costs. *J Health Econ* 1991; **10**: 292–311.

13. Roth J, Figlio DN, Chen Y, *et al*. Maternal and infant factors associated with excess kindergarten costs. *Pediatrics* 2004; **114**: 720–8.

14. Botting N, Powls A, Cooke RWI, *et al*. Cognitive and educational outcome of very-low-birthweight children in early adolescence. *Dev Med Child Neurol* 1998; **40**: 652–60.

15. Buck GM, Msall ME, Schisterman EF, *et al*. Extreme prematurity and school outcomes. *Paediatr Perinat Epidemiol* 2000; **14**: 324–31.

16. Hille ETM, den Ouden AL, Bauer L, *et al*. School performance at nine years of age in very premature and very low birth weight infants: perinatal risk factors and predictors at five years of age. *Pediatrics* 1994; **125**: 426–34.

17. Saigal S, Szatmari P, Rosenbaum P, *et al*. Cognitive abilities and school performance of extremely low birth weight children and matched term control children at age 8 years: a regional study. *J Pediatr* 1991; **118**: 751–60.

18. Anderson P, Doyle LW and the Victorian Infant Collaborative Study Group. Neurobehavioral outcomes of school-age children born extremely low birth weight or very preterm in the 1990s. *JAMA* 2003; **289**: 3264–72.

19. D'Angio CT, Sinkin RA, Stevens TP, *et al*. Longitudinal, 15-year follow-up of children born at less than 29 weeks gestation after introduction of surfactant therapy into a region: Neurologic, cognitive, and educational outcomes. *Pediatrics* 2002; **46**: 812–15.

20. Hagen EW, Palta M, Albanese A, *et al*. School achievement in a regional cohort of children born very low birthweight. *Dev Behav Pediatr* 2006; **27**: 112–20.

21. Vohr BR, Msall ME. Neuropsychological and functional outcomes of very low birth weight infants. *Semin Perinatol* 1997; **21**: 202–20.

22. Saigal S, den Ouden L, Wolke D, *et al*. School-age outcomes in children who were extremely low birth weight from four international population-based cohorts. *Pediatrics* 2003; **112**: 943–50.

23. Johnson A, Bowler U, Yudkin P, *et al*. Health and school performance of teenagers born before 29 weeks gestation. *Arch Dis Child Fetal Neonatal Ed* 2003; **88**: F190–8.

24. O'Callaghan MJ, Burns YR Gray PH. School performance of ELBW children: A controlled study. *Dev Med Child Neurol* 1996; **38**: 917–26.

25. Taylor HG, Klein N, Minich N, *et al*. Middle school-age outcomes in children with very low birthweight. *Child Dev* 2000; **71**: 1495–511.

26. Pinto-Martin J, Whitaker A, Feldman J, *et al*. Special education services and school performance in a regional cohort of low-birthweight infants at age nine. *Paediatr Perinatal Epidemiol* 2004; **18**: 120–9.

27. Saigal S, Hoult LA, Streiner DL, *et al*. School difficulties at adolescence in a regional cohort of children who were extremely low birthweight. *Pediatrics* 2000; **105**: 325–31.

28. Avchen RN, Scott KG, Mason CA. Birth weight and school-age disabilities: a population-based study. *Am J Epidemiol* 2001; **154**: 895–901.

29. Feder KP, Majnemer A, Bourbonnais D, *et al.* Handwriting performance in preterm children compared with term peers at age 6 to 7 years. *Dev Med Child Neurol* 2005; **47**: 163–70.

30. Grunau RE, Whitfield MF, Fay TB. Psychosocial and academic characteristics of extremely low birth weight (≤800 g) adolescents who are free of major impairment compared with term-born subjects. *Pediatrics* 2004; **114**: e725–32.

31. Whitfield MF, Grunau RVE, Holsti L. Extremely premature (≤800 g) schoolchildren: multiple areas of hidden disability. *Arch Dis Child* 1997; **77**: F85–90.

32. Johnson EO, Breslau N. Increased risk of learning disabilities in low birthweight boys at age 11 years. *Biol Psychiatry* 2000; **47**: 490–500.

33. Klein N, Hack M, Breslau N. Children who were very low birthweight: Developmental and academic achievement at nine years of age. *J Dev Behav Pediatr* 1989; **10**: 32–7.

34. Taylor HG, Burant C, Holding PA, *et al.* Sources of variability in sequelae of very low birth weight. *Child Neuropsychol* 2002; **8**: 164–78.

35. Taylor HG, Hack M, Klein N, *et al.* Achievement in children with birth weights less than 750 grams with normal cognitive abilities: evidence for specific learning disabilities. *J Pediatr Psychol* 1995; **20**: 703–19.

36. Litt J, Taylor HG, Klein N, *et al.* Learning disabilities in children with very low birth weight: Prevalence, neuropsychological correlates, and educational interventions. *J Learn Disabil* 2005; **38**: 130–41.

37. Hintz SR, Kendrick DE, Vohr BR, *et al.* Gender differences in neurodevelopmental outcomes among extremely preterm, extremely-low-birthweight infants. *Acta Paediatr* 2006; **95**: 1239–48.

38. Samuelsson S, Bylund B, Cervin T, *et al.* The prevalence of reading disabilities among very-low-birth-weight children at 9 years of age – dyslexics or poor readers? *Dyslexia* 1999; **5**: 94–112.

39. Samuelsson S, Finnstrom O, Leijon I, *et al.* Phonological and surface profiles of reading difficulties among very low birth weight children: converging evidence for the developmental lag hypothesis. *Sci Stud Read* 2000; **4**: 197–217.

40. Halsey CL, Collin MF, Anderson CL. Extremely low birth weight children and their peers: A comparison of preschool performance. *Pediatrics* 1993; **91**: 807–11.

41. Luoma L, Herrgard E, Martikainen A, *et al.* Speech and language development of children born at < 32 weeks gestation: a 5-year prospective follow-up study. *Dev Med Child Neurol* 1998; **40**: 380–7.

42. Msall ME, Tremont MR. Measuring functional outcomes after prematurity: Developmental impact of very low birth weight and extremely low birth weight status on childhood disability. *Ment Retard Dev Disabil Res Rev* 2002; **8**: 258–72.

43. O'Brien F, Roth S, Stewart A, *et al.* The neurodevelopmental progress of infants less than 33 weeks into adolescence. *Arch Dis Child* 2004; **89**: 207–11.

44. Pharoah POD, Stevenson CJ, West CR. General certificate of secondary education performance in very low birthweight infants. *Arch Dis Child* 2003; **88**: 295–8.

45. Breslau N, Paneth NS, Lucia VC. The lingering academic deficits of low birth weight children. *Pediatrics* 2004; **114**: 1035–40.

46. Cohen SE, Beckwith L, Parmelee AH, *et al.* Prediction of low and normal school achievement in early adolescents born preterm. *J Early Adolesc* 1996; **16**: 46–70.

47. Samuelsson S, Finnstrom O, Flodmark O, *et al.* A longitudinal study of reading skills among very-low-birthweight children: is there a catch-up? *J Pediatr Psychol* 2006; **31**: 967–77.

48. Tideman E. Longitudinal follow-up of children born preterm: cognitive development at age 19. *Early Hum Dev* 2000; **58**: 81–90.

49. Saigal S, Stoskopf B, Boyle M, *et al.* Comparison of current health, functional limitations, and health care of young adults who were born with extremely low birth weight and normal birth weight. *Pediatrics* 2007; **119**: E562–73.

50. Hack M, Flannery DJ, Schluchter M, *et al.* Outcomes in young adulthood for very-low-birth-weight infants. *N Engl J Med* 2002; **346**: 149–57.

51. Cooke RWI. Health, lifestyle, and quality of life for young adults born very preterm. *Arch Dis Child* 2004; **89**: 201–6.

52. Ericson A, Kallen B. Very low birthweight boys at the age of 19. *Arch Dis Child Fetal Neonatal Ed* 1998; **78**: F171–4.

53. Lefebvre F, Mazurier E, Tessier R. Cognitive and educational outcomes in early adulthood for infants weighing 1000 grams or less at birth. *Acta Paediatr* 2005; **94**: 733–40.

54. Taylor HG, Klein N, Schatschneider C, *et al.* Predictors of early school age outcomes in very low birthweight children. *Dev Behav Pediatr* 1998; **19**: 235–43.

55. Gross SJ, Mettelman BB, Dye TD, *et al.* Impact of family structure and stability on academic outcome in preterm children at 10 years of age. *J Pediatr* 2001; **138**: 169–75.

56. Hollomon HA, Dobbins DR Scott KG. The effects of biological and social risk factors on special education

placement: birthweight and maternal education as an example. *Res Dev Disabil* 1998; **19**: 281–94.

57. Msall ME, Buck GM, Rogers BT, *et al.* Risk factors for major neurodevelopmnental impairments and need for special education resources in extremely premature infants. *J Pediatr* 1991; **119**: 606–14.

58. Vohr B, Allan WC, Westerveld M, *et al.* School-age outcomes of very low birth weight infants in the Indomethacin Intraventricular Hemorrhage Prevention Trial. *Pediatrics* 2003; **111**: e340–6.

59. Breslau N, Johnson EO, Lucia VC. Academic achievement of low birth-weight children at age 11: the role of cognitive abilities at school entry. *J Abnorm Child Psychol* 2001; **29**: 273–9.

60. Dieterich SE, Assel MA, Swank P, *et al.* The impact of early maternal verbal scaffolding and child language abilities on later decoding and reading comprehension skills. *J Sch Psychol* 2006; **43**: 481–94.

61. Halsey CL, Collin MF, Anderson CL. Extremely low-birth-weight children and their peers: a comparison of school-age outcomes. *Arch Pediatr Adolesc Med* 1996; **150**: 790–4.

62. Downie ALS, Frisk V, Jakobson LS. The impact of periventricular brain injury on reading and spelling abilities in the late elementary and adolescent years. *Child Neuropsychol* 2005; **11**: 479–95.

63. Short EJ, Kirchner L, Asaad GR, *et al.* Developmental sequelae in preterm infants having a diagnosis of brochopulmonary dysplasia. *Arch Pediatr Adolesc Med* 2007; **161**: 1082–7.

64. Msall MD, Phelps DL, DiGaudio KM, *et al.* Severity of neonatal retinopathy of prematurity is predictive of neurodevelopmental functional outcome at age 5.5 years. *Pediatrics* 2000; **106**: 998–1005.

65. Stathis SL, O'Callaghan M, Harvey J, *et al.* Head circumference in ELBW babies is associated with learning difficulties and cognition but not ADHD in the school-aged child. *Dev Med Child Neurol* 1999; **41**: 375–80.

66. Vohr BR, Garcia-Coll CT. Neurodevelopmental and school performance of very low birth weight infants: a seven year longitudinal study. *Pediatrics* 1985; **76**: 345–50.

67. Peterson J, Taylor HG, Minich N, *et al.* Subnormal head circumference in very low birth weight children: neonatal correlates and school-age consequences. *Early Hum Dev* 2006; **82**: 325–34.

68. Hall A, McLeod A, Counsell C, *et al.* School attainment, cognitive ability, and motor function in a total Scottish very-low-birthweight population at eight years: a controlled study. *Dev Med Child Neurol* 1995; **37**: 1037–50.

69. Stewart AL, Rifkin L, Amess PN, *et al.* Brain structure and neurocognitive and behavioural function in adolescents who were born very preterm. *Lancet* 1999; **353**: 1653–7.

70. Allin M, Matsumoto H, Santhouse AM, *et al.* Cognitive and motor function and the size of the cerebellum in adolescents born very pre-term. *Brain* 2001; **124**: 60–6.

71. Isaacs EB, Edmonds CJ, Lucas A, *et al.* Calculation difficulties in children of very low birthweight: A neural correlate. *Brain* 2001; **124**: 1701–7.

72. Downie ALS, Jakobson LS, Frisk V, *et al.* Auditory temporal processing deficits in children with periventricular brain injury. *Brain Lang* 2002; **80**: 208–25.

73. Holsti L, Grunau RVE, Whitfield MF. Developmental coordination disorder in extremely low birth weight children at nine years. *J Dev Behav Pediatr* 2002; **23**: 9–15.

74. Taylor HG, Hack M, Klein N. Attention deficits in children with < 750 gm birth weight. *Child Neuropsychol* 1998; **4**: 21–34.

75. Hansen BM, Dinesen J, Hoff B, *et al.* Intelligence in preterm children at four years of age as a predictor of school function: a longitudinal controlled study. *Dev Med Child Neurol* 2002; **44**: 517–21.

76. Cohen SE, Parmelee AH, Sigman M, *et al.* Antecedents of school problems in children born preterm. *J Pediatr Psychol* 1988; **13**: 493–508.

77. Sullivan MC, McGrath MM. Perinatal morbidity, mild motor delay, and later school outcomes. *Dev Med Child Neurol* 2003; **45**: 104–12.

78. McCormick M, Gortmaker S, Sobol A. Very low birth weight children: behavior problems and school difficulty in a national sample. *J Pediatr* 1990; **117**: 688–93.

79. O'Callaghan MJ, Harvey JM. Biological predictors and co-morbidity of attention deficit and hyperactivity disorder in extremely low birthweight infants at school. *J Paediatr Child Health* 1997; **33**: 491–6.

80. Klebanov PK, Brooks-Gunn J, McCormick MC. Classroom behavior of very low birth weight elementary school children. *Pediatrics* 1994; **94**: 700–8.

81. Saigal S, Rosenbaum P. What matters in the long term: Reflections on the context of adult outcomes versus detailed measures in childhood. *Semin Fetal Neonatal Med* 2007; **12**: 415–22.

82. Baron IS, Litman FR, Ahronovich MD, *et al.* Neuropsychological outcomes of preterm triplets discordant for birthweight: a case report. *Clin Neuropsychol* 2007; **21**: 338–62.

83. Ment LR, Peterson BS, Vohr B, *et al.* Cortical recruitment patterns in children born prematurely compared with control subjects during a passive

listening functional magnetic resonance imaging task. *J Pediatr* 2006; **149**: 490–8.

84. Noble KG, Wolmetz ME, Ochs LG, *et al.* Brain-behavior relationships in reading acquisition are modulated by socioeconomic factors. *Dev Sci* 2006; **9**: 642–54.

85. McCormick M, Brooks-Gunn J, Buka SL, *et al.* Early intervention in low birth weight premature infants: results at 18 years of age for the Infant Health and Development Program. *Pediatrics* 2006; **117**: 771–80.

86. Landry SH, Miller-Loncar CL, Smith KE, *et al.* The role of early parenting in children's development of executive processes. *Dev Neuropsychol* 2002; **21**: 15–41.

87. Wilson-Costello D. Is there evidence that long-term outcomes have improved with intensive care? *Semin Fetal Neonatal Med* 2007; **12**: 344–54.

Pathways of risk and resiliency after prematurity: role of socioeconomic status

Michael E. Msall, Mary C. Sullivan, and Jennifer Park

Introduction

Long-term survival for infants born very preterm (VPT < 32 weeks' gestation) increased dramatically with the regionalization of neonatal intensive care and resulted in decreased rates of major neurodevelopmental disabilities in survivors. For those born extremely preterm (EPT, < 28 weeks' gestation), survival has also increased dramatically, but there remains high rates of cognitive impairment and intellectual disability. However, despite these biomedical advances, environmental and social conditions that can deleteriously affect the health and well-being of these already vulnerable children have not improved in the USA. There are major gaps in accessing comprehensive family supports and quality early childhood experiences for recent cohorts of children at the highest biomedical and social risks. The purpose of this chapter is to examine the role of social and environmental factors in aggravating or moderating neonatal risks for suboptimal developmental and behavioral outcomes after VPT and EPT birth. We will also discuss available evidence from both longitudinal studies and community interventions for children at psychosocial disadvantage. This evidence offers important lessons to critically consider in evaluating developmental and educational trajectories for recent cohorts of children with the double jeopardy of VPT/EPT birth and social adversity.

Neonatal and social risks

The rate of preterm birth has risen in the past decade with approximately 1 in 7 infants in the USA born preterm each year[1]. Currently, 15 per 1000 US live births, more than 60 000 infants annually, are born with very low birth weight status (< 1500 g). These infants have high risks for long-term neurodevelopmental disabilities such as intellectual disability, blindness, sensory-neural hearing loss, and cerebral palsy [2]. There can be several biomedical reasons behind this increase, such as the increased rate of multiple births (twins, triplets, or quadruplets) due to assisted reproductive technologies and increased maternal age. Other biomedical factors include maternal uterine or cervical abnormalities and maternal chronic health conditions, including diabetes, high blood pressure, epilepsy, and cardiac disorders (see also Chapter 1). Another factor which has been associated with VPT/EPT birth is teenage pregnancy, although this has been decreasing over the past decade [1,2]. However, it is very critical to remember that both VPT and EPT are heterogeneous, and our understanding of causal pathways that lead to successful intervention is at an early scientific stage.

Another variable that contributes to preterm birth is social risk. Social risk factors include suboptimal home and community environments. Poverty, domestic violence, drug addiction (e.g., opiates, cocaine, and methamphetamine), crime, hunger, and poor quality housing are some of the features of social risks [3]. Mothers who live in such environments experience multiple stressors, are prone to nutritional deficiency, often receive suboptimal prenatal care, more likely are a single-parent, and have a higher exposure to tobacco and alcohol compared to mothers from non-poor backgrounds [2]. Several studies have also shown that rates of marijuana, cocaine, tobacco, and alcohol use are higher for women who are unmarried, unemployed, and have less than a college education, indicating that substance abuse and poverty are closely related [4,5]. It has been suggested that the prevalence of substance abuse, illicit drug use, and smoking among women from impoverished or low socioeconomic status (SES) background is largely due to the sense of helplessness, low self-esteem, difficulties coping with stress, and pressure from coping with difficult financial situations in everyday living [4,6].

Neurodevelopmental Outcomes of Preterm Birth, ed. Chiara Nosarti, Robin M. Murray, and Maureen Hack. Published by Cambridge University Press. © Cambridge University Press 2010.

Such social adversity is a large contributing factor in preterm birth, especially when mothers receive late prenatal care (or not at all) to identify maternal reproductive complications or health problems that jeopardize fetal growth. Also, late or no prenatal care decreases the chances of maternal access to educational and support services (such as counseling, community health, and educational services) [2].

The negative effects of maternal low SES almost always translate into neonatal risks, and since ethnicity in the USA is closely related to SES, it is not surprising to see discrepancies in preterm births amongst ethnic groups. African-American infants are more than 1.5 times more likely than whites to be born preterm and 2.5 times more likely to be very premature than their white peers [2]. These data on preterm births correlate with disparity in wealth distribution, with African-American families experiencing the lowest 3-year average median income (2003–5) among US racial groups [7]. These data on higher rates of prematurity in women experiencing social disadvantage from poverty and minority status also hold across both developing and developed countries.

Physical outcomes of prematurity

As the survival rates of VPT and EPT infants dramatically increased, so did the awareness of long-term vulnerability of these children on multiple outcomes, including physical and developmental health, behavioral and adaptive well-being, as well as social functioning. Of the neurodevelopmental outcomes, cerebral palsy has received the most attention. In the Swedish Cerebral Palsy registry, rates of cerebral palsy for the birth years 1995–8 were 77 per 1000 for < 28 weeks' gestation, 40 per 1000 for 28–31 weeks' gestation, and 6.7 per 1000 for 32–36 weeks' gestation. These high rates of cerebral palsy across all degrees of preterm birth are substantial, considering that cerebral palsy occurs in only 1.1 per 1000 live births for > 36 weeks' gestation [8]. Although there are many types of cerebral palsy with varying degrees of difficulty with motor control and higher cortical function, the two most common types among preterm infants are spastic diplegia and spastic hemiplegia. These cerebral palsy syndromes affect the motor control of lower extremities or one side of the body, respectively, and increase risks for communicative, perceptual, learning, and attention disorders [9]. However, an examination of these broader outcomes for recent VPT and EPT cohorts at ages 5–8 years has not occurred in large regional or multicenter cohorts.

Another physical disability preterm infants are susceptible to is visual loss or blindness caused by retinopathy of prematurity (ROP). This disorder primarily affects premature infants weighing 1250 g or less and those that are born before 31 weeks of gestation and reaches its severe stages in those who are most immature and medically frail. In a multicenter cryosurgery for ROP study, increased severity of ROP was linked to motor, self-care, and communicative disability at kindergarten entry [10]. Children with severe ROP but with favorable visual acuity had a motor disability rate of 5% compared to 43% of children with severe ROP but with unfavorable visual acuity (i.e., eyesight worse than 6.4 cycles per degree on Teller Cards, includes legal and total blindness). In this cohort, neonatal risk factors for severe disability involving multiple motor, self-care, and communicative domains included severe ROP, gestational age < 27 weeks, birth weight < 750 g, and poverty as reflected by absence of private health insurance. Protective factors that were associated with a significant risk reduction for severe disability were African-American ethnicity. In middle childhood, children with severe ROP had substantial differences in cognitive and educational outcomes [11]. Children with severe ROP and unfavorable visual status had a 3 in 5 chance of intellectual disability (57%) and a 3 in 5 chance of needing special education services. Children with severe ROP and favorable visual skills had a 1 in 5 chance of intellectual disability (22%) and a 1 in 4 chance of needing special education. More than 4 in 5 children with unfavorable vision (84%), but less than half of children with favorable vision (48%), were below grade level in school performance. However, lower SES and minority status were associated with lower grade performance and special education services across both visual outcome groups.

Preterm infants also have a higher risk for rehospitalization. Morris and colleagues examined 1591 surviving infants from the National Institute of Child Health and Human Development (NICHD) Neonatal Network. They reported that 49% of extremely low birth weight (ELBW) infants from this cohort were rehospitalized by 18–22 months' corrected age. Low family income, insurance type, and medical morbidities of chronic lung disease and hydrocephalus increased the odds of rehospitalization [12]. Thus, both SES and medical morbidity interact in increasing risks for suboptimal health outcomes in ELBW survivors.

Cognitive outcomes of prematurity

Preterm infants are often diagnosed with cognitive impairment, whether by using the Bayley, Griffith, or Battelle Scales during the first 3 years of life or the Weschler Scales or similar assessments in middle childhood. Although not all preterm survivors experience intellectual disability (IQ <70), research suggests that degrees of prematurity are linked to adverse cognitive outcome. Studies have suggested that while infants born at 32–36 weeks' gestation have a 1.4-fold increased risk of intellectual disabilities compared to term infants, this figure jumps to a 7-fold risk for infants born before 32 weeks' gestation [13]. Approximately 23–30% of children born at 27–32 weeks' gestation had cognitive scores consistent with intellectual disability, while that figure was 21–42% and 27–44% for children born at 26 weeks' gestation and 24 weeks' gestation, respectively. For children born before 24 weeks' gestation, 27–52% of them had cognitive scores consistent with intellectual disability [9]. Despite these concerns about increased rates of intellectual disability among preterm infants, very few recent studies have systematically examined biomedical and social factors that are associated with intellectual disability once children with severe neurosensory disorders are excluded. Even among those without intellectual disability, there are high rates of cognitive impairments, defined as cognitive scores 1–2 standard deviations below the mean.

Poor cognitive aptitude can lead to poor academic performance, learning disability, and poor executive functioning [14–17]. The average academic performance of children who were born prematurely and/or with low birth weight is reported to be significantly lower than that of their term peers, especially in reading, spelling, and mathematics [16,18–20]. In their 10-year follow-up of infants who were born VPT, Gross and colleagues found that 41% of their study population of preterm infants were performing at grade level as opposed to 70% of the control population of term children. Preterm children were also more likely to receive special education and classroom assistance, and three times as many preterm children were diagnosed with learning disabilities compared to their term peers. However, these differentials were substantially altered by parental social status. Parental marital status and parental educational attainment were significantly related to educational outcome. Among preterm children whose parents were married, 1 in 2 (52%) had grade level performance and 9% received special education services. In contrast, among those children whose mothers were single, only 1 in 5 (18%) had optimal school outcome and 1 in 4 (25%) required special education services. Special education placement increased from 10% of children whose parents finished high school to greater than 25% for children whose parents had not finished high school [19].

Behavioral/emotional outcomes of prematurity

Behavioral and emotional disorders are more prevalent among children born premature compared with their term-birth peers. Meta-analysis on behavioral outcomes by Bhutta and colleagues revealed that children born preterm have a 2.65-fold risk for developing attention deficit hyperactivity disorder (ADHD) during school age [15]. These children are also at high risk for externalizing problems, such as exhibiting aggression and disruptive behavior, which are major obstacles in establishing friendships or other social relationships (e.g., lack of patience in waiting for their turn in group play, such as team sports) [21,22]. In these studies, birth weight, family function, gender, and SES predicted the behavioral adjustment of adolescents who survived ELBW status in the 1980s or the middle childhood behavioral and childhood behavioral and social adjustment of children who survived 23–25 weeks' gestation in the 1990s.

Population data from prospectively followed children at 5, 17, 30, and 42 months in Montreal showed that over half of the children (58%) had modest physical aggression, but learned to use alternative behaviors prior to elementary school [23]. However, 1 in 7 had a trajectory of escalating physical aggression. Most of these children were males (59%), living in low-income households with young mothers who did not complete high school. The neonatal and five month variable that predicted escalating aggression included high family dysfunction and maternal coercive parenting [23]. In a separate Montreal study, Boisjoli et al. examined the 15-year follow-up of a large sample of boys attending inner city kindergarten who had low SES backgrounds. Interventions were multimodal, including social skills training of the child, parent training in effective child rearing using the Oregon Social Learning Center model, and teacher support for high-risk boys. At age 24 years, 2 in 3 of those in the control had dropped out of high school and 1 in 3 had a criminal record. This compared to high school graduation rates of 47% in the non-behavior group and 55% of the intervention group. In addition, 1 in 6 of the inner city adults without childhood aggression had a criminal record, while 1 in 5 (22%) of the intervention group had a criminal record. Thus, access to appropriate parenting supports in conjunction with early childhood and early elementary intervention can reduce trajectories whereby disruptive behavior in males with social disadvantage, increases risk for suboptimal educational, behavioral, and social outcomes [24]. In a similar manner, Reynolds and colleagues demonstrated that combined preschool and after-school intervention substantially reduced grade retention and special education and had a long-term effect on high school completion and avoidance of juvenile arrest in low income, minority Chicago children [25]. To date, access to preschool and educational supports similar to those provided to high-risk children living in social adversity in Montreal or in Chicago has not occurred for VPT/EPT survivors.

Postnatal and social risks

The effects of poverty and low SES on infants born prematurely often increase their vulnerability to suboptimal health, and developmental, behavioral, and educational outcomes. For example, a child born at 25 weeks' gestation with diplegic cerebral palsy will have greater risks for intellectual disability and academic underachievement if they do not access appropriate educational programs. However, if the family's social background inhibits the parents from accessing such assistance (e.g., lack of transportation, frequent moves, other family members with disability), that child's community success and quality of life will be severely reduced.

The degree of poverty and low SES impact on low birth weight and premature infants was dramatically shown in a follow-up study in Edinburgh over 50 years ago [26,27]. In these studies, Drillien found that in families with a high level of SES, an infant's birth weight only had a slight impact on his/her intellectual performance. In families of the lowest level of SES, moderately low birth weight (> 1500–2499 g) had little or no effect on the children's intellectual performance. However, a combination of low SES and very low birth weight (VLBW, < 1500 g) has resulted in a significant decrease in intellectual function. In particular, Drillien noted that the development quotient (DQ) improved with age among VLBW children from high SES families, but declined among VLBW children with low SES background. This study dramatically illustrates that biological factors alone do not determine a child's long-term outcome.

There are several possible reasons to explain these differences. First is the familial factor, since it has been demonstrated that parents who have cognitive and educational disability have an increased likelihood of having children who have cognitive and education challenges [28]. However, recent analysis using data on monozygotic and dizygotic twins in the collaborative perinatal project who were raised with or without poverty exposure demonstrated that the contribution to cognitive outcomes as measured by Weschler IQ at age 7 years is related to shared environment, not genetics, in children with low SES background [29]. In addition, this situation is reversed in affluent families.

Another important factor is the adverse effects of poverty on access to quality schools. Among both VLBW and ELBW survivors, disproportionate numbers live in communities with high rates of school drop-outs and poorly performing schools. This will result in barriers to accessing quality early and middle childhood educational experiences. The combination of low birth weight and preterm birth with social and family distress has shown to increase adverse developmental outcomes. In an 8- to 10-year follow-up study of infants who were the sickest, tiniest, and with the most medical complications in the newborn period, Msall and colleagues found that not only favorable vision and functional motor status at kindergarten entry were associated with significantly lower rates of special education and below-grade-level educational achievement, but higher SES was also associated with positive academic and developmental outcomes. Factors that were strongly associated with increased risk for special education services included minority status, poverty, lack of access to a car, and Supplemental Social Security income because of disability and poverty [11].

The adverse effects of economic and social disadvantages on child development have been well documented, with several studies suggesting that suboptimal outcomes of poverty and SES on child development have the most impact during preschool years [30,31]. Between the ages of 18 months and 5 years, US children in poverty experience fragmented medical, developmental, and educational supports. Postnatal outcomes of social risk include lead poisoning due to older and poor-quality housing, child abuse and neglect, and poor nutrition and lack of access to medical care. These in turn lead to increased rates of accidental injuries, visual impairment due to untreated strabismus, undetected hearing problems, mild intellectual disability due to limited learning experiences, and emotional impairments.

Bradley and Corwyn have noted that indicators of SES were significantly related to cognitive outcomes in both infancy and middle childhood. Evidence suggests a particularly strong relationship between SES and verbal skills, as well as developmental learning experiences [31]. Children from low SES background disproportionately lack access to cognitively stimulating resources and activities such as books, audio tapes, educational toys, visits to the museum, and parent–child learning activities [4,31,32]. A study by Hart and Risley further demonstrated the gaps in interaction and communication between parents and their children from different SES backgrounds [33]. In their analysis of verbal communication between parents and children, Hart and Risley found out that children in middle-class families receive verbal input exceeding 30 000 000 words by age 3 with 83% being educational and positive in content, while 17% were negative and disciplinary in content. In contrast, children from poor minority families received inputs of 10 000 000 words by age 3 with 29% being educational and positive in content while 71% were negative and disciplinary. These differences resulted in less verbal abilities, lower IQ, more behavioral difficulties, and poorer educational achievement throughout childhood for children from low SES background [33]. In a more recent study by Bradley and colleagues, during infancy and early childhood non-poor mothers were shown to be twice as likely to read to their children times a week compared to poor mothers. More well-to-do mothers were more likely than their poor counterparts to speak to their children or respond to their children verbally [32]. Thus, VPT and EPT children living in households with stressors of poverty and social capital experience missed opportunities for experiencing rich verbal and social modeling experience.

In their prospective follow-up study of neonatal intensive care unit (NICU) graduates, Resnick and colleagues attempted to measure the effects of birth weight, medical conditions, and SES on educational disabilities from a Florida state-wide sample of over 24 000 children [34]. The results suggested a correlation between birth weight and special education services. Among children who survived birth weights of 500–750 g, 40% required special education, compared with 24% of those who weighed ≥ 2500 g at birth. Mild intellectual disability (IQ 55–69) was most related to male gender, black race, and mother's educational

achievement of less than high school completion. Specific learning disabilities, emotional handicaps, and speech and language impairment were strongly tied to sociodemographic factors, especially lower family income. Of all the outcomes, only physical impairment (i.e., cerebral palsy), sensory impairment (i.e., blindness, deafness), and profound mental handicap (i.e., IQ < 30) were associated with biomedical factors [34]. In a subsequent evaluation of the links between regional neonatal databases and educational databases for public school students in Florida, Roth and colleagues estimated that total excess cost to the state associated with risk factors of any degrees of low birth weight status, congenital anomaly, complications of labor, no prenatal care, poverty at birth, and low levels of maternal education (< high school) to be around US$160 million per year. Of these risk factors, combination of poverty at birth (US$80.8 million) and low maternal education (US$43.0 million) accounted for over three quarters of the total excess costs for kindergarten costs. With the reduction of public funding in recent years and lack of human and other resources available to medical and educational professionals, the importance of prenatal and early childhood education as preventive interventions for late prematurity and moderate prematurity, as well as comprehensive programs for VPT and EPT children experiencing social adversity is critical [35].

Neighborhood conditions (e.g., accessibility to day care, museums, library, playgrounds, healthcare facilities, and after-school programs) also have a large affect on child development. Poor or low SES neighborhoods are also often characterized by social disorganization such as poor-quality schools, crime, unemployed adults, and high dropout rates from high school [36]. This often exposes children to both domestic and community violence, which adversely impact social and emotional developmental pathways. It is, therefore, not surprising to see that children growing up in neighborhoods of low SES have an increased rate of both suboptimal health and behavioral status compared to children from high SES and middle-class families [37,38].

Low SES is considered to impact on behavioral problems and disorders in children and adolescents with increased rates of ADHD, disruptive behavior, depression, and anxiety [30]. Considering also that behavioral and emotional disorders occur at high rates for school-age children who survived VPT/EPT birth [15,21,22,39], the additive environmental vulnerability for these children is especially high. In settings of limited access to behavioral intervention and educational supports, these disorders have a tendency to adversely impact on learning and educational attainment.

Protective factors within the individual, family, and community

There are many personal, familial, and neighborhood challenges that face VPT/EPT and low birth weight survivors from low SES. However, there are several protective factors that can work towards these children's advantage to enhance their chances for successful adolescent and adult outcomes [40,41].

Personal resilience can be a defining characteristic of a child, who, under adverse circumstances, can withstand the impact of environmental adversity. These environmental risks include economic hardships, born to a single-parent who has not finished high school, experiencing parental mental illness or parental substance abuse, exposure to violence, neglect, teenage motherhood, perinatal complications, death of a parent, and break-up of parents' marriages [40,41]. In early childhood, resilient children are often described as active, alert, socially responsive, and well regulated. They are also easy to soothe, affectionate, cuddly, and good-natured with very few feeding or sleeping problems. In preschool years, they become more cheerful and self-confident compared to their less resilient peers experiencing adversity. By middle childhood, the characteristics of resilient children include well-developed problem-solving and communication skills, social skills, and inner directed achievement motivation. These skills help children concentrate on school work amid their suboptimal home life and engage in activities or hobbies that give them a sense of mastery and increase their self-esteem. As adolescents, youths that coped successfully with their suboptimal environment had higher sense of self-worth and internal locus of control, and were more responsible, independent, and socially mature than their peers who did not [41].

Protective factors can come from the child's environment, such as within the family and the community, that help shield the child from detrimental effects of poverty and low SES. One common trait among children who are identified as resilient is the close bond they develop with a caregiver that provides them with nurturing, responsive structure, and attention during the first few years of their life. These caregivers include not only their mothers, but alternative caregivers such as grandparents and older siblings [41]. Such relationships not only provide healthy attachment and security, but also safety and structured opportunities for exploration. These reciprocal interactions help infants regulate their emotions and offer a smoother transition to learning, communication, and social skills [40].

Other protective factors from the community include religion (promoting a sense of cohesiveness and stability, as well as providing a moral guide), friends (enhancing socialization skills and providing emotional support), school (providing rules, structure, organization, and responsibility), and a teacher or a mentor (providing academic advice and being a positive role model).

Although all is not lost for children growing up in poverty, failure to have supports that address behavioral difficulties and promote positive experiences can have multiple adverse impacts on educational and social successes. With proper care and assistance, children experiencing adversity can grow up to be healthy adults, responsible parents, and positive members of our community. However, in order to understand the factors that promote resiliency, it is important to examine lessons learned from previous studies of effective early intervention for children growing up with or without biological risk who experienced domestic and social adversity.

Learning from previous studies

If one considers that there are a large number of children in the US experiencing combinations of serious indicators of social disadvantage in conjunction with biological risks, then one begins to understand that at a population level, it is critically important to implement community lessons from model intervention programs. Although the additive effects of biomedical and social risks can substantially increase suboptimal outcomes and decrease positive development, these adverse effects can be reduced or minimized with early preventive educational and social interventions. This is especially important, considering that in many cases biomedical risks caused by prenatal effect of poverty and low SES (such as prematurity and low birth weight) can be worsened by conditions of suboptimal postnatal social and familial environments. We will highlight lessons learned from longitudinal studies of children identified in the nursery with biomedical risks, and the importance of human capital in early childhood with respect to positive adult outcomes.

Lesson 1: The Abecedarian Project

Established in 1972, the Abecedarian Project took place at the Frank Porter Graham Child Development Center in North Carolina. Their target population was children born between 1972 and 1977 who were considered to be at high risk for developmental impairment. These empirical risk factors included parental education status, family income, father's involvement and work record, maternal or paternal cognitive disability, household composition, and ties with extended family members. The cohorts were randomly assigned to either an intensive developmental preschool educational curriculum (n = 57) or basic care (n = 54) group. The overall characteristic of the cohort included being born in poverty to mothers who had not graduated from high school (100%), single parenthood (75%), and African-American ethnicity (99%). It should be noted that information on the children's background, ethnicity, and parental educational achievement are readily available during prenatal visits and in the newborn nursery [42].

Children from both intervention and control groups received basic care, free nutritional supplements, social services, and health care. However, the children from the intervention group received an intense, high-quality early child education curriculum from the first months of life until the age of 5. The program consisted of cognitive and fine motor developmental activities, structured learning for social and adaptive skills, and games to promote communicative and exploration skills. After age 3 the program shifted the precursors of activities that create the foundation for learning to reading, calculating numbers, remembering songs, playing music, and understanding cause and effect. The children learned in a small group setting, and the day care was for 6–8 hours a day, 50 weeks per year. Progress for both groups (intervention and contrast) was monitored at ages 3, 4, 5, 6.5, 8, 12, 15, and 21 years [43].

The difference between two groups was apparent as early as 18 months of age. At every age of assessment from 18–54 months, the intervention group scored significantly higher on measures of cognitive development than the basic care group. These differences carried over to academic achievement and grade level success into middle childhood and adolescence: children in the intervention group had significantly higher scores on reading and math tests from age 8 through 21; less than 1 in 3 (31%) of the intervention group subjects had been retained at the age 15, compared with more than 1 in 2 (54.5%) of the basic care group; 1 in 4 (25%) of the intervention group had been placed in special education, compared with almost 1 in 2 (48%) of the basic group. At age 21, more than 1 in 3 (35%) of the treatment group had graduated from or were enrolled in a four-year college course, compared with 1 in 7 (14%) of the control group.

Another key component of the Abecedarian Project was the fact that half of each group was randomly assigned to an additional intervention program lasting from kindergarten to second grade upon school entry. This resulted in four groups: (1) birth–second grade intervention group, (2) early intervention only (birth–5 years), (3) late intervention only (kindergarten–second grade), and (4) neither early nor late intervention. The continuing intervention program consisted of educational support for children in school and at home, learning supports over the summer, and teaching parents how to enhance their children's education at home. The outcomes at the end of second grade showed that children who attended both early and continuing intervention had the highest scores on measures of intelligence and standardized achievement tests in reading and math. The early intervention only group also performed better than the late intervention group [44].

The Abecedarian Project thus demonstrated that a comprehensive early developmental intervention not only benefits the children in the short term (i.e., through second grade), but that its positive effects last throughout young adulthood. It is important to realize that this comprehensive program for mothers with limited education who were single minority parents living in poverty is not currently accessible for the majority of VLBW and ELBW survivors.

Lesson 2: The Kauai Longitudinal Study

Half a century ago, a team of medical and social scientists examined biological and socio-environmental factors in 700 Asian and Polynesian children born in 1955 on the Island of Kauai in Hawaii. The children were monitored from prenatal period (as early as fourth week of pregnancy) through middle childhood and then reassessed at age 18, 32, and then at middle age. Approximately half of the children lived in poverty and were raised by parents who had not graduated from high school. Close to 1 in 3 of the surviving children experienced moderate to severe degrees of perinatal stress, or grew up in chronic poverty or experienced family dysfunction. Ten percent of the children were exposed to moderate prenatal stress, including preeclampsia, renal insufficiency, poorly controlled diabetes, partial placental abruption, breech presentation, mid or high forceps delivery, or requiring supplemental oxygen for less than 5 minutes. Three percent experienced eclampsia, renal or diabetic coma, complete abruption, emergency Cesarian section, and greater than 5 minutes of oxygen supplementation [45,46].

By the time the children reached age 2 years, the effect of socio-environmental factors was beginning to show: the rate of early cognitive disability (Cattell, DQ < 70) among children from impoverished backgrounds was significantly higher. Later, two thirds of the children at risk showed signs of learning and behavioral problems. One in 6 children had a special healthcare need requiring ongoing medical, developmental, or custodial care. One in 5 developed sensory-learning and behavioral disorder. However, at age 10 years, ten times more children had problems attributed to their environment rather than the effects of perinatal biological stressors. This finding led to the conclusion that adverse outcomes due to socio-environmental factors have a more severe impact on developmental and behavioral outcomes. In fact, once severe neurodevelopmental disability is excluded, children with biological risk experience suboptimal educational and behavioral outcome only if there is concurrent caregiving adversity. By age 18 years, 15% had problems with the police and 10% required mental health service. A follow-up at age 32 years revealed variables that contributed significantly to maladaptive adult outcomes (e.g., crime) included being raised by a single mother, prolonged disruption of family life (e.g., unemployment of primary caregiver, parental illness, etc.), and prolonged absence of mother.

It is important to note that there were 72 children in the study who developed normally, despite being exposed to high rates of adversity (perinatal complications, parental psychopathology, family instability, and chronic poverty). These "resilient" children, however, also had other protective biomedical and environmental factors such as positive temperament, positive parental attitudes, low levels of family conflicts, reduced life stress, access to counseling and remedial services, and smaller family size. Other protective factors included emotional ties with parent substitutes (grandparents, older siblings, etc.) and an external support system such as church, youth groups, or school. In addition, these resilient children shared the following characteristics: (1) they were liked by their peers as well as adults; (2) cognitively they were predominately reflective, not impulsive; (3) they demonstrated internal locus of control; and (4) they used flexible coping strategies in overcoming adversities [41]. These elements provided the children with stability and competence in their lives and, in most cases, were carried into adulthood. Personal competence and determination, support from a spouse or mate, and reliance on religion were some of the shared qualities among resilient individuals in their early 30s.

The Kauai Longitudinal Study demonstrates that positive socio-environmental factors have both short-term and long-term benefits that outweigh the adversity of biomedical factors and poverty. Again, in examining neonatal outcomes, supports for enhancing children's access to these protective factors has not routinely occurred in VPT and EPT populations.

Lesson 3: The Infant Health and Development Program (IHDP) Study

The Infant Health and Development Program (IHDP) was a multicenter study designed to evaluate the effects of early intervention on health and developmental outcomes of low birth weight survivors. Almost 1000 (n = 985) premature low birth weight infants from Boston, Dallas, Little Rock, Miami, New Haven, New York, Philadelphia, and Seattle were recruited between the years 1985 and 1986. The methodology and outcomes of this Program are described in detail in Chapter 18. In brief, 377 infants were randomly assigned to the intervention group while 608 were assigned to the follow-up only group (i.e., control group). Throughout the duration of the program, children from both groups were given medical care and received a series of developmental and social assessments [47].

The IHDP intervention group received quality home visits and center-based early educational interventions, addressing cognitive, fine motor, language, gross motor, social, and self-help skills, which lasted until the children were 3 years of age.

The assessment of cognitive and behavioral outcomes and health of the participants at 3 years of age showed that children in the intervention group had significantly higher scores on the intelligence test and receptive vocabulary test than the control group. The intervention group also scored lower on reported behavior problems than the control group. In addition, the program's greatest impact occurred among children whose mothers had low IQs. Approximately 40% of children from the control group whose mothers had cognitive disability had intellectual disability at age 3 compared with 15% of intervention children whose mothers also had cognitive disability.

Overall, the short-term benefit of the IHDP intervention was that psychosocial mental retardation in early childhood could be prevented among children at double jeopardy because of prematurity and parents with limited income and education. However, the sustainability of these results, especially for VLBW and ELBW survivors was not demonstrated at age 5, 8, and 18 years. Whether this reflects additional adversity that both groups experienced in contemporary urban schools or the need for more extensive supports between ages 5 and 8 years similar to the Abecedarian study or under- resourced communities throughout childhood and adolescence is not known.

Lesson 4: Growth and developmental outcomes of Dutch children born very preterm and very low birth weight

A nationwide collaborative follow-up study of Dutch infants born very premature and/or with VLBW was done by Hille and colleagues during 1983. A total of 1338 infants were enrolled in the study and were followed up at age 2, 5, and 9 years. The children were divided into the following four groups: (1) children in the mainstream education at the appropriate level for age without special assistance; (2) children in mainstream education at the appropriate level for age but with special assistance; (3) children one or more grades below the appropriate level for age, with or without special assistance; and (4) children in special education [48].

At age 5 years, 12% of the children were in special education, mainly in schools for children with physical (i.e., cerebral palsy) and/or intellectual disability. At 9 years of age, approximately 19% of children were receiving special education, with approximately half (47%) of them having already been in special education since age 5 years. Of the children who were in mainstream education, 80% were not performing up to their age-appropriate academic standards: 32% were in a grade below the level appropriate for their age and 38% were receiving special assistance in school [48].

Several risk factors were seen to be associated with school outcome, namely, gestational age, birth weight, gender, and SES. Over half of the VPT survivors in this study (58%) and approximately 66% of ELBW survivors were in a grade below their appropriate level or in special education. Twice as many boys as girls were in special education, and children from low SES were five times more likely to be in special education (35%) compared with their high SES counterparts (7%). In fact, both low SES and male gender disproportionately required special education placement. Less than 1 in 5 (19%) of low SES survivors were at grade level compared with 3 in 5 (57%) of their high SES peers. Socioeconomic status and gender more substantially contributed to suboptimal school outcomes rather than degree of VPT/EPT or ELBW/VLBW [48].

The same cohort was followed up at age 19 years through standard assessments using examinations and questionnaires. The outcomes echoed those of the results found 10 years prior: twice as many young adults who survived VPT birth and/or VLBW had poor education achievement compared to the general Dutch population, and three times as many were neither employed nor in school. Approximately one third (31.7%) of the study population had moderate to severe problems in functioning, activities, and participation. The researchers also found out that parental education level had a large impact on these young adults' outcome. Among VPT birth and VLBW survivors: the lower the parental education level, the higher the proportion of problems in education, functioning, participation, or cognitive ability. Approximately 1 in 6 of adult survivors of VPT whose parents had not finished high school had severe problems in cognitive and neurosensory functioning. Among those children whose parents had completed college, 1 in 14 had severe cognitive and neurosensory dysfunction at age 19. These disparities were more dramatic in overall activities and participation. Only 1 in 8 of 19-year-old VLBW survivors with high SES had moderate to severe problems in activities or participation; 2 in 5 of the youths whose parents had not completed high school had moderate to severe problems in activities and participation [49].

Effective interventions

Based on cumulative research in child development, early intervention, educational achievement, school readiness, and adolescent outcomes, several guidelines and essential factors that yield the developmental supports that address social adversity in young children start to emerge. What components are necessary in reducing risk, increasing competencies, and promoting self-efficacy?

Firstly, as parents are children's first teachers, the role of caregiver and the child's attachment to his/

her caregiver have a very large impact on the child's well-being, especially among young or isolated parents. Not only should fostering strong interactions and healthy relationships between parent and child (or caregiver and child) be an integral part of the intervention, but also promoting parental stress management and better parenting styles (e.g., consistent, warm, and firm instead of impulsive, inconsistent, and assertive methods of controlling through violence) should be strongly encouraged [40]. Some assert that home-based interventions are the optimal way to influence parents of children in poverty and those who have children with disability. Studies of US home-based interventions with parents of infants and young children of low income/low SES illustrate benefits to infants and young children. Landry and colleagues trained facilitators and community mentors to address responsive parenting: behavioral support, language stimulation, and support of attentional skills. Mothers demonstrated more responsive behaviors if they stayed in the program, while children showed change in social and emotional skills with greater gains in VLBW children [50].

Secondly, a successful program should focus on strengthening both children's cognitive skills as well as socioemotional skills. As we have seen in this chapter, behavioral and emotional health is just as important as cognitive performance for classroom success. By ensuring that both these elements are present then there is increased likelihood of success throughout middle childhood and adolescence.

Thirdly, intervention programs should encourage children's pro-social behavior and stimulate their curiosity. These interventions strongly decrease rates of aggression and disruptive behaviors which jeopardize children's classroom, educational, and social success.

Fourthly, in order to create the best possible opportunities for learning, the teachers should be well trained in the areas of child development that promote literacy, social skills, and problem-solving, as well as in dealing with families under stress resulting from suboptimal living conditions. In this way, the additive effects of the Abecedarian and Chicago projects might be extended.

Fifthly, to ensure the best possible outcome, intervention programs must start early and need to be intensive, especially throughout early childhood and preschool years. Although a 4-year-old child enrolled in a 2–3 hours a day program is better than being enrolled in no early intervention at all, the same child could have been better prepared for school cognitively, developmentally, socially, and behaviorally if he/she had a more comprehensive, structured full day intervention program since the age of 2 years.

Sixthly, the focus of the programs should be prevention, not remedial education or crisis special education. As we have seen from the Abecedarian Project, the effects of suboptimal learning environments can be long lasting and harder to mend. The fact that remedial intervention programs at school age have proven less effective than model early intervention programs indicates that once the damage of adverse environmental factors has been done, it is very difficult to completely reverse those negative effects. Heckman, in his meta-analysis, examined how early family environments are major predictors of both cognitive and non-cognitive abilities in children. Environments that fail to stimulate and cultivate these skills in children place them at a significant disadvantage from an early age that only increases through their middle childhood and adolescence [51].

Lastly, successful intervention programs should ensure the continuity of educational supports, even after the designated preschool program is finished. Children continue to require the experiences and supports that promote learning, academic, and social competencies. Since cognitive, linguistic, social, and emotional competencies are interdependent, it is important to highlight both basic and advanced skills. These abilities are formed in a predictable sequence of developmental opportunities throughout childhood and adolescence.

Conclusion

Both VPT/EPT infants born into poverty and low SES will have numerous hurdles to go through in terms of their physical, developmental, and emotional health. Unlike their middle-class or affluent counterparts, these children will have less access to medical care, parent–child interactions, quality early education, and extracurricular activities. Although potentially detrimental to a child's future, the status of his/her gestation age and birth weight are rarely the major determining factors when long-term educational, social, and behavioral outcomes are examined. In this chapter we have examined several research studies that emphasized the importance of environmental factors, which can either aggravate or moderate neonatal risks caused by VPT or EPT birth. With so much to lose while living under suboptimal conditions, it is of critical importance that both health and educational professionals create systems for enhancing access to early childhood learning experiences, parenting supports, and quality preschool education services. These will insure that VLBW and ELBW survivors do not miss out on the critical experiences that lead to the developmental and behavioral competencies essential to long-term adult success.

Acknowledgments

This work was supported by National Institute of Health (NIH) Grant NICHD RO3 37627. Additional support was provided by the Grant Healthcare Foundation, "Passport to Developmental Health." We would also like to thank Angela Berger, Susan Troyke, Penny Huddlestone, Colette Gatling, and Heather Reeves for their commitments and overtime to children at highest risk.

References

1. Hamilton BE, Miniño AM, Martin JA, *et al.* Annual summary of vital statistics: 2005. *Pediatrics.* 2007; **119**(2): 345–60.

2. March of Dimes. *Data Book for Policy Makers. Maternal, Infant, and Child Health in the United States*; 2005.

3. Holzmann R, Jorgensen S. *Social Risk Management: A New Conceptual Framework for Social Protection, and Beyond*. Washington, DC: The World Bank; 2000.

4. Huston, AC (ed.). *Children in Poverty: Child Development and Public Policy*. Cambridge, UK: Cambridge University Press; 1991.

5. Hans SL. Demographic and psychosocial characteristics of substance-abusing pregnant women. *Clin Perinatol* 1999; **26**(1): 55–74.

6. Weitzman M, Byrd RS, Aligne CA, Moss M. The effects of tobacco exposure on children's behavioral and cognitive functioning: implications for clinical and public health policy and future research. *Neurotoxicol Teratol* 2002; **24**(3): 397–406.

7. US Census Bureau. *Income, Poverty, and Health Insurance Coverage in the United States: 2005. 2006.* Available from: www.census.gov/prod/2006pubs/p60–231.pdf. Accessed August 2009.

8. Himmelmann K, Hagberg G, Beckung E, Hagberg B, Uvebrant P. The changing panorama of cerebral palsy in Sweden. IX. Prevalence and origin in the birth-year period 1995–1998. *Acta Paediatr* 2005; **94**(3): 287–94.

9. Allen MC. Prematurity. In: Accardo PJ, ed. *Capute & Accardo's Neurodevelopmental Disabilities in Infancy and Childhood,* Vol. 1, *Neurodevelopment Diagnosis and Treatment*, 3rd edn. Baltimore, MD: Paul H Brookes Publishing Co. 2008; 199–226.

10. Msall ME, Phelps DL, DiGaudio KM, *et al.* Severity of neonatal retinopathy of prematurity is predictive of neurodevelopmental functional outcome at age 5.5 years. Behalf of the Cryotherapy for Retinopathy of Prematurity Cooperative Group. *Pediatrics* 2000; **106**(5): 998–1005.

11. Msall ME, Phelps DL, Hardy RJ, *et al.*; Cryotherapy for Retinopathy of Prematurity Cooperative Group. Educational and social competencies at 8 years in children with threshold retinopathy of prematurity in the CRYO-ROP multicenter study. *Pediatrics* 2004; **113**(4): 790–9.

12. Morris BH, Gard CC, Kennedy K, NICHD Network. Rehospitalization of extremely low birth weight (ELBW) infants: are there racial/ethnic disparities? *J Perinatol* 2005; **25**(10): 656–63.

13. Stromme P, Hagberg G. Aetiology in severe and mild mental retardation: a population study of Norwegian children. *Dev Med Child Neurol* 2000; **42**(2): 76–86.

14. Hack M, Taylor HG, Klein N, Mercuri-Minich N. Functional limitations and special health care needs of 10- to 14-year-old children weighing less than 750 grams at birth. *Pediatrics* 2004; **106**(3): 554–60.

15. Bhutta AT, Cleves MA, Casey PH, Cradock MM, Anand KJ. Cognitive and behavioral outcomes of school-aged children who were born preterm: a meta-analysis. *JAMA* 2002; **288**(6): 728–37.

16. Grunau RE, Whitfield MF, Fay TB. Psychosocial and academic characteristics of extremely low birth weight (≤800 g) adolescents who are free of major impairment compared with term-born control subjects. *Pediatrics* 2004; **114**(6): e725–32.

17. Gibson AT. Outcome following preterm birth. *Best Pract Res Clin Obstet Gynaecol* 2007; **21**(5): 869–82.

18. Salt A, Redshaw M. Neurodevelopmental follow-up after preterm birth: follow up after two years. *Early Hum Dev* 2006; **82**(3): 185–97.

19. Gross SJ, Mettelman BB, Dye TD, Slagle TA. Impact of family structure and stability on academic outcome in preterm children at 10 years of age. *J Pediatr* 2001; **138**(2): 169–75

20. Hagen EW, Palta M, Albanese A, Sadek-Badawi M. School achievement in a regional cohort of children born very low birthweight. *J Dev Behav Pediatr* 2006; **27**(2): 112–20.

21. Saigal S, Pinelli J, Hoult L, Kim MM, Boyle M. Psychopathology and social competencies of adolescents who were extremely low birth weight. *Pediatrics* 2003; **111**(5 Pt 1): 969–75.

22. Farooqi A, Hagglof B, Sedin G, Gothefors L, Serenius F. Mental health and social competencies of 10- to

12-year-old children born at 23 to 25 weeks of gestation in the 1990s: a Swedish national prospective follow-up study. *Pediatrics* 2007; **120**(1): 118–33.

23. Tremblay RE, Nagin DS, Séguin JR, *et al.* Physical aggression during early childhood: trajectories and predictors. *Pediatrics* 2004; **114**(1): e43–50.

24. Boisjoli R, Vitaro F, Lacourse E, Barker ED, Tremblay RE. Impact and clinical significance of a preventive intervention for disruptive boys: 15-year follow-up. *Br J Psychiatry* 2007; **191**: 415–19.

25. Reynolds AJ, Temple JA, Robertson DL, Mann EA. Long-term effects of an early childhood intervention on educational achievement and juvenile arrest: a 15-year follow-up of low-income children in public schools. *JAMA* 2001; **285**(18): 2339–46. Erratum in: *JAMA* 2001; **286**(9): 1026.

26. Drillien CM. A longitudinal study of the growth and development of prematurely and maturely born children. II. Physical development. *Arch Dis Child* 1958; **33**(171): 423–31.

27. Drillien CM, Thomson AJ, Burgoyne K. Low-birthweight children at early school-age: a longitudinal study. *Dev Med Child Neurol* 1980; **22**(1): 26–47.

28. Zigler E, Hodapp RM. *Understanding Mental Retardation*. New York, NY: Cambridge University Press; 1986.

29. Turkheimer E, Haley A, Waldron M, D'Onofrio B, Gottesman II. Socioeconomic status modifies heritability of IQ in young children. *Psychol Sci* 2003; **14**(6): 623–8.

30. Brooks-Gunn J, Duncan GJ. The effects of poverty on children. *Future Child* 1997; **7**(2): 55–71.

31. Bradley RH, Corwyn RF. Socioeconomic status and child development. *Annu Rev Psychol* 2002; **53**: 371–99.

32. Bradley RH, Corwyn RF, McAdoo HP, Coll CG. The home environments of children in the United States Part I: variations by age, ethnicity, and poverty status. *Child Dev* 2001; **72**(6): 1844–67.

33. Hart B, Risley TR. In vivo language intervention: unanticipated general effects. *J Appl Behav Anal* 1980; **13**(3): 407–32.

34. Resnick MB, Gueorguieva RV, Carter RL, *et al.* The impact of low birth weight, perinatal conditions, and sociodemographic factors on educational outcome in kindergarten. *Pediatrics* 1999; **104**(6): e74.

35. Roth J, Figlio DN, Chen Y, *et al.* Maternal and infant factors associated with excess kindergarten costs. *Pediatrics* 2004; **114**(3): 720–8.

36. Hertzman C, Wiens M. Child development and long-term outcomes: a population health perspective and summary of successful interventions. *Soc Sci Med* 1996; **43**(7): 1083–95.

37. Msall ME, Avery RC, Msall ER, Hogan DP. Distressed neighborhoods and child disability rates: analyses of 157,000 school-age children. *Dev Med Child Neurol* 2007; **49**(11): 814–17.

38. Palfrey JS. *Child Health in America. Making a Difference Through Advocacy*. Baltimore, Maryland: The Johns Hopkins University Press; 2006.

39. Gardner F, Johnson A, Yudkin P, *et al.* Extremely Low Gestational Age Steering Group: behavioral and emotional adjustment of teenagers in mainstream school who were born before 29 weeks' gestation. *Pediatrics* 2004; **114**(3): 676–82.

40. Masten AS, Coatsworth JD. The development of competence in favorable and unfavorable environments. Lessons from research on successful children. *Am Psychol* 1998; **53**(2): 205–20.

41. Werner EE. Protective factors and individual resilience In: Shonkoff JP, Meisels SJ, eds. *Handbook of Early Childhood Intervention*, 2nd edn. New York, NY: Cambridge University Press. 2000; 115–34.

42. Bryant D, Maxwell K. The effectiveness of early intervention for disadvantaged children In: Guralnick MJ, ed. *The Effectiveness of Early Intervention*. Baltimore, MD: Paul Brookes Publishing Co. 1997; 23–46.

43. Campbell F A, Pungello EP, Miller-Johnson S, Burchinal M, Ramey CT. The development of cognitive and academic abilities: growth curves from an early childhood educational experiment. *Dev Psychol* 2001; **37**(2): 231–42.

44. Ramey CT, Campbell FA, Burchinal M, *et al.* Persistent effects of early intervention on high-risk children and their mothers. *Appl Dev Sci* 2000; **4**: 2–14.

45. Lester BM, Miller-Loncar CL. Biology versus environment in the extremely low-birth weight infant. *Clin Perinatol* 2000; **27**(2): 461–81

46. Werner EE, Smith RS. *Overcoming the Odds: High Risk Children from Birth to Adulthood*. Ithaca, NY: Cornell University Press; 1992.

47. Gross T, Spiker D, Haynes C. (eds.) *Helping Low Birth Weight, Premature Babies. The Infant Health and Development Program*. Stanford, California: Stanford University Press; 1997.

48. Hille ET, den Ouden AL, Bauer L, *et al.* School performance at nine years of age in very premature and very low birth weight infants: perinatal risk factors and predictors at five years of age. Collaborative Project on Preterm and Small for Gestational Age (POPS) Infants in The Netherlands. *J Pediatr* 1994; **125**(3): 426–34.

49. Hille ET, Weisglas-Kuperus N, van Goudoever JB, *et al.*; Dutch Collaborative Pops 19 Study Group. Functional outcomes and participation in young adulthood for very preterm and very low birth weight infants: the Dutch Project on Preterm and Small for Gestational Age Infants at 19 years of age. *Pediatrics* 2007; **120**(3): e587–95.

50. Landry SH, Smith KE, Swank PR. Responsive parenting: establishing early foundations for social, communication, and independent problem-solving skills. *Dev Psychol* 2006; **42**(4): 627–42.

51. Heckman JJ. Skill formation and the economics of investing in disadvantaged children. *Science* 2006; **312**(5782): 1900–2.

Cognitive and behavioral interventions

Marie C. McCormick and Beth McManus

Introduction

With the success of neonatal intensive care in increasing the survival of very premature infants [1] came the recognition that some developmental intervention was needed for infants whose hospital stays might last several months until they were mature enough to go home [2]. Early observations revealed both the nature of the behavioral and physiological reactions of very preterm infants to their surroundings, and the characteristics of neonatal intensive care as it impinged on these immature infants. In particular, the milieu of the hospital vastly contrasted with the intrauterine environment, and the neurologically immature neonate was ill-prepared to contend with these physiological, motoric, and interactional demands [2]. As a response to these observations, investigators and caregivers began to develop modifications of their approaches to premature infants in the hospital and to consider post-discharge interventions to foster neurodevelopment. In this chapter, we will consider what is known about these cognitive and behavioral interventions and their effectiveness in the short and long term.

Theoretical perspectives

From a variety of theoretical perspectives, it would be anticipated that preterm infants might experience difficulty in achieving developmental milestones compared to their full-term peers. *Neural-maturational theory* posits that behavior results from an unfolding of predetermined brain function. That is, development occurs predictably as a result of integration of primitive reflexes, which allow for the initiation of higher-level cognitive function [3,4]. From this perspective, preterm infants would be expected to experience later neurodevelopmental difficulties because adverse perinatal and neonatal events such as intraventricular bleeding and damage to the white matter (periventricular

leukomalacia) disrupt neural maturation [5]. Indeed, the data are supportive, at least in part, of a neuromaturational approach. Risk of neurological insult in preterm infants is negatively associated with gestational age. The rate of cerebral palsy ranges from 1.4/1000 in infants greater than 36 weeks to 80/1000 in infants less than 28 weeks [5]. Furthermore, frank neurological damage, that is, grade 3 or 4 intraventricular hemorrhage, is associated with a threefold increased risk of cerebral palsy and a 60% increased risk of poor cognitive skills [5].

However, even in the absence of overt biological damage, experience suggests that the neural maturation of preterm infants may be compromised compared to full-term infants. Although preterm infants are typically discharged from the hospital at or close to when they would have been born, the behavior of preterm infants differs substantially from their full-term counterparts [5] with difficulties with organized state transition, oral feeding skills, and motor skills. Thus, a broader theoretical framework is needed to explain the disparity between diagnosed biological damage and clinical presentation. That is, some children with neonatal injury will develop within typical ranges while others with no brain damage will present with persistent neurological difficulties.

Neuromaturational approaches tend to consider development to be a fixed result of physical insults with virtually no role for remediation. However, recent evidence regarding early brain development of young children suggests that creation and refinement of synaptic connections in the developing brain is quite sensitive to the environment, that is, opportunities for cognitive, social, and motor development [2]. These observations reinforce the importance of experience as suggested by cognitive theories, which recognize the influence of individual thought processes in the emergence of new behavior. Both Behavioral and

Neurodevelopmental Outcomes of Preterm Birth, ed. Chiara Nosarti, Robin M. Murray, and Maureen Hack. Published by Cambridge University Press. © Cambridge University Press 2010.

Piagetian Theories argue that behavior is a result of not only genetic makeup and biologic potential, but also an individual's reaction – perceptions and memory – of his/her environment [6]. Specifically, skills are gained based upon the integration of previous experiences with an environmental stimuli and operant conditioning, where consequences manipulate behavior. Thus, development is a series of feedback processes where the individual interacts constantly with environment continuously adjusting to its demands and challenges. Premature infants might have difficulty in initiating and responding in such a reciprocal way, in part, due to their neuromaturational immaturity. For example, delayed mobility, immature self-soothing skills, and deficits in age-appropriate social interaction skills may affect an infant's capacity to explore his/her environment in order to create the cognitive impressions necessary for learning [6]. However, as noted below, other factors (namely broader social forces) may impede this relationship between cognitive processing and the environment as they relate to the neurodevelopment of preterm infants and, therefore, a more comprehensive theoretical model is warranted.

A final perspective on the development of preterm infants can be gleaned from the emergence of the life course model of human development [7], which argues that physical, psychosocial, and behavioral processes from conception to old age act additively and interactively to create risk and resilience, and thus, health and disease. This notion of cumulative risk is particularly relevant to preterm infants who not only experience early physical health problems, and have early interactional difficulties, but who also may disproportionately live in relative socioeconomic disadvantage, with the latter reflecting the fact that poverty is a risk factor for both prematurity and poor subsequent development regardless of gestational age [8]. Moreover, mothers of immature infants may be less able to respond to the demands of their infant due to an increased risk of depression [9]. Strong empirical evidence supports the effect of cumulative risk on child development [4].

These theoretical perspectives suggest that the provision of environments that support the immature infant and education of caregivers to promote enriched experiences for optimal brain development early in life will translate into improved neurodevelopment. However, the empiric support for many developmental strategies is highly variable. These will be detailed in the following sections.

Hospital-based interventions

Hospital-based interventions can be considered in two categories. First is modifying the hospital environment to reduce stress on the infant from noise, bright lights, and frequent caretaking activities. Second is the provision of various types of supplemental stimulation, either singly or in some combination. In addition, more recent work has focused on parental stress and coping.

Modification of the environment

As in any intensive care environment, the infant is subjected to a number of aversive stimuli. These would include the processes related to mechanical ventilation; frequent monitoring with blood-drawing, electrode placement, and checking of vital signs; and frequent feeding often with gavage tube placement. Further, infant movement to other settings may be required for diagnostic testing such as X-rays or even surgery.

An early report from the Joint Committee on High-Risk Environment, Intervention and Follow-up noted several differences between the fetal environment and the neonatal intensive care unit (NICU). These included:

- Excessive noise from incubators and other equipment, and caretaker talking that might not be contingent to the infant's state. The effect of noise might be potentially exacerbated by the use of drugs known to harm hearing, for example gentamicin.
- Bright lights without day–night cycling.
- Thermal regulation that does not mimic the fetal environment and lacks circadian rhythms.
- Variations in air quality of isolettes due to pollutants in internal and "fresh air" [10].

The report goes on to list recommendations for environmental modification and further research. These include sound-absorbing ceiling, wall, and floor tiles; not placing items on top of incubators; implementing vibrating mobile phones for staff; and moving infants away from noisy sinks and trash receptacles. While many of the recommendations have been implemented, the net effect of these changes on the development of preterm infants is unclear. Later recommendations have focused on reducing fetal and neonatal exposure to low frequency and loud noises [11].

Supplemental stimulation

While some characteristics of the neonatal intensive care environment would seem to overwhelm the infant with multiple sources of stimulation, others would suggest a relative impoverishment of the sensory environment. For example, early ICUs often restricted parental visiting. In addition, caretaking might involve multiple rotating nurses who performed nursing duties according to strict schedules rather than being responsive to infant state (i.e., infant was calm, awake, and alert, and demonstrating attempts at self-soothing and interaction with his/her environment), schedules that might not allow time for holding, rocking, and sucking non-nutritively during a gavage feeding, for example. Further, the physical constraints required for intensive care meant that the infant often did not experience these usual movements and aspects of infant care. Intensive care units with open floor plans that were often crowded by numerous pieces of equipment impeded the opportunity for infants to be held, soothed, and appropriately stimulated by professional or intimate caregivers. In response, infant-focused stimulation programs were developed to foster more mature state organization and self-regulation and to provide some combination of visual, auditory, or vestibular-kinesthetic stimuli [2].

Single modality interventions

In a systematic review, Symington and Pinelli [12] examined four different types of interventions: positioning, clustering of nursery care activities, modification of external stimuli, and individualized developmental care interventions. The last will be considered in more detail below. In addition, no studies of clustering of nursery care activities could be identified. Outcomes included weight gain, length of hospital stay, length of mechanical ventilation, physiological parameters such as heart rate, and other clinically relevant outcomes. A total of 36 studies were reviewed.

Positioning studies included intentional positioning, nesting, prone vs. supine position, and swaddling. The available studies addressed nesting and swaddling. No evidence was found that nesting shortened length of stay or led to greater weight gain. One study found that swaddling was associated with more mature performance on a standard neurobehavioral examination.

Modifications of external stimuli involved vestibular, auditory, visual or tactile stimulation either alone or in some combination. They concluded that tactile stimulation was associated with improvements in short-term growth and reduced length of stay. All four modes of stimulation were associated with faster transition to full nipple feeding and reduced length of stay. However, only

one study examined a combination of different types of stimulation, vestibular and auditory. Other combinations had not been studied. Further, the authors raised the question about the clinical significance of the interventions even when statistical significance was reported. In addition, no study addressed the costs or personnel required to administer the intervention.

Vickers et al. reviewed studies on the use of massage in preterm infants [13]. Their definition of massage included gentle, slow stroking of various parts of the infant's body. Although they expected to find massage as part of multimodal interventions, they were able to locate 14 studies, only 2 of which included other stimulatory modalities. Two of these involved gentle, still touch rather than stroking. Infants receiving massage interventions gained more weight per day, had shorter lengths of stay, better performance on the Brazelton scales (habituation, motor maturity and range of state), and possibly fewer postnatal complications, although interpretation of these scales was difficult. Gentle touch did not confer any of these benefits. Vickers et al. [13] conclude that the literature provides some support for a modest effect on weight gain and length of stay, but the evidence of effectiveness is weak due to the methodological concerns about the studies reviewed.

Reviews of these early studies [2] indicate that, although the investigators generally reported positive results, design weaknesses precluded understanding the clinical utility of these interventions or to what populations of premature infants they might apply. Among these weaknesses were:

- Differences in onset, frequency, and duration of stimulation across various studies.
- Variations in when infants were thought to be sensitive to the stimulation.
- Samples of small number of infants of widely varying gestational ages with varying sensitivity to different types of stimuli and failure to differentiate among infants with potentially different developmental challenges such as those born small for gestational age.
- Multiple outcome measures varying from physiological observations, to the rates of neonatal complications, to parent interaction.
- Relatively brief periods of follow-up so that the stability of any advantages attributed to the intervention cannot be assessed.
- Lack of knowledge of the functional organization of the premature brain and, therefore, varying theoretical rationales for the intervention.

- Lack of methodological rigor including use of non-randomized designs and failure to characterize the care given the controls.

Multimodal interventions

Two types of interventions can be considered to combine various types of the interventions above. These include kangaroo or skin-to-skin care, and individualized developmental care.

Kangaroo or skin-to-skin care

Conde-Agudelo et al. examined 14 trials of kangaroo mother care (KMC) for its effects on mortality and morbidity [14]. Kangaroo mother care was defined as including skin-to-skin contact (SSC) between the mother's breasts, frequent and exclusive or nearly exclusive breast-feeding, and early discharge from the hospital regardless of gestational age. Kangaroo mother care was found to reduce the risk of nosocomial infection at 41 weeks, and severe illness and lower respiratory tract infection at 6 months. In addition, KMC was associated with higher rates of exclusive breast-feeding, higher weight gain and larger head circumferences by discharge, higher maternal satisfaction with the method of care, and greater sense of maternal competence in the care of the child. Kangaroo mother care did not alter mortality, the risk of gastrointestinal disease at 6 months, readmission to the hospital, or psychomotor development. In one study, KMC actually resulted in lower scores on a social support questionnaire administered during the neonatal stay. Data on hypo- and hyperthermia, and on costs were difficult to interpret. It should be noted that all the available trials were conducted in developing countries, and that none included long-term follow-up and adequate cost data. While the evidence suggests that KMC may be associated with reductions in clinically important outcomes, the methodological base is weak.

The application of KMC to preterm infants in developed countries has focused on the effect of SSC, although breast-feeding remains an important outcome. In an early review, Anderson [15] identified four randomized trials of SSC and at least an additional seven have subsequently been published. Skin-to-skin contact was associated with better breast-feeding rates, duration and/or milk production in three of the trials cited by Anderson and three subsequent ones [15–18], but not a fourth [19]. Despite the evidence that SSC may improve breast-feeding, growth outcomes have been variable with one of Anderson's studies reporting

improved growth, and one later trial [18] reporting no difference in weight or length but a small advantage in head circumference and no difference in length of stay. Studies have reported on the effect of SSC on infant vital signs [16,20], but the results are difficult to summarize, as different parameters were observed. Two studies have attempted to assess the longer-term effect of SSC on maternal and infant outcomes. Feldman et al. [21] observed improved mother–infant interaction at discharge and six months, lower maternal depression at discharge, improved HOME scores (a standardized assessment of how developmentally supportive a home environment is) at three months, and higher Bayley scores (Bayley Scales of Infant Development; a standardized assessment of child development with psychomotor and cognitive subscales) at six months for infants with SSC compared to controls. In contrast, Miles et al.[19] found no differences across a broad array of measures of infant behavior, reactivity to distress and pain, and cognitive and socioemotional development up to one year of age [19]. In addition, they demonstrated no difference in maternal mental health, parenting stress, or attachment. Thus, the evidence base supporting SSC for preterm infants is limited, but it appears to be a popular mode of intervention with almost all the NICUs in a recent survey reporting that they use kangaroo care [22].

Contingency-based developmental care

With the recognition that the newborn already had competencies to engage its caretakers, investigators began to assess the capabilities of premature infants, and to develop quantitative assessments of their responses [23]. These types of assessments revealed the more limited repertoire of independent self-regulatory skills among premature infants, thus suggesting the need for developmental programs to be developed and tailored to respond to the cues of the individual child. Thus, the response of the caretaker was contingent on specific infant behavior.

In a recent systematic review, Jacobs et al.[24] reviewed five randomized trials and three phase-lag studies of the Newborn Individualized Developmental Care and Assessment Program (NIDCAP), developed by Als et al. [25] to provide such tailored, responsive care. Using an explicit scoring system, they rated all the trials as of poor methodological quality with numerous flaws and questions about the methods. No study reported long-term (school-age) neurodevelopmental outcomes, and the effect of NIDCAP on short-term neurodevelopmental outcomes was inconclusive. In the meta-analyses, there was no significant reduction of intraventricular hemorrhage (IVH), patent ductus arteriosus, necrotizing enterocolitis, or retinopathy of prematurity. The only consistent pulmonary outcome favoring NIDCAP was a significant reduction in the need for supplemental oxygen; the results for other pulmonary conditions either varied across studies or showed no reduction (pneumothorax or pulmonary interstitial emphysema). The effects were also conflicting with regard to growth, although, where reported, NIDCAP was associated with earlier full oral feeds. No statistical differences were seen in the length of hospital stay or gestational age at discharge. Although four trials and two cohort studies reported reduced costs associated with NIDCAP, only one was judged to have specified how the costs were assessed. They conclude that, although modification of the infant's environment in response to the infant's behavioral responses makes intuitive sense, the data do not support NIDCAP as the framework for doing so.

Subsequently, Als et al. have published results of a three-site randomized trial [25]. The results favored the individualized developmental care, and a variety of interrelated factors such as shorter times on parenteral feeding and shorter lengths of stay contributed to the positive effects. However, the statistical technique, multiple analysis of variance, does not permit an easy assessment of how the outcomes might be mediated by earlier results of the intervention. Moreover, no assessment of the potential savings in neonatal intensive care costs versus the costs of the program was provided, and this intervention is very labor-intensive for highly trained personnel.

Parental stress and coping

While not focused on the infant, other investigators have considered interventions for parents to reduce the stress of having a premature infant and improve coping. Kaaresen et al. provided a seven-day intervention prior to discharge to the parents of 71 randomly selected preterm infants < 2000 g, and compared their outcomes with 69 preterm and 74 term controls [26]. The intervention consisted of an initial session during which parents were encouraged to express their feelings about the hospital stay and possible grief reactions. This was followed by seven consecutive daily sessions with a trained neonatal nurse who taught the parents to be sensitive and respond to the infant's cues. Follow-up visits in the home were conducted at 3, 14,

30, and 90 days after discharge. The primary outcome measure was the Parenting Stress Index. This instrument has both child and parent domains. The former elicit parental stress as a function of the child's individual characteristics; the latter, stress associated with the parental role. At 6 and 12 months, the intervention parents (both mothers and fathers) reported lower scores (less stress) in both child and parent domains. The effect sizes were considered small to moderate. The potential effects of reduced parental stress on infant development, however, remain to be assessed.

Melnyk et al. selected 260 singleton infants who were born between 26 and 34 weeks of gestation and less than 2500 g cared for in two NICUs [27]. They were randomly assigned to one of two conditions. The intervention, Creating Opportunities for Parent Empowerment (COPE), was administered in four phases: (1) 2–4 days after admission, parents received an audiotaped introduction to infant behavior and parent information; (2) 2–4 days later, they received an audiotape reinforcing the first session and providing suggestions about how the parents might participate in their infant's care; (3) 1–4 days before discharge, parents again received an audiotape that reviewed infant states and parental interactions, and the transition to home; and (4) one week following discharge, parents received audiotaped information with anticipatory guidance on parent–infant relationships and activities to foster development. The comparison group received audiotaped material at the same rate, but this information was more general on hospital services, discharge services, and immunization schedules. Outcome data were collected at the various phases of the intervention and at 2-months corrected for duration of gestation. The primary infant outcome was length of stay, and the primary parental outcomes were measures of parental emotional and functional coping. At 2 months of age corrected for duration of gestation, intervention mothers reported fewer symptoms of anxiety and depression, but no difference was seen for intervention fathers compared to controls. Intervention infants averaged 3.8 days fewer than controls in the initial neonatal stay, but no information on other infant outcomes was provided.

Despite the limited evidence of effectiveness, developmental interventions appear to be used widely in NICUs. In a survey of neonatologists and nurses, Field et al. [22] found that the majority of NICUs had instituted environmental changes, namely containment or swaddling, blankets on the isolette, and music.

Developmental interventions frequently used included kangaroo care, non-nutritive sucking, breast-feeding, and rocking.

Post-discharge intervention

Research indicates that neurodevelopmental vulnerability, particularly germane to cognitive and behavioral outcomes, persists long after the newborn period. The available data indicate that rates of cognitive deficits increase with decreasing birth weight with the smallest babies exhibiting the highest rates of adverse outcomes. Approximately 8–13% of infants born less than 1000 g have cognitive deficits while about 1 in 5 infants born less than 750 g do. Behavioral outcomes, namely attention deficits, conduct disorders, and hyperactivity, are increasingly prevalent with decreasing birth weight and thought to be primarily biological in etiology [5].

Effect of early intervention in other groups.

Assessing the effectiveness of "early intervention" is complicated by the fact that no consistent model of service delivery of cognitive and behavioral interventions for at risk-children exists [28,29]. In fact, even the term "early intervention" has many meanings [30]. For example, the term has been used to describe not only early in life, but also early in the manifestation of a disease process, that is, neurological or developmental disability. Early intervention programs vary in their target population, mode of service delivery, the profession of service providers, and the frequency and duration of services [4,28].

Nonetheless, a growing body of empirical evidence supports the conclusion that intervention in the preschool period may enhance development and improve the chances of success in school and beyond. Much of this evidence involves samples of healthy, socioeconomically disadvantaged children. Summaries of this experience [31–33] indicate improvements in cognitive development (IQ), and these positive findings are more consistently seen with small, center-based educational programs than with programs based on home-visiting models or large, school-district-wide programs. At least four of these successful programs have documented persistence of the effect of the program into adolescence and adulthood without further intervention [34–37].

Less evidence has accumulated with regard to children with established developmental disabilities. However, Shonkoff and Hauser-Cram have conducted a meta-analysis of 31 studies of early intervention for children with Down syndrome and other types of developmental delay, and documented substantial effects at the end of the program in favor of early intervention [38]. Specifically, early intervention was associated with a clinically significant improvement in developmental outcome, greater than one half standard deviation in whatever assessment instrument was used. Successful programing was associated with presumed capacity for amelioration (i.e., model of developmental delay versus mental retardation, which moves away from the assumption that children with disabilities cannot benefit from services); clearly delineated curriculum; and high levels of parental involvement. However, the authors note that the study data are limited by lack of comprehensive outcome measures and few measures of parent–child interaction or family function.

Early intervention for premature infants

The relevance of this experience to preterm infants is uncertain. Although preterm infants are more likely to come from disadvantaged families, not all preterm and/or low birth weight infants do. Moreover, most preterm infants will not have established biological injuries to lead to developmental difficulties at the time of discharge home. Nonetheless, in view of the established vulnerability of preterm infants, a variety of early intervention strategies have been studied. As with the studies of inpatient interventions, considerable variability in sample sizes, onset of the intervention, intervention modalities, and duration of intervention make this literature difficult to assess. They also vary in the outcomes assessed and the timing of these assessments.

Spittle *et al.* have recently prepared a systematic review of this literature [39]. The primary focus of their review is to identify studies that assessed the effect of early intervention during the period 0–2 years with follow-up into the preschool and early school periods compared with standard follow-up care. The outcomes of interest are cognitive and motor development. They were able to locate 16 studies involving 2408 subjects of which 6 were randomized trials, and the remainder quasi-experimental designs. One of these studies has previously been described in this chapter [27], and two of their studies [40,41] will be described in more detail below because of their sample size (1289 subjects of the total in all studies) and rigor.

Most studies aimed to improve both cognitive and motor outcomes, with the exception of five studies involving physical therapy for motor skills, and one focused solely on cognitive outcomes. The focus of the interventions varied from direct attention to the child to enhancing parent–child interactions. The underlying theoretical models differed substantially, as did the personnel delivering the intervention. Onset, modality and frequency of interventions sessions varied, with some beginning before discharge, employing home visits vs. center-based interventions, lasting up to 3 years of age.

In general, they found that these types of interventions resulted in treatment effect on cognitive outcomes of a half standard deviation favoring the intervention, a clinically significant effect. No effects were seen for motor development, nor were rates of cerebral palsy different among intervention and control groups. The results for different birth weight/gestational age groupings under 37 weeks and 2500 g were inconsistent, with some studies finding greater effects among smaller or immature infants, and others finding that heavier infants benefited more from the interventions. Interventions that began in the hospital before discharge and those that began after discharge were effective in the short term in improving cognitive performance. Interventions that also focused on improving parent–child relationships were more effective than those that focused solely on child development or parent support. While concluding that the literature supports the effectiveness of early intervention programs in improving the short- and medium-term cognitive outcomes of preterm infants, the literature is too heterogeneous to provide guidance on what is the optimal duration and intensity of the intervention. Moreover, there is little information on the cost-effectiveness of such programs.

Other studies not included in this systematic review also contribute to the literature on the effects of early intervention in terms of other outcomes or types of intervention. Meyer et al. completed a randomized trial with 34 infants < 1500 g at birth of an individualized family-based intervention during hospitalization [42]. The intervention focused on infant behavior and characteristics, family organization and functioning, the caregiving environment, and home discharge and community resources. Intervention mothers reported less stress and depressive symptoms, and showed better-quality interaction with their infants during feeding. Intervention infants demonstrated fewer adverse feeding behaviors such as grimacing and gagging. Mothers in both groups made gains in self-esteem over time.

Sajaniemi et al. conducted a randomized study of weekly home-based occupational therapy interventions from 6 to 12 months of life for 100 extremely low birth weight infants designed to enhance parent–child interactions and improve motor control and coordination [43]. No differences in cognitive outcomes at age 4 were seen between the two groups, but the control group exhibited more atypical patterns of attachment than the intervention group.

Two studies have focused on making mothers more observant of and responsive to infant behavioral cues. Koldewijn et al. [44] performed a pilot trial of The Infant Behavioral Assessment and Intervention Program (IBAIP) [45], an extension of the neurobehavioral approach developed by Als for the inpatient environment [25]. The 20 intervention infants (mean gestational age: 29.2 weeks, mean birth weight: 1232 g) received six to eight IBAIP intervention sessions at home from discharge until 6 months of age. At the time, intervention infants demonstrated less stress and more approach behaviors than the 20 control subjects of similar gestational age and birth weight.

However, the discipline and training of the home visitor and the content of the home visits are not clear. Moreover, assignment to the study arm was not random, and assessors were not masked to study status and the study curriculum was not implemented by clinicians independent of the study. The authors are currently conducting a larger trial.

The second study [46] employed a complex design for 327 preterm infants based on maternal educational attainment. High education mothers (> 13 years of education) were randomly assigned to a hospital-based program of state modulation (SM), which focused on teaching mothers to read the infant's cues and modulate the states of consciousness during feedings. The control group received a program on car seats. Low education mothers (< 12 years of education) were randomly assigned to an intervention group that received the SM program plus an established nurse home visiting intervention, Nursing Systems for Effective Parenting-Preterm. The control group received the car seat program and standard public health nursing home visits. At 5 months of age corrected for duration, both intervention groups demonstrated more sensitivity to their infants' cues and provided more stimulation during teaching interactions. The authors conclude that SM is effective regardless of educational attainment, but adding the nursing home visiting component is needed for less well-educated women.

Avon Premature Infant Project (APIP)

This project [40] is the first of the two larger post-discharge studies to be presented in more detail. Both were rated as high-quality study by Spittle *et al.* [39]. The APIP was a randomized controlled trial with three arms to assess the effect of a developmental intervention and to isolate its effect from general parental support. Eligible infants were < 32 completed weeks of gestation born to mothers in the greater Bristol area. Of the 328 randomized subjects, 274 completed the study and were assessed. The two intervention arms were designed to be as similar as possible in the number of workers, visiting frequency, and supervision. The developmental intervention arm received a standardized curriculum, Portage, designed for infants with developmental delay, modified to be introduced earlier than in usual practice and delivered through home visits by trained nurses. The parental support arm consisted of support provided by parental advisors. Both arms had weekly home visits for the first few months, reduced to every 2–4 weeks for the next year, and monthly thereafter. The controls received standard care. The primary outcome was the child's development as measured by the Griffiths Scales at 2 years of age. Despite randomization, the study arms were unbalanced for socioeconomic factors. After controlling for these factors, cognitive development scores were higher for both Portage and parental support groups as compared with controls. In addition, for infants < 1251 grams at birth (a preplanned stratum), the scores were higher for the Portage group compared to controls, as were scores for children with abnormal ultrasound scans.

However, these gains in cognitive skills among the intervention group were not sustained at 5 years of age [47]. In fact, at age 5, the intervention group demonstrated lower cognitive skills, a reversal of what was observed at age 2. Sub-analyses by birth weight strata revealed that these differences were statistically significant for the higher (> 1250 g) birth weight group. The authors attribute the lack of positive findings, in part, to response bias. Substantially more socioeconomically advantaged parents in the preterm control group as compared to the intervention group responded to follow-up, thus biasing the data toward more positive developmental gains.

Infant Health and Development Program (IHDP)

The Infant Health and Development Program (IHDP) [41] was a randomized, multisite program that enrolled a diverse cohort of preterm, low birth weight (< 2500 g)

infants in eight sites. The IHDP stratified 985 infants by birth weight group into heavier low birth weight (HLBW, > 2000 g) or lighter low birth weight (LLBW, ≤ 2000 g). All participants received high-risk pediatric follow-up care consisting of pediatric visits every four to six months with regular developmental assessments and referral for any services available in the community.

One third of the infants in each stratum were randomly assigned to the educational intervention. The intervention consisted of weekly home visits (until 12 months of age) by personnel well trained in the intervention curriculum (standardized activities and materials adapted to individualized, development needs of participants), high-quality center-based visits (5 days/week, from ages 12 to 36 months) that included transportation, and monthly parent support meetings.

The outcomes of interest consisted of measures of cognitive development and behavior. Because infants known to be at risk for infectious conditions were being placed in center-based care at 12 months, health outcomes were assessed to ascertain that no adverse events occurred. At major outcome assessments (3, 5, 8, and 18 years of age), the assessors were masked to study status. Details about instruments and timing of assessments, as well as summaries of other analyses, have been published [41,48], so that only a brief summary will be provided here.

Cognitive outcomes

At age 3 years cognitive scores were statistically and clinically significantly higher in the intervention group (INT) for both birth weight strata than those in the follow-up only group (FUO). In the HLBW group, INT children demonstrated an advantage of greater than 13 IQ points compared to those in the FUO group; in the LLBW group, the difference was nearly 7 points [49]. Further analyses [50] revealed that the difference in cognitive scores was seen for all infants in the LLBW group, including those ≤ 1000 g. In addition, intervention effects were seen for all but those infants coming from homes in which the mother had some or more college education [51], those from more socially disadvantaged families experienced greater gains in cognitive skills at age 3 than control counterparts. Assessments at later ages [52–54] showed that cognitive differences favoring the INT group persisted in the HLBW group, although the difference was now in the range of 4 points, and these cognitive advantages were paralleled by better academic achievement in the INT group [53,54]. The gains in IQ in the LLBW group associated with the intervention at age 3 were not sustained at any follow-up period. Rates of children requiring special education placement or repeating a grade did not differ among the study groups at age 8, but were suggestive of substantial difference at age 18 among the HLBW group[53,54].

Behavioral outcomes

Early assessments of behavior relied on maternal reports of behavior problems. At age 18, youths were asked to report on their own behavior, as well as the extent to which they engaged in risky behaviors such as substance use, delinquent behavior, and risky sexual practices. As with cognition, differences favored the INT group in having fewer behavior problems than the FUO group at age 3 in both birth weight strata [49]. However, in neither group did the differences persist in maternal reports of behavior [52–54]. Among the HLBW group, the intervention was protective of risky behaviors with fewer of these behaviors being reported by the INT group [54].

Health outcomes

At the end of the intervention period at age 3, infants in the INT group were reported to have experienced a slightly higher number of episodes of non-severe illnesses, but no difference in severe illnesses characterized by needing emergency or hospital care, growth, or parental rating of child health were seen [49]. No differences in measures of health status between the two groups were seen at any other assessment period [52–54].

Diffusion into practice

Despite the heterogeneity of interventions, the literature would support the utility of early interventions for preterm infants. While many countries are providing services to preschool children, the theoretical perspective and target groups vary substantially.

United States: Part C of IDEA

Over the past 20 years, the United States has developed a national program of early intervention (EI) as part (Part C) of the legislation for educating individuals with disability, now known as the Individuals with Disability Education Act (IDEA). As the service model has evolved, it has included elements such as:

- An Individualized Family Service Plan to specify the goals and services for the child and encourage family participation in decision-making.

- A service coordinator to facilitate communication and evaluation across different providers.
- Integration of the child and family into the community.
- Interagency councils to coordinate service providers.
- A transition plan at age 3.
- Provision of services in child's natural environment [55–57].

Little empirical evidence exists to support the effectiveness of Part C services. In part, this lack of evidence reflects the fact the EI is not a single program. Each state sets its own eligibility criteria and develops its own organizational model. In addition, although federal law requires that each state have an EI program and allocates dollars to the states for these services, states are free to use additional funds, either out of state revenues or through health insurance plans to provide a variety of elements of EI [58]. Thus, it is no surprise that states vary considerably in who is eligible to receive services at one point and over time, lead agency, models of service coordination and other aspects of the program, including within-state variation [28,29,59,60]. These data reflect variations in children who are already enrolled in EI, but say nothing about those who might be eligible but might not be enrolled. However, data from one state [61] (one of the more generous) reveals that 12% of children, eligible by virtue of their birth weight, were not receiving services. In an observational cohort study of children in EI [62], their parents reported some improvement in motor function and substantial improvement in speech and language. However, other observational studies [63] raise questions as to whether this improvement is more than would be expected with the usual patterns of maturation.

Other early intervention efforts

Odom *et al.* [64] have described global early intervention practices. The authors did not focus on preterm infants, but this population would likely be included in young children receiving services, although this is largely variable. Internationally, early intervention programs vary from those with a focus on children with physical disabilities such as cerebral palsy (e.g., China, India, and Egypt) to those with specialized, segregated services for a variety of diagnoses (e.g., Ethiopia, Germany, and Korea). Other countries utilize a more ecological model that fosters community advocacy and inclusion of high-risk children (e.g., Germany, Portugal, Sweden, and Australia). Two countries, Jamaica and Israel, have specific cognitive and behavioral intervention for high-risk newborns, although the results of these programs were not reported.

Conclusion

The developmental management of premature infants has changed dramatically from the early days of effective intensive care in the late 1960s and early 1970s. As noted above, early intensive care units represented a harsh environment for fragile infants, one that was insensitive to their developmental needs. In the intervening years, modifications of the neonatal intensive care environment have appeared to include three main trends. The first is the reduction of adverse environmental stimuli and greater approximation of the usual environment of preterm infants with day–night cycles of light, for example. The second reflects greater sensitivity to the developmental states of preterm infants and means to reduce stress and enhance self-soothing techniques. The third involves greater parental, especially maternal, participation in the care of the infant, including close physical contact.

However, the evidence base for the optimal combination of interventions remains sparse. As the systematic reviews of single intervention modalities indicate, the small number of heterogeneous studies makes it difficult to assess the effectiveness of any single intervention. In addition, most studies of in-hospital interventions provide little sense of the context of the study or other care practices in the unit. It is now well documented that care practices vary substantially among different units with implications for variations in outcomes [65,66]. Thus, it is unclear whether even those interventions for which some evidence exists might work as well in a different unit with different practices. In view of the shift in developmental care practices over the past three decades, it is unlikely that stronger evidence will emerge, as it would more than likely be considered unethical to engage in randomized trials with an untreated control group. Thus, the most that might happen would be comparisons of various interventions against each other.

Likewise, the multimodal interventions require further assessment. For example, it should be possible to investigate various aspects of skin-to-skin care to understand what may be optimal in the modern intensive care unit. As with the single modality studies, studies of multimodal care, even if multisite, do

not provide much information on other care practices, so that it is unclear whether variations in outcomes might reflect other aspects of the care. For example, if substantial differences in nutritional practices among NICUs result in differential weight gain, the intervention that improves weight gain in one setting with less aggressive nutritional practices may not prove to be so successful in a unit with greater attention to fostering growth. Other aspects of these interventions also deserve further study. For example, it is unclear what burden is placed on both caregivers and nurses in providing more intensive developmental therapy. However, NIDCAP [24] requires extensive behavioral assessments and documentation of these assessments to support the developmental intervention. In hospitals already feeling pressures to reduce costs, such labor-intensive efforts may not be feasible.

An emerging area of inquiry and intervention is providing support to enhance parental coping (although enhancing parental skills may also be implicit in other types of interventions). For the most part, these interventions have focused on strengthening parents' abilities to recognize and respond to their infants' cues, and improving caretaking confidence. Such interventions rest on the assumption that infant–parent interactions are the source of parental stress among the parents of NICU patients. Evidence that other factors may place a stress on NICU parents comes from the economics literature. In a recent review, Zupancic [67] notes the dearth of studies of direct non-medical costs for parents before and after discharge for out-of-pocket expenditures for such activities as visiting and travel, and productivity loss due to reductions in work, although the studies available indicate a significant financial burden. Remarkably little empiric investigation addresses the sources of stress and resiliency among the families of NICU parents. In consequence, we lack a research base for addressing other sources of stress in these families.

The data on the effectiveness of early childhood interventions post-discharge are stronger and more consistent in demonstrating cognitive and behavioral gains. The difficulty here is that the strongest data come from two research projects (APIP and IHDP) with attention to the fidelity and quality of the intervention, although the heterogeneity of the sites in IHDP provides evidence of generalizability. An often-encountered critique of such efforts, especially IHDP, is that the intensity of the intervention is too costly for implementation of a larger scale. Fewell and Scott have argued that much of the increased costs reflects the cost of research, and that an IHDP-like intervention could be implemented for amounts closer to those of routine center-based care[68]. What this concern points to, however, is the need for continued investigation into the appropriate intensity and curricula that might lead to similar results with lower cost, if possible.

What the data on the implementation of these programs through IDEA suggest, however, is that it is not clear that the enormous variability across different programs may limit the effectiveness of these programs in improving child outcomes. For example, variable state eligibility requirements for Part C services suggest that some preterm infants may not receive developmental intervention post hospital discharge. In the same vein, the life course model and some sparse empirical data would suggest that programing commencing in the hospital and following children until school age would be most efficacious in terms of ameliorating neurodevelopmental risk.

Thus, these results would suggest that further program evaluation and social policy implementation should include standardized measures of children's global abilities (i.e., community integration and school achievement) rather than impairment-specific assessments, address quality of services, address cost-effectiveness of various hospital and post-discharge protocols and implement quasi-experimental comparisons of existing programs to understand what may be best practices for this vulnerable group of infants.

In addition, the lack of sustained intervention effect in both APIP and IHDP suggests the importance of other elements of the educational experience. More vulnerable infants may need continued support to achieve their optimal outcomes. A preschool program, no matter how intense, does not "inoculate" a child with developmental vulnerabilities against the adverse effects of under-performing in kindergartens and elementary and high schools. Thus, more work is needed to identify the appropriate supports and methods of transition among different levels of education.

Regardless of the limitations and further work needed, what this review has demonstrated is that at every stage of the early career of the premature infant, development is malleable and can be enhanced. Unlike the impression gleaned from the early follow-up literature on these infants that seemed to suggest a fixed and irreversible quantum of developmental disability, the literature that is emerging now suggests that much can be accomplished. That is not to say that some neonates survive with such significant impairments that independent living and academic accomplishments will be severely limited. However, even in these cases, specific interventions can improve functioning and reduce nursing burden. For the majority of surviving premature infants, however, early and probably ongoing interventions will provide significant improvement in outcomes.

References

1. Horbar JD, Lucey JF. Evaluation of neonatal intensive care technologies. *Future Child* 1995; **5**: 139–61.

2. Gilkerson L, Gorski PA, Panitz P. Hospital-based intervention for preterm infants and their families. In: Mesels SJ, Shonkoff JP, eds. *Handbook of Early Childhood Intervention*, 1st edn. Cambridge: Cambridge University Press. 1990; 3–31.

3. Campbell SK. The child's development of functional movement. In:Campbell SK, Vander Linden DW, Palisano R, eds. *Physical Therapy for Children*. St. Louis, MO: Elsevier. 2006; 33–76.

4. Meisels S, Shonkoff J. Early childhood intervention: a continuing evolution. In: Shonkoff J, Samuels M, eds. *Handbook of Early Childhood Intervention*, 2nd edn. New York, NY: Cambridge University Press. 2000; 3–34.

5. Board on Health Sciences Policy, Committee on Understanding Premature Birth and Assuring Healthy Outcomes, Institute of Medicine of the Academies. Neurodevelopmental, health, and family outcomes for infants born preterm In: Behrman RE, Butler AS, eds. *Preterm Birth Causes, Consequences, and Prevention*. Washington, DC: The National Academies Press. 2006; 346–97.

6. Shonkoff JP, Phillips DA, eds. *From Neurons to Neighborhoods. The Science of Early Childhood Development*. Washington, DC: National Academy Press; 2000.

7. Ben-Shlomo Y, Kuh D. A life course approach to chronic disease epidemiology: conceptual models, empirical challenges and interdisciplinary perspectives. *Int J Epidemiol* 2002; **31**: 285–93.

8. Brooks-Gunn J, Duncan G. The effects of poverty on children. *Future Child* 1997; **7**: 55–71.

9. Gennaro S, York R, Brooten D. Anxiety and depression in mothers of low birth weight and very low birth weight infants: birth through 5 months. *Issues Comp Pediatr Nurs* 1990; **31**: 97–109.

10. Graven SN, Bowen FW, Brooten D, *et al.* The high-risk infant environment. Part 1. The role of the neonatal intensive care unit in the outcome of high-risk infants. *J Perinatol* 1992; **12**: 164–72.

11. Graven SN. The full-term and premature newborn. Sound and the developing infant in the NICU: conclusions and recommendations for care. *J Perinatol* 2000; **20**: S88–S93.

12. Symington A, Pinelli J. Developmental care for promoting development and preventing morbidity in preterm infants. *Cochrane Database Syst Rev* 2006; (2): CD001814. DOI: 10.1002/14651858.CD001814. pub2.

13. Vickers A, Ohlsson A, Lacy JP, Horsley A. Massage for promoting growth and development of preterm and/ or low birth-weight infants. *Cochrane Database Syst Rev* 2004; (2): CD000390.pub2.DOI:10.1002/14651858. CD000390.pub.2

14. Conde-Agudelo A, Diaz-Rossello JL, Belizan JM. Kangaroo mother care to reduce morbidity and mortality in low birthweight infants. *Cochrane Database Syst Rev* 2003; (2): CD002771. DOI: 10.1002/14651858. CD002771.

15. Anderson GC. Current knowledge about skin-to-skin (kangaroo) care for preterm infants. *J Perinatol* 1991; **11**: 216–26.

16. Bier JB, Ferguson AE, Morales Y, *et al.* Comparison of skin-to-skin contact with standard contact in low-birth-weight infants who are breast-fed. *Arch Pediatr Adolesc Med* 1996; **150**: 1265–9.

17. Hurst NM, Valentine CJ, Renfro L, Burns P, Ferlic L. Skin-to-skin holdings in the neonatal intensive care unit influences maternal milk volume. *J Perinatol* 1997; **17**: 213–17.

18. Rojas MA, Kaplan M, Quevedo M *et al.* Somatic growth of preterm infants during skin-to-skin care versus traditional holding: a randomized, controlled trial. *J Dev Behav Pediatr* 2003; **24**: 163–8.

19. Miles R, Cowan F, Glover V, Stevenson J, Modi N. A controlled trial of skin-to-skin contact in extremely preterm infants. *Early Hum Dev* 2006; **82**: 447–55.

20. Bergman N, Linley LL, Fawcus SR. Randomized controlled trial of skin-to-skin contact from birth versus conventional incubator for physiological stabilization in 1200- to 2199-gram newborns. *Acta Paediatr* 2004; **93**: 779–85.

21. Feldman R, Eidelman AI, Sirota L, Weller A. Comparison of skin-to-skin (kangaroo) and traditional care: parenting outcomes and preterm infant development. *Pediatrics* 2002; **110**: 16–26.

22. Field T, Hernandez-Reif M, Feijo L, Freedman J. Prenatal, perinatal and neonatal stimulation: a survey of neonatal nurseries. *Infant Behav Dev* 2006; **29**: 24–31.

23. Brazelton TB. The behavioral competence of the newborn. In: Taylor PM, ed. *Parent-Infant Relationships.* New York: Grune and Stratton. 1980; 69–85.

24. Jacobs SE, Sokol J, Ohlsson A. The Newborn Individualized Developmental Care and Assessment Program is not supported by meta-analyses of the data. *J Pediatr* 2002; **140**: 699–706.

25. Als H, Gilkerson L, Duffy FH, *et al.* A three-center, randomized, controlled trial of individualized developmental care for very low birth weight preterm infants: medical, neurodevelopmental, parenting and caregiving effects. *J Dev Behav Pediatr* 2003; **24**: 399–408.

26. Kaaresen PI, Ronning JA, Ulvund SI, Dahl LB. A randomized, controlled trial of the effectiveness of an early-intervention program in reducing parenting stress after preterm birth. *Pediatrics* 2006; **118**: e9–19.

27. Melnyk BM, Feinstein NF, Alpert-Gillis L *et al.* Reducing premature infants' length of stay and improving parents' mental health outcomes with the Creating Opportunities for Parent Empowerment (COPE) neonatal intensive care unit program: a randomized, controlled trial. *Pediatrics* 2006; **118**: e1414–27. DOI:10.11542/peds.2005–2580.

28. Spiker D, Hebbeler K, Wagner M, Cameto R, McKenna P. A framework for describing variation in state early intervention systems. *Top Early Child Spec Educ* 2000; **20**: 195–207.

29. Scarborough A, Hebbler K, Spiker D. Eligibility characteristics of infants and toddlers entering early intervention services in the United States. *J Policy Practice in Intellect Disabilities* 2006; **3**: 57–64.

30. Blaw-Hospers CH, Hadders-Algra M. A systematic review of the effects of early intervention on motor development. *Dev Med Child Neurol* 2005; **47**: 421–32.

31. Simeonsson RJ, Cooper DH, Scheiner AP. A review and analysis of the effectiveness of early intervention programs. *Pediatrics* 1982; **69**: 635–41.

32. Barnett W. Long-term effects of early childhood programs on cognitive and social outcomes. *Future Child* 1995; **5**: 25–50.

33. Karoly L, Kilburn M, Bigelow J, Caulkins J, Cannon J. Benefit-cost findings for early childhood intervention programs. In: *Assessing Costs and Benefits of Early Childhood Programs: Overview and Application to the Starting Early Starting Smart Program.* Santa Monica, CA: RAND. 2001; 49–71.

34. Schweinhart LJ, Barnes HV, Weikart DP. *Significant Benefits: The High/Scope Preschool Study Through Age 27,* Monographs of the High/School Education Research Foundation, 10. Ypsilianti, MI: High/Scope Press; 1993.

35. Campbell F, Ramey C. Effects of early intervention on intellectual development and academic achievement: a follow-up study of children from low-income families. *Child Dev* 1994; **65**: 884–98.

36. Reynolds AJ. *The Chicago Child–Parent Centers: Longitudinal Study of Extended Early Childhood*

Interventions. Institute for Research on Poverty. Discussion Paper no. 1126–97. Available from: www.irp.wisc.edu/publications/dps/pdfs/dp112697.pdf. Accessed June 24, 2007.

37. Olds DL, Kitzman H. Review of research on home visiting for pregnant women and parents of young children. *Future Child* 1993; **3**: 53–92.

38. Shonkoff J, Hauser-Cram P. Early intervention for disabled infants and their families: a quantitative analysis. *Pediatrics* 1987; **80**: 650–8.

39. Spittle AJ, Orton J, Doyle LW, Boyd R. Early developmental intervention programs post hospital discharge to prevent motor and cognitive impairments in preterm infants (Review). *Cochrane Database Syst Rev* 2007; (2): CD005495.

40. Avon Premature Infant Project. Randomised trial of parental support for families with very preterm children. *Arch Dis Child Fetal Neonatal Ed* 1998; **79**: F4–11.

41. Gross RT, Spiker D, Haynes CW, eds. *Helping Low Birth Weight, Premature Babies. The Infant Health and Development Program.* Stanford, CA: Stanford University Press; 1997.

42. Meyer EC, Coll CT, Lester BM, *et al.* Family-based intervention improves maternal psychological well-being and feeding interaction of preterm infants. *Pediatrics* 1994; **93**: 241–6.

43. Sajaniemi N, Makela J, von Wendt L, Hamalainen T, Hakamies-Blomqvist L. Cognitive performance and attachment patterns at four years of age in extremely low birth weight infants after early intervention. *Eur Child Adolesc Psychiatry* 2001; **10**: 122–9.

44. Koldewijn K, Wolf MJ, van Wassenaer A, *et al.* The Infant Behavioral Assessment and Intervention Program to support preterm infants after hospital discharge: a pilot study. *Dev Med Child Neurol* 2005; **47**: 105–12.

45. Infant Behavioral Assessment and Intervention Program. An Education and Training Program for Health Care and Early Intervention Professionals. Available from: www.ibaip.org. Accessed July 25, 2007.

46. Kang R, Barnard K, Hammond M, *et al.* Preterm infant follow-up project: a multi-site field experiment of hospital and home intervention programs for mothers and preterm infants. *Public Health Nurs* 1995; **12**: 171–80.

47. Johnson S, Ring W, Anderson P, Marlow N. Randomized trial of parental support for very preterm children: outcome at 5 years. *Arch Dis Child* 2005; **90**: 909–15.

48. McCormick MC, McCarton C, Brooks-Gunn J, Belt P, Gross RT. The Infant Health and Development Program: interim summary. *J Dev Behav Pediatr* 1998; **19**: 359–70.

49. The Infant Health and Development Program. Enhancing the outcome of low-birth-weight, premature infants: a multi-site, randomized trial. *JAMA* 1990; **262**: 3035–42.

50. McCormick MC, McCarton C, Tonascia J, Brooks-Gunn J. Early educational intervention for very low birth weight infants: results from the Infant Health and Developmental Program. *J Pediatr* 1993; **123**: 527–33.

51. Brooks-Gunn J, Gross RT, Kraemer HC, Spiker D, Shapiro S. Enhancing the cognitive outcomes of low birth weight, premature infants: for whom is the intervention most effective? *Pediatrics* 1992; **89**: 1209–15.

52. Brooks-Gunn J, McCarton CM, Casey PH, *et al.* Early intervention in low-birth-weight premature infants. Results through age 5 from the Infant Health and Development Program. *JAMA* 1994; **272**: 1257–62.

53. McCarton CM, Brooks-Gunn J, Wallace IF, *et al.* Results at age 8 years of early intervention for low birth-weight premature infants. The Infant Health and Development Program. *JAMA* 1997; **277**: 126–32.

54. McCormick MC, Brooks-Gunn J, Buka SL, *et al.* Early intervention in low birth weight premature infants. Results at 18 years for the Infant Health and Development Program. *Pediatrics* 2006; **117**: 771–80.

55. Widerstrom A. Newborns and infants at risk for or with disabilities. In: Widerstrom A, Mowder B, Sandall S, eds. *Infant Development and Risk,* 2nd edn. Baltimore, MD: Paul H. Brookes Publishing Co., Inc. 1997; 3–24.

56. Hurth J. Service Coordination Caseloads in State Early Intervention Systems. *NECTAS Notes* 1998; **8**: 1–6. Available from: www.nectac.org/~pdfs/pubs/nnotes8.pdf. Accessed July 25, 2007.

57. Silverstein R. *A User's Guide to the 2004 IDEA Reauthorization* (P.L. 108–446 and the Conference Report). Center for the Study and Advancement of Disability Policy 2005. Available from: www.ccd.org/task_forces/education/IdeaUserGuide.pdf. Accessed July 25, 2007.

58. Greer M, Taylor A, Andrews S. A Framework for Developing and Sustaining a Part C Finance System. *NECTAC Notes* 2007; Issue 23. Available from: www.nectac.org/~pdfs/pubs/nnotes23.pdf. Accessed July 25, 2007.

59. Dunst C, Hamby D. States' Part C eligibility definitions account for differences in the percentage of children participating in early intervention programs. *Snapshots* 2004; **1**: 1–5. Available from: www.puckett.org/. Accessed February 17, 2007.

60. Dunst C, Hamby D, Fromewick J. Status and trends in the number of infants and toddlers in the IDEA Part C early intervention program (1994–2002). *Snapshots* 2004; **1**: 1–5. Available from: www.puckett.org/. Accessed February 17, 2007.

61. Clements K, Barfield W, Kotelchuck M, Lee K, Wilbert N. Birth characteristics associated with early intervention referral, evaluation for eligibility, and program eligibility in the first years of life. *Matern Child Health J* 2006; **10**: 433–41.

62. Hebbeler K, Spiker D, Bailey D, *et al. Early Intervention for Infants and Toddlers with Disabilities and Their Families: Participants, Services, and Outcomes.* Final Report of the National Early Intervention Longitudinal Study (NEILS). Jan 2007. Available from: www.sri.com /neils/pdts/neils_report_02_07_final2.pdf. Accessed July 25, 2007.

63. Mahoney G, Robinson C, Fewell RR. The effects of early motor intervention on children with Down syndrome or cerebral palsy: a field-based study. *J Dev Behav Pediatr* 2001; **22**: 153–62.

64. Odom SL, Hanson MJ, Blackman JA, Kaul S. (eds). *Early Intervention Practices Around the World.* Baltimore, MD: Paul H. Brookes Publishing Co., Inc.; 2003.

65. Lee SK, McMillan DD, Ohlsson A, *et al.* Variations in practice and outcomes in the Canadian NICU network: 1996–1997. *Pediatrics* 2000; **106**: 1070–9.

66. Vohr BR, Wright LL, Dusick AM, *et al.* Center differences and outcomes of extremely low birth weight infants. *Pediatrics* 2004; **113**: 781–9.

67. Zupancic JAF. A systematic review of costs associated with preterm birth. In: Behrman RE, Butler AS, eds. *Preterm Birth. Causes, Consequences, and Prevention.* Appendix D. Washington, DC: The National Academies Press 2006; 688–724.

68. Fewell RR, Scott KG. The cost of implementing the intervention. In: Gross RT, Spiker D, Haynes CW, eds. *Helping Low Birth Weight, Premature Babies. The Infant Health and Development Program.* Stanford, CA: Stanford University Press. 1997; 479–502.

Integrative summary and future directions

Chiara Nosarti, Robin M. Murray, and Maureen Hack

Whilst preterm birth represents the single largest factor worldwide in terms of infant mortality [1], mortality rates associated with preterm birth have decreased in recent decades thanks to advances in perinatal and neonatal care [2,3]. However, the improved survival of very preterm and very low birth weight infants has been associated with an increase in the prevalence of neonatal problems (including periventricular hemorrhage, chronic lung disease, retinopathy of prematurity (ROP), and septicemia) and neurodevelopmental sequelae [4]. Therefore, attention has increasingly focused on the quality of life of survivors, who are at greater risk of brain damage and consequent neurological disorders, and neuropsychological and behavioral impairments in childhood and later in life [5–8].

In this volume, leading experts from multiple disciplines, investigating various aspects of the long-term consequences of very preterm birth, have presented a comprehensive and updated summary of research in their field. As well as extending existing knowledge of the neurodevelopmental sequelae following very preterm birth, a shared aim of this burgeoning body of research is to identify the mechanisms underlying variations in outcome and thus recognize subgroups of children who are at increased risk of neurodevelopmental problems, who can then be referred early to appropriate intervention services.

Preterm birth occurs in a substantial percentage of the population: just less than 13% of US live births are reported as being preterm (< 37 completed weeks of gestation). Very preterm births, occurring before 32 completed gestational weeks, account for about 15% of preterm births, which is equivalent to 1–2% of all pregnancies [9]. In addition to preterm birth, in this volume we have often referred to the neurodevelopmental outcome of individuals who were born with a very low birth weight, the vast majority of whom are small

for gestational age (SGA) [10], and many of whom have also experienced varying degrees of intrauterine growth failure.

Preterm birth has been associated with numerous risk factors, described in Chapter 1, including previous family history of obstetric complications, maternal infections, non-white ethnicity, maternal characteristics such as age at delivery (low and high), short interpregnancy interval and other adverse outcomes in previous pregnancies (i.e., induced or spontaneous abortions and one or more other very preterm deliveries), socioeconomic disadvantage, maternal smoking and substance abuse (including narcotics and alcohol), and environmental factors, such as exposure to a variety of air pollutants. While efforts aimed at reducing maternal exposure to risk factors associated with preterm birth have sometimes proved efficacious, e.g., smoking cessation [11], the etiology of many of the risk factors listed above may be partly explained by complex biological mechanisms, including genetic effects and neuroendocrine stress response. For instance, there is evidence that allelic variations in certain genes involved in the immune system (e.g., interleukin-6) may influence the physiological processes leading to preterm delivery [12]. Regarding hypothalamic–pituitary–adrenal (HPA) axis activation, it has been observed that mothers who go on to deliver before term tend to have cortisol levels that are higher than those in mothers who deliver at term [13]. Studies investigating interactions between environmental, genetic, and biological risk factors may help to devise primary preventative strategies, aimed at decreasing the number of pregnancies ending before term, and associated morbidities.

When considering secondary prevention, the aim is to identify factors associated with disease, and in the context of this volume, adverse neurodevelopmental outcome, as early as possible, even before problems become manifest. The study of the mechanisms of brain injury in vulnerable populations could provide a powerful means to inform the formulation of secondary preventative strategies. Developments in neonatal care for extremely preterm infants have been associated with a wide spectrum of insults in the neonatal period, sometimes even resulting in iatrogenic complications [14]. Changes in the type of neonatal care hence need to be taken into account when studying the outcome of ex-very preterm populations differing in year of birth and/or geographical location of the neonatal care unit. It is of interest to note that factors emphasized as being central to the care of preterm infants as early as 1907 by the pioneering French obstetrician Pierre Budin, such as nutrition, have been later revisited and found to be associated with childhood and adolescent outcome. A recent study by Isaacs and colleagues not only found cognitive effects of early nutrition when comparing two groups of adolescents, assigned a standard- or high-nutrient 4-weeks diet after preterm birth, but also observed an increased volume of the caudate nucleus and higher verbal IQ in those individuals assigned a high-nutrient diet [15].

The mechanisms of brain injury need to be studied in relation to specific phases of brain maturation that take place between the twenty-fourth and the fortieth week of gestation, involving pre-myelinating oligodendrocytes, microglia, axons, subplate neurons, the proliferative cerebral dorsal subventricular zone, thalamus, cortex, and cerebellum. Due to their rapidly developing and complex characteristics, these neurodevelopmental processes are likely to be vulnerable to exogenous and endogenous insults [16]. To provide an example, the germinal matrix (GM) is a transient embryonic structure that proliferates the neuroblasts and glioblasts which provide the basis for the organization of the cortex, and during the third trimester of gestation is also a source of primitive glial cells. Anatomically, the GM is located adjacent to the lateral ventricles, with the majority of tissue lying between the ventricles and the caudate nucleus in the telencephalon. It is separated from the cerebrospinal fluid of the lateral ventricles only by a single layer of ependyma [17], hence initial bleeding within the GM may spread throughout the ventricular system and cause intraventricular hemorrhage (IVH). As neuronal cell migration to the cortex is completed by the twenty-fourth gestational week, GM/IVH hemorrhage may destroy the migrating glial precursor cells and affect subsequent brain development [17,18]. The incidence of IVH,

which occurs in approximately 20% of preterm infants, has been found to be reduced by administration of antenatal steroids [19], and postnatal indomethacin [20], both possibly exerting a protective effect on the cerebral microvasculature. Another common lesion observed in preterm infants has been recently labeled "encephalopathy of prematurity," and refers to periventricular leukomalacia (PVL; a frank necrosis in white matter) and accompanying neuronal/axonal deficits involving the cerebral white matter, thalamus, basal ganglia, cerebral cortex, brainstem, and cerebellum, occurring in approximately 50% of infants with very low birth weight. Encephalopathy of prematurity has been described as a "complex amalgam of primary destructive disease and secondary maturational and trophic disturbances" [16]. Please refer to Chapter 2 for a detailed description of mechanisms of brain injury and Chapter 4 for discussion of the prognostic significance of neonatal brain injury as detected by neuroimaging techniques.

As well as benefits, treatment-related side effects have been also noted. For instance, bronchopulmonary dysplasia is the most common pulmonary morbidity in ex-preterm infants and is associated with chronic hypoxia. Longer duration on oxygen in survivors of bronchopulmonary dysplasia has been found to be associated with impaired cognitive function at school age [21]. Administration of postnatal steroids has been also associated with increased neurodevelopmental impairment in extremely low birth weight infants (1000 g or less) [22]. However, duration on oxygen, as well as postnatal steroids administration, may represent a proxy for the severity of the infant's medical condition, and the contribution of other neurological risk factors that are common in those individuals receiving the intervention to neurodevelopmental outcome needs to be taken into account.

While neuronal proliferation is predominantly complete by the end of the second trimester, during the third trimester neuronal migration, glial cell proliferation, synaptogenesis and pruning, myelination and cortical connectivity have yet to be established [23]. The vast majority of brain development in fact occurs in the third trimester of gestation, with the volume of whole brain more than doubling and the volume of cortical gray matter increasing approximately fourfold [24]. During this time period, subcortical gray matter increases 70% [25], and cortical folding and gyrification emerge [26]. It is therefore not surprising that very preterm birth has been associated with altered brain growth and structural and functional brain abnormalities later in life. Characteristic patterns of brain injury detected by neonatal cranial ultrasound (CUS) are all likely to directly or indirectly affect white matter structure and there is evidence that white matter injury and impaired GM development may be associated [27]. Various neuroimaging techniques have been used to study brain structure (CUS, computed tomography [CT], magnetic resonance imaging [MRI], diffusion tensor imaging [DTI]) and function (positron emission tomography [PET], functional MRI [fMRI]) following preterm birth.

Neonatal neuroimaging studies in preterm neonates, summarized in Chapter 4, have described total white matter and cortical gray matter reductions [28], as well as reduced gray matter volumes in sensorimotor and parieto-occipital regions [8]. Neonatal MRI studies have also shown that severely abnormal findings may be moderately accurate for predicting an adverse outcome, particularly in relation to neurological sequelae including disorders of the motor system (see Chapter 3). These disorders include spasticity, dykinesia, and ataxia, which are commonly referred to as cerebral palsy (CP), which has a prevalence of 40–100 per 1000 live births in very low birth weight and very preterm individuals compared with 1 per 1000 in term infants [29] and increases with lower birth weight and lower gestational age. Cerebral palsy is thought to be associated with a pathomechanism specifically affecting the immature brain. Some studies have found as many as 90% of preterm-born children with CP to have major abnormalities detected on CUS (i.e., grade 3 and 4 hemorrhage, cystic PVL, and focal infarction) [30] and 90% to have periventricular white matter lesions [31]. The extent and topography of the periventricular white matter lesion determine the clinical subtype of CP (e.g., unilateral or bilateral form), as well as the presence and severity of associated complications, such as mental retardation or cerebral visual problems. The prediction of childhood cognitive outcome from CUS results has proven more difficult, especially for subtle cognitive changes [32,33]. However, it is interesting to note that abnormalities on CUS may not be always associated with an adverse outcome, as shown by results from a large multicenter cohort study of extremely low birth weight children, 14% of whom had a history of grade 3–4 IVH and 3% had a history of PVL, but all had a normal neurological assessment at 18 months of age [34].

A non-invasive technique which has been available for the past 20 years is MRI, which when obtained at term equivalent, near the time of discharge of the preterm infant from the neonatal unit, has been shown to have prognostic significance. For instance, Valkama and colleagues found that the presence of parenchymal lesions gave a sensitivity of 100% and specificity of 79% for motor abnormality in a study of very preterm-born infants, approximately 20% of whom had neurological deficits at follow-up [35]. Cognitive delay has also been found to be predicted by moderate to severe cerebral white matter injury on term-equivalent MRI, whether cystic or diffuse in nature, which was a further predictor of motor delay, CP, and neurosensory impairment [36]. Useful guidelines for the use of the various imaging techniques are provided in Chapter 4.

An increased risk of structural brain alterations in ex-preterm individuals has been described from childhood into young adulthood (see Chapters 5 and 6). Smaller cortical volumes and larger lateral ventricles have been reported in ex-very preterm and very low birth weight individuals compared to controls [37–40]. Reduced gray matter volumes in sensorimotor and parieto-occipital regions have been shown in 8-year-old prematurely born children [8]. In adolescence, reductions in total cortical gray matter have been demonstrated [40] and specifically in temporal, frontal, and occipital cortices [7]. White matter alterations in several brain regions, including frontal, parietal, temporal, and occipital lobes have been documented [7,41]. Magnetic resonance imaging studies looking at specific regions of interest have demonstrated decreases in size in ex-very preterm and very low birth weight individuals compared to controls in hippocampus [40], cerebellum [42], corpus callosum [43,44], caudate nucleus [45], and thalamus [46]. Diffusion tensor imaging studies, summarized in Chapter 8, provide an index of white matter microstructure, influenced by the coherence of the white matter, its organization, and the density and degree of myelination of fiber bundles, and have revealed altered white matter microstructure in preterm neonates [47,48], and failure of developmental changes in microstructure to occur [49]. White matter disturbances in the internal capsule and corpus callosum have been described in children [50], which seem to persist into adolescence and early adulthood [51,52].

The nature of the differences reported in the literature suggests that the brains of preterm-born individuals are substantially different in structure, a finding which would be compatible with plastic reorganization of structure in response to early brain lesions. Such an interpretation would be consistent with the hypothesis put forward by Thomas and Karmiloff-Smith, who posited that developmental disorders may be associated with altered development of the entire brain, so that the end-state functional architecture of developmentally altered systems may possess modules that are not to be found in the normally developing brain, or in other words are characterized by "different functional structures" [53]. Following this line of thought, altered patterns of structure–function relationships may be observed following early brain injury because functions are remapped onto other undamaged areas of the brain [54].This hypothesis would explain why some of the observed cortical and subcortical abnormalities have been associated with cognitive difficulties often observed among very preterm-born individuals [7,43,44,46,55,56], whereas other studies have failed to determine the specific pattern of brain abnormality underlying selective neuropsychological impairments in adolescence and adult life [38,40]. In relation to structural MRI findings, the neurodevelopmental outcomes which have been most frequently investigated include neurological outcome, such as CP [31,57] and minor motor impairment [58,59], cognitive measures such as spatial, attention, and executive function [7,60,61], memory [55,56], language [42,43], and behavioral problems [62,63].

Several studies have reported that very preterm/low birth weight individuals compared to controls in childhood and adolescence are at increased risk of manifesting behavioral abnormalities (see Chapter 9), including externalizing and attentional problems [64,65], attention deficit hyperactivity disorder (ADHD) [66], early autistic behaviors [67], separation anxiety and enuresis [65], anxiety disorder [68], and depressive disorder [69,70]. Only a few studies have investigated behavioral and psychiatric outcome of very preterm/low birth weight individuals in adulthood (see Chapter 10). Increased rates of psychopathology have been reported [71], including mood disorder [72], anxiety, and depression [73,74]. Preterm birth and being SGA were recently found to be associated with an increased risk of psychiatric hospitalization during late adolescence and early adulthood with a variety of diagnoses [75].

A different approach to the investigation of the possible association between pre- and perinatal complications (often collectively termed obstetric complications or OCs) and later psychiatric disorders has been adopted by studies which selected patients with a specific psychiatric diagnosis and then investigated whether patients with this diagnosis were more likely to have experienced obstetric complications than healthy controls. The focus has particularly been on schizophrenia [76,77] and anorexia nervosa [78]. Most other psychiatric disorders have not been fully investigated. An historical and meta-analytic review published by Cannon *et al.* summarized the results of eight population-based studies and identified three groups of complications which were significantly associated with schizophrenia, although the effect sizes tended to be small, with odds ratios of less than 2 [76]. These were (1) complications of pregnancy, including preeclampsia; (2) abnormal fetal growth and development, including low birth weight; and (3) complications of delivery, including birth asphyxia. Results from a large population-based, case-control study of girls aged 10–21 years reported an increased risk of anorexia nervosa in girls with a cephalhematoma and preterm birth (gestational age $\leq$ 32 weeks). Furthermore, amongst preterm births, those who were SGA were 5.7 times more likely to have a diagnosis of anorexia than girls with higher birth weight for gestational age [78].

In terms of cognitive outcome, several studies have demonstrated that individuals who were born very preterm and those with a very low birth weight tend to have lower IQ than age-matched controls and to experience academic difficulties in childhood and adolescence [56,79–82]. Other studies reported that the differences between very preterm-born individuals and controls in terms of educational performance and IQ scores disappeared by adulthood/late adolescence, suggesting a developmental delay with subsequent "catch-up" in performance [83,84], although other studies have reported lower IQ scores in very preterm-born adults [82]. Perinatal variables may mediate longitudinal changes in cognitive performance, as Taylor *et al.* reported that between the ages of 7 and 14 years, children with < 750 g birth weight showed increased impairments over time compared to controls, whereas those with > 750 g birth weight showed fewer deficits and no specific impairments [85]. However, it is of interest to note that despite the reported significant differences in cognitive performance compared with term-born controls, the scores obtained by ex-very preterm individuals and those with a very low birth weight almost invariably fall within the normal range, when compared with standardized data [82,86].

One of the cognitive domains which has been studied in ex-preterm samples is executive functioning (see Chapter 15), which refers to a variety of processes which are responsible for goal-directed or future-oriented behavior. Several studies have suggested that ex-very preterm preschoolers and school-age children and those with a very low birth weight exhibit impaired executive function [61,87,88]. Specific deficits have been reported in object working memory, planning abilities, motor sequencing and inhibition, verbal conceptual reasoning, spatial conceptualization and organization, and visual reasoning [61,88–90]. There is evidence that some impairments in executive functioning persist into adolescence and early adulthood and include attention, perceptual-motor, and organizational abilities [91], visuomotor skills and memory [85], response inhibition and mental flexibility [82]. A gradient relationship between spatial organization and cognitive flexibility and birth weight has been reported [85,87]. Executive processes are regarded as "higher-order" cognitive operations, and, as such, may be dependent on "lower-order" operations such as information processing, perception, and memory. Given that deficits in lower-order processes have been described in preterm/low birth weight samples [91,92], it can be hypothesized that executive deficits may reflect underlying impairments in the "building blocks" of executive functioning.

Selective language impairments have been observed in individuals who were born very preterm/very low birth weight (see Chapter 13). From infancy onwards the described deficits have involved verbal delays in language development [93], as well as specific problems in articulation and correct use of grammar [94] and lexical morphology [95]. Slight delays in the development of lexicon and grammar have been observed in a study of very preterm-born two-year-old children, but only in those individuals who had an extremely low birth weight, whereas a typical linguistic development was reported in healthy very preterm-born participants [96]. At school age, developmental language delays [97], as well as deficits in reading skills [98], naming [99], speech, motor function, interaction and motivation [100], have been observed. As differences in processing speed have been observed between very preterm-born individuals and controls [92], it remains to be established whether these may be one of the underlying mechanisms associated with the observed language deficits, or whether language difficulties may indicate general cognitive functional difficulties [101].

Regarding memory and learning (see Chapter 14), published evidence suggests that spatial [88,102] and phonological working memory [61], and verbal learning [56,91] may be impaired in children born preterm and with a very low birth weight, whereas data concerning long-term explicit memory and procedural learning are less conclusive. It is to be ascertained whether these deficits reflect primary deficits in memory systems and alterations in brain areas that are thought to be associated with memory such as the middle temporal gyrus [7], or whether they are a consequence of deficits in executive functions and damage to the neural substrates of these functions [44]. Furthermore, it is important to note that children born preterm can often experience difficulties in cognitive domains involving perceptual-motor and organizational skills [91], which could be affecting their performance on working memory tasks. It would be useful in the future to attempt to dissociate possible memory deficits from other cognitive impairments observed in very preterm groups, as well as to investigate the associations between different cognitive abilities in order to elucidate how a domain-specific deficit may affect the development of others, or possibly how sparing of a domain-specific function may occur at the expense of other cognitive skills.

The study of the neural correlates, developmental course, and cognitive source of impairments in working memory, language, and executive function may help to understand the academic problems reported in ex-preterm individuals, as for instance working memory skills have been shown to be a predictor of academic achievement [103]. Problems in academic achievement and school performance in very preterm/very low birth weight children are apparent soon after school entry [104], and include grade repetition and/or the need for special education assistance, parent and teacher reports of poor school performance, and low scores on tests of academic skills, such as those evaluating reading, spelling, mathematics, and writing (see Chapter 16). Findings from studies of academic outcomes have shown a "gradient" relation between the degree of low birth weight/low gestational age and educational outcomes [81]. The social impact of the described academic problems is substantial, and economic costs associated with educational resources aimed at children with low birth weight (LBW, < 2500 g) in the United States in 1989 was estimated as approximating US$370.8 million [105]. Furthermore, children who need to repeat grades or require special education assistance in primary school are at greater risk than other children for long-term learning and behavior problems, including school dropout [106].

Innumerable environmental factors may interact with and impact educational as well as neurodevelopmental outcome [107] (see Chapter 17). These include maternal education, family income, type of health insurance, and access to early intervention services, and can account for variability in outcomes independent of biological risks [108]. Higher rates of special education and learning disabilities have been associated with lower parental educational level, unmarried parental status, and lower family income [109–112]. As early as 1958 Drillien noted the impact of poverty and low socioeconomic status on low birth weight and ex-preterm infants [113]: a combination of low socioeconomic status and very low birth weight (< 1500 g) resulted in a significant decrease in intellectual function in the infant, while development quotient improved with age among very low birth weight children from high socioeconomic backgrounds, but declined among very low birth weight children from a low socioeconomic background.

As well as having the potential to aggravate the neonatal risks posed by preterm birth, environmental factors can exert a protective effect, as they may increase a child's likelihood of unimpaired adult outcome. These include personal resilience, a characteristic of a child, who, under adverse circumstances, is able to withstand the impact of environmental adversity [114]. Children who are identified as being resilient are characterized by the capacity to establish close bonds with the caregivers that provide them with nurturing during the first years of life. This skill may facilitate the creation of emotionally supportive friendships and the choice of positive role models, such as a mentor, which are regarded as representing social protective factors. It could be speculated that personality characteristics of very preterm-born individuals, who have been found to have significantly lower extraversion scores, higher neuroticism scores, and higher lie scores than term-born controls [115], may not always be compatible with resilient traits.

If a variety of environmental factors can adversely affect neurodevelopmental outcome, it follows that the provision of environments that support the immature infant and promote enriched experiences for optimal brain development early in life has the potential to result in improved neurodevelopmental outcome (see Chapter 18). Hospital-based interventions have attempted to modify the hospital environment to reduce stress on the infant from noise, bright lights, and routine caretaking activities. Other interventions have consisted in providing various types of supplemental stimulation. Clinical trials such as the Neonatal Individualized Developmental Care and Assessment Program (NIDCAP) [116] were developed to provide a tailored response to the cues of preterm infants. However, the empiric support for short-term benefits on neurodevelopmental outcome was inconclusive.

Tertiary prevention programs, aimed at improving the neurodevelopmental outcome of ex-very preterm/very low birth weight individuals by limiting cognitive and behavioral complications, and providing cognitive enhancers, have been conducted after hospital discharge, encouraged by the success of programs improving cognitive development in healthy socioeconomically disadvantaged children [117]. These have overall demonstrated improvements in cognitive and behavioral outcomes. The Infant Health and Development Program (IHDP) was a randomized trial of early educational intervention after discharge from the hospital on the health and developmental status of very low birth weight (≤ 1500 g) infants. The "intervention" group had higher cognitive scores and fewer behavioral problems at age 3 compared to the non-intervention group [118], although these improvements decreased with increasing age at follow-up, at age 8 [119] and 18 years [120]. Spittle and colleagues [121] in a review of early developmental intervention programs post hospital discharge to prevent motor and cognitive impairments in preterm infants, found these types of interventions resulted in treatment effect on cognitive outcomes of a half standard deviation favoring the intervention, which was regarded as representing a clinically significant effect. However, positive effects were reported at infant and preschool age, but were not sustained at school age. No significant effects were observed for motor development, or rates of CP. The results for different birth weight/gestational age groupings were inconsistent, with some studies finding greater effects among smaller or immature infants, and others finding that heavier infants benefited more from the interventions. Interventions starting in the hospital before discharge and those beginning after discharge were associated with improved cognitive performance in the short term. Interventions targeting the improvement of parent–child relationships were more effective than those that focused exclusively on child development or parent support. This suggests that published studies support the effectiveness of early intervention programs in improving the short- and medium-term cognitive outcomes of preterm infants, but they may be too heterogeneous to provide guidance on what is the optimal duration and intensity of the intervention.

Other studies have used MRI to investigate longitudinal brain growth in relation to neurodevelopmental outcome (see Chapter 6). Between the ages of 8 and 12 years ex-preterm individuals showed brain volumes increases of 2–3% which were similar to changes observed in controls. During the same time period, ex-preterm children showed a smaller decrease in cerebral gray matter compared to controls (2.5% vs. 9.5%, respectively), and a smaller increase in cerebral white matter volumes (>26% vs. 10%, respectively) [122]. Between mid to late adolescence (14–19 years) other changes have been observed, such as a 3% decrease in cerebellar volume in very preterm-born individuals compared to no significant change in controls [123], as well as greater increases in the size of the corpus callosum (13% in preterm-born individuals vs. 3% in controls) [124]. As with the cerebellum, this growth had functional consequences, as it was associated with cognitive outcome (the greater the growth, the higher the IQ scores at age 19). These studies suggest that adult neurodevelopmental outcome ought to be investigated in relation to processes of brain development, with a focus on how these processes may mediate the development of cognitive functions. These studies also suggest that very preterm birth is associated with alterations in the trajectory of cerebral development at least up to late adolescence. These alterations may represent developmental delays, although their magnitude suggests that the normal patterns of brain development following very preterm birth may be both different and delayed [7].

When interpreting documented associations between neurodevelopmental outcome and structural brain correlates, caution is needed as many of these associations may not be directly causal, but simply both resulting from preterm birth itself and its associated complications, such as the quality of an individual's hearing, vision, neurological status, functional skills in daily living, and behavior. It is therefore not surprising that comorbidities such as ROP [111] and congenital anomalies [125] have been found to be associated with an even more unfavorable neurodevelopmental outcome. The number of neonatal morbidities seem to have an additive effect on outcome, and in a study by Schmidt et al. there was a fivefold increase in the rates of neurodevelopmental impairments in children with a history of three neonatal morbidities compared to children with no history of morbidities [126]. However, a large body of literature suggests that even

mild neurological impairment may affect cognitive processes [127]. Learning disabilities are associated with minor neurological abnormalities in ex-very preterm children [128], and mild motor delay with lower academic achievement scores [129]. Associations between neurological outcome and IQ in very preterm/very low birth weight samples of different ages have been reported [64,127]. Problems in educational achievement and school performance in very preterm/very low birth weight children have been associated with biological risk, including IVH and other brain abnormalities as detected on neonatal CUS, chronic lung disease, necrotizing enterocolitis, meningitis, and postnatal corticosteroid treatment, length of neonatal hospitalization, and numbers of neonatal complications [104,112,130,131]. A potentially explanatory hypothesis concerning the role of neuropsychological skills as mediators of the effects of biological risk on school-age educational achievement has been supported [108]. This model showed associations of very low birth weight with specific cognitive skills which, in turn, were associated with achievement in reading and mathematics, independently of the effects of socioeconomic factors.

In addition to cause–effect inferences, methodological consideration, which readers may need to take into account when interpreting the results of outcome studies of individuals born very preterm/very low birth weight, have been summarized in Chapter 12 as falling into four main categories: (1) conceptualization/design issues (for instance, mediators/moderators, selection of control groups), (2) study populations (definition of birth weight and gestational age, use of broad, geographically representative groups, comparable age cohorts, factors associated with changes in medical procedures), (3) procedural issues (inclusion of possible confounding factors, adjustment for gestational age, consideration of biological risk issues), and (4) measurement/outcome (lack of a developmental "gold standard," lack of consistency in terms of diagnostic criteria, duration of follow-up, comparability of tests, inclusion/exclusion of children with major handicap) [132–134].

Studies investigating the neurodevelopmental sequelae of individuals born very preterm and those with a low birth weight suggest that these groups experience significant cerebral structural alterations compared with term-born controls, and often show cognitive deficits in childhood and adolescence. However, a proportion of individuals who were born at the extreme limits of viability (e.g., < 1000 g) seem to have relatively unimpaired neurodevelopmental outcomes [86]. The presence of alterations in key structural brain regions following very preterm birth may result in functional changes in distributed brain systems, which may underlie the development of alternative neural pathways which enable the compromised individuals to maintain competent performance of specific cognitive tasks. In samples with a variety of pathologies, and in subjects with suspected cerebral abnormalities, fMRI techniques may provide a characterization of the damage in a way that may not be deduced from structural scans (i.e., residual responsiveness within the regions of partial brain damage, or abnormal responses distant to the damaged area). Therefore, in very preterm-born adolescents and young adults, investigations on functional neuroanatomy, summarized in Chapter 7, can provide important insights into the neurobiological mechanisms that support recovery from brain injury.

Published fMRI data in preterm-born adolescent cohorts compared to controls have reported differential neural activation patterns during a variety of cognitive tasks, including spatial memory [135], response inhibition, and selective attention allocation processing [136]. A few fMRI studies have selected very preterm groups on the basis of known structural brain alterations. Ex-very preterm adolescent males with callosal thinning or atrophy have shown differential neural activation while carrying out auditory and visual tasks [137] and during phonological and orthographic processing [138]. Recently, Lawrence *et al.* [139] reported altered patterns of brain activation during tasks involving attention allocation and inhibitory control in very preterm-born young adults (mean age 20 years). These authors showed reduced activation in a fronto-parietal-cerebellar network during attention allocation, and increased activation in posterior brain regions during inhibitory control in very preterm-born subjects compared to controls. Another cognitive task which has been used in functional brain imaging studies with very preterm samples is the learning of paired associates, such as face–name associations, which represents an essential cognitive operation carried out in everyday life. A study by Giménez *et al.* [140] investigated the neural correlates of declarative memory (e.g., conscious explicit memory) using a face–name association task. Results revealed differential neural activation during the encoding phase of the experiment with increased blood-oxygen-level-dependent (BOLD)

signal response in the right hippocampus in very preterm adolescents compared to controls, a region of the brain which has been found to be also structurally altered in similar subject samples [40].

Environmental effects have been recently studied in relation to the development of the central nervous system. For instance, the physical environment of the neonatal intensive care unit can have a long-lasting impact on neuroendocrine functions, including nociceptive circuits and alterations in behavioral responses to pain [141]. Clinical trials such as the NIDCAP have been found to affect not only neurodevelopmental outcome but brain development. This has been demonstrated with respect to white matter in frontal and occipital cortices, which showed increased coherence (measured by electroencephalogram) and higher relative anisotropy (measured by DTI) in the internal capsule in the experimental group compared to the control group [142]. This demonstrates the potential for application of anisotropy measures as a biomarker to evaluate the short-term impact of potential neurological-based interventions.

Finally, there is initial evidence that biological risk (e.g., gestational age) may interact with genetic factors to contribute to increased susceptibility for cognitive and behavioral outcome. Genetic factors may account for almost half of the maternal liability to have SGA births [143]. A recent study found that brain-derived neurotrophic factor (BDNF) showed lower levels amongst individuals born with a gestational age < 37 weeks compared to term controls [144]. Brain-derived neurotrophic factor plays a critical role in protecting against the adverse consequences of fetal hypoxia by promoting growth and differentiation of new neurons, hence a dysregulation of neurotrophic signaling may lead to dendritic atrophy and disruption of synaptogenesis in the fetus. A differential BDNF response to birth hypoxia between individuals with schizophrenia and controls suggests that the expression of this critical cell-signaling mechanism may not be associated with increased vulnerability to schizophrenia in the absence of a particular biological risk. In addition, genetic factors may be associated with neurodevelopmental outcome. A recent study investigated the relationship between the val108/158met polymorphism of the catechol-O-methyl transferase (COMT) gene and corpus callosum development in young adults who were born very preterm and found that the met allele was associated with greater growth and more organized callosal microstructure [145]. This allele produces a lower-activity form of the enzyme, suggesting that COMT genotype may confer resilience to the effects of perinatal white matter damage in individuals who were born very preterm. It would be therefore important for future studies to disentangle the maternal genetic, fetal genetic, and environmental effects for the study of the relationship between preterm birth and low birth weight and adult neurodevelopmental outcome.

With reference to the discipline of developmental psychopathology, Cicchetti and Cannon emphasized the importance of understanding the differentiation, integration, and organization of biological, cognitive, and behavioral development in order to place the individual investigated in its environmental context, and thus facilitate the identification of the etiology, course, outcomes, and therapeutic intervention for high-risk conditions and pathologies [146]. Similar paradigms could be applied to the study of the neurodevelopment of very preterm/very low birth weight infants.

We propose advances in neurodevelopmental research, which could inform the design and implementation of appropriate intervention services for individuals at risk of short- and long-term sequelae, will be provided by continuing research into the following:

1. Furthering the understanding of the pathophysiology of perinatal brain injury and plasticity during development via sophisticated/newer MRI and fMRI techniques. In this respect, novel forms of compact and mobile MRI techniques with enhanced sensitivity and time resolution are currently being piloted [147] and could provide an invaluable research tool for the study of the very preterm neonate.
2. Furthering the understanding of the molecular basis and genetic contribution to susceptibility to brain injury.
3. Perinatal research into methods to prevent neonatal brain injury and/or to ameliorate its effects when unavoidable.
4. Furthering the understanding of the effects of early childhood intervention, especially in infants at greater biological (the extremely immature and low birth weight infants) and environmental (the socioeconomically disadvantaged) risk.
5. Increasing awareness of behavioral problems and the development of psychopathology during childhood and the development of appropriate primary and secondary intervention strategies.
6. Improvements in the overall sociodemographic environment in which very preterm/low birth weight infants grow and develop, including wider availability of and accessibility to intervention programs, which have the potential to improve some of the adverse developmental sequelae described in this volume.

References

1. Bryce J, Boschi-Pinto C, Shibuya K, Black RE. WHO estimates of the causes of death in children. *Lancet* 2005; **365**: 1147–52.

2. Richardson DK, Gray JE, Gortmaker SL, *et al.* Declining severity adjusted mortality: evidence of improving neonatal intensive care. *Pediatrics* 1998; **102**: 893–9.

3. Fanaroff AA, Hack M, Walsh MC. The NICHD neonatal research network: changes in practice and outcomes during the first 15 years. *Semin Perinatol* 2003; **27**: 281–7.

4. Wilson-Costello D, Friedman H, Minich N, Fanaroff AA, Hack M. Improved survival rates with increased neurodevelopmental disability for extremely low birth weight infants in the 1990s. *Pediatrics* 2005; **115**: 997–1003.

5. Botting N, Powls A, Cooke RW, Marlow N. Cognitive and educational outcome of very-low-birthweight children in early adolescence. *Dev Med Child Neurol* 1998; **40**: 652–60.

6. Breslau N, Chilcoat HD. Psychiatric sequelae of low birth weight at 11 years of age. *Biol Psychiatry* 2000; **47**: 1005–11.

7. Nosarti C, Giouroukou E, Healy E, *et al.* Grey and white matter distribution in very preterm adolescents mediates neurodevelopmental outcome. *Brain* 2008; **131**: 205–17.

8. Peterson BS, Anderson AW, Ehrenkranz R, *et al.* Regional brain volumes and their later neurodevelopmental correlates in term and preterm infants. *Pediatrics* 2003; **111**: 939–48.

9. Hamilton BE, Minino AM, Martin JA, *et al.* Annual summary of vital statistics: 2005. *Pediatrics* 2007; **119**: 345–60.

10. United Nations Children's Fund and World Health Organization. *Low Birthweight: Country, Regional and Global Estimates.* New York: UNICEF; 2004.

11. Cnattingius S, Granath F, Petersson G, Harlow BL. The influence of gestational age and smoking habits on the risk of subsequent preterm deliveries. *N Engl J Med* 1999; **341**: 943–8.

12. Hartel C, Finas D, Ahrens P, *et al.* Polymorphisms of genes involved in innate immunity: association with preterm delivery. *Mol Hum Reprod* 2004; **10**: 911–15.

13. Sandman CA, Glynn L, Schetter C D, *et al.* Elevated maternal cortisol early in pregnancy predicts third

trimester levels of placental corticotropin releasing hormone (CRH): priming the placental clock. *Peptides* 2006; **27**: 1457–63.

14. Stark AR, Carlo WA, Tyson JE, *et al*. Adverse effects of early dexamethasone in extremely-low-birth-weight infants. National Institute of Child Health and Human Development Neonatal Research Network. *N Engl J Med* 2001; **344**: 95–101.

15. Isaacs EB, Gadian DG, Sabatini S. The effect of early human diet on caudate volumes and IQ. *Pediatr Res* 2008; **63**: 308–14.

16. Volpe JJ. Brain injury in premature infants: a complex amalgam of destructive and developmental disturbances. *Lancet Neurol* 2009; **8**: 110–24.

17. Volpe JJ. Intracranial hemorrhage. In: *Neurology of the Newborn* 4th edn. Philadelphia, PA: W.B. Saunders Company. 2001; 397–496.

18. Ment LR, Schneider KC, Ainley MA, Allan WC. Adaptive mechanisms of developing brain. The neuroradiologic assessment of the preterm infant. *Clin Perinatol* 2000; **27**: 303–23.

19. Roberts D, Dalziel S. Antenatal corticosteroids for accelerating fetal lung maturation for women at risk of preterm birth. *Cochrane Database Syst Rev* 2006; (3): CD004454.

20. Fowlie PW, Davis PG. Prophylactic indomethacin for preterm infants: a systematic review and meta-analysis. *Arch Dis Child Fetal Neonatal Ed* 2003; **88**: F464–6.

21. Anderson PJ, Doyle LW. Neurodevelopmental outcome of bronchopulmonary dysplasia. *Semin Perinatol* 2006; **30**: 227–32.

22. Vohr BR, Wright LL, Poole WK, McDonald SA. Neurodevelopmental outcomes of extremely low birth weight infants < 32 weeks' gestation between 1993 and 1998. *Pediatrics* 2005; **116**: 635–43.

23. Volpe JJ. Neuronal proliferation, migration, organization and myelination. In: *Neurology of the Newborn* 4 edn. Philadelphia, PA: W.B. Saunders Company. 2001; 45–99.

24. Hüppi PS, Warfield S, Kikinis R. Quantitative magnetic resonance imaging of brain development in premature and mature newborns. *Ann Neurol* 1998; **43**: 224–35.

25. Mewes AU, Hüppi PS, Als H, *et al*. Regional brain development in serial magnetic resonance imaging of low-risk preterm infants. *Pediatrics* 2006; **118**: 23–33.

26. Dubois J, Benders M, Cachia A, *et al*. Mapping the early cortical folding process in the preterm newborn brain. *Cereb Cortex* 2008; **18**: 1444–54.

27. Inder TE, Warfield SK, Wang H, Hüppi PS, Volpe JJ. Abnormal cerebral structure is present at term in premature infants. *Pediatrics* 2005; **115**: 286–94.

28. Inder TE, Hüppi PS, Warfield S, *et al*. Periventricular white matter injury in the premature infant is followed

by reduced cerebral cortical gray matter volume at term. *Ann Neurol* 1999; **46**: 755–60.

29. Himmelmann K, Hagberg G, Beckung E, Hagberg B, Uvebrant P. The changing panorama of cerebral palsy in Sweden. IX. Prevalence and origin in the birth-year period 1995–1998. *Acta Paediatr* 2005; **94**: 287–94.

30. de Vries LS, Van HI, Caastert, Rademaker KJ, Koopman C, Groenendaal F. Ultrasound abnormalities preceding cerebral palsy in high-risk preterm infants. *J Pediatr* 2004; **144**: 815–20.

31. Krageloh-Mann I, Horber V. The role of magnetic resonance imaging in elucidating the pathogenesis of cerebral palsy: a systematic review. *Dev Med Child Neurol* 2007; **49**: 144–51.

32. Sherlock RL, Anderson PJ, Doyle LW. Neurodevelopmental sequelae of ntraventricular haemorrhage at 8 years of age in a regional cohort of ELBW/very preterm infants. *Early Hum Dev*, 2005; **81**: 909–16.

33. Krageloh-Mann I, Toft P, Lunding J, *et al*. Brain lesions in preterms: origin, consequences and compensation. *Acta Paediatr* 1999; **88**: 897–908.

34. Vohr BR, Msall ME, Wilson D, *et al*. Spectrum of gross motor function in extremely low birth weight children with cerebral palsy at 18 months of age. *Pediatrics* 2005; **116**: 123–9.

35. Valkama AM, Pääkko EL, Vainionpaa LK, *et al*. Magnetic resonance imaging at term and neuromotor outcome in preterm infants. *Acta Paediatr* 2000; **89**: 348–55.

36. Woodward LJ, Anderson PJ, Austin NC, Howard K, Inder TE. Neonatal MRI to predict neurodevelopmental outcomes in preterm infants. *N Engl J Med* 2006; **355**: 685–94.

37. Allin M, Henderson M, Suckling J, *et al*. Effects of very low birthweight on brain structure in adulthood. *Dev Med Child Neurol* 2004; **46**: 46–53.

38. Cooke RW, Abernethy LJ. Cranial magnetic resonance imaging and school performance in very low birth weight infants in adolescence. *Arch Dis Child Fetal Neonatal Ed* 1999; **81**: F116–21.

39. Kesler SR, Ment LR, Vohr B, *et al*. Volumetric analysis of regional cerebral development in preterm children. *Pediatr Neurol* 2004; **31**: 318–25.

40. Nosarti C, Al Asady MH, Frangou S, *et al*. Adolescents who were born very preterm have decreased brain volumes. *Brain* 2002; **125**: 1616–23.

41. Gimenez M, Junque C, Narberhaus A, *et al*. White matter volume and concentration reductions in adolescents with history of very preterm birth: A voxel-based morphometry study. *Neuroimage* 2006; **32**: 1485–98.

42. Allin M, Matsumoto H, Santhouse AM, *et al*. Cognitive and motor function and the size of the cerebellum in adolescents born very pre-term. *Brain* 2001; **124**: 60–6.

43. Nosarti C, Rushe TM, Woodruff PW, *et al.* Corpus callosum size and very preterm birth: relationship to neuropsychological outcome. *Brain* 2004; **127**: 2080–9.

44. Narberhaus A, Segarra D, Caldu X, *et al.* Corpus callosum and prefrontal functions in adolescents with history of very preterm birth. *Neuropsychologia* 2008; **46**: 111–16.

45. Abernethy LJ, Palaniappan M, Cooke RW. Quantitative magnetic resonance imaging of the brain in survivors of very low birth weight. *Arch Dis Child* 2002; **87**: 279–83.

46. Gimenez M, Junque C, Narberhaus A, *et al.* Correlations of thalamic reductions with verbal fluency impairment in those born prematurely. *Neuroreport* 2006; **17**: 463–6.

47. Counsell SJ, Shen Y, Boardman JP, *et al.* Axial and radial diffusivity in preterm infants who have diffuse white matter changes on magnetic resonance imaging at term-equivalent age. *Pediatrics* 2006; **117**: 376–86.

48. Hüppi PS, Maier SE, Peled S, *et al.*. Microstructural development of human newborn cerebral white matter assessed in vivo by diffusion tensor magnetic resonance imaging. *Pediatr Res* 1998; **44**: 584–90.

49. Miller SP, Vigneron DB, Henry RG, *et al.* Serial quantitative diffusion tensor MRI of the premature brain: development in newborns with and without injury. *J Magn Reson Imaging* 2002; **16**: 621–32.

50. Nagy Z, Westerberg H, Skare S, *et al.* Preterm children have disturbances of white matter at 11 years of age as shown by diffusion tensor imaging. *Pediatr Res* 2003; **54**: 672–9.

51. Kontis D, Catani M, Cuddy M, *et al.* Diffusion tensor MRI of the corpus callosum and cognitive function in adults born preterm. *Neuroreport* 2009; **20**: 424–8.

52. Skranes J, Vangberg TR, Kulseng S, *et al.* Clinical findings and white matter abnormalities seen on diffusion tensor imaging in adolescents with very low birth weight. *Brain* 2007; **130**: 654–66.

53. Thomas M, Karmiloff-Smith A. Are developmental disorders like cases of adult brain damage? Implications from connectionist modelling. *Behav Brain Sci* 2002; **25**: 727–50.

54. Stiles J, Reilly J, Paul B, Moses P. Cognitive development following early brain injury: evidence for neural adaptation. *Trends Cogn Sci* 2005; **9**: 136–43.

55. Gimenez M, Junque C, Narberhaus A, *et al.* Hippocampal gray matter reduction associates with memory deficits in adolescents with history of prematurity. *Neuroimage* 2004; **23**: 869–77.

56. Isaacs EB, Lucas A, Chong WK, *et al.* Hippocampal volume and everyday memory in children of very low birth weight. *Pediatr Res* 2000; **47**: 713–20.

57. Spittle AJ, Boyd RN, Inder TE, Doyle LW. Predicting motor development in very preterm infants at 12 months' corrected age: the role of qualitative magnetic resonance imaging and general movements assessments. *Pediatrics* 2009; **123**: 512–17.

58. Rademaker KJ, Lam JN, Van Haastert, I, *et al.* Larger corpus callosum size with better motor performance in prematurely born children. *Semin Perinatol* 2004; **28**: 279–87.

59. Vohr BR, Wright LL, Dusick AM, *et al.* Neurodevelopmental and functional outcomes of extremely low birth weight infants in the National Institute of Child Health and Human Development Neonatal Research Network, 1993–1994. *Pediatrics* 2000; **105**: 1216–26.

60. Atkinson J, Braddick O. Visual and visuocognitive development in children born very prematurely. *Prog Brain Res* 2007; **164**: 123–49.

61. Anderson PJ, Doyle LW. Executive functioning in school-aged children who were born very preterm or with extremely low birth weight in the 1990s. *Pediatrics* 2004; **114**: 50–7.

62. Nosarti C, Allin M, Frangou S, Rifkin L, Murray R. Decreased caudate volume is associated with hyperactivity in adolescents born very preterm. *Biol Psychiatry* 2005; **13**: 339.

63. Stewart AL, Rifkin L, Amess PN, *et al.* Brain structure and neurocognitive and behavioural function in adolescents who were born very preterm. *Lancet* 1999; **353**: 1653–7.

64. Breslau N, Chilcoat HD, Johnson EO, Andreski P, Lucia VC. Neurologic soft signs and low birthweight: their association and neuropsychiatric implications. *Biol Psychiatry* 2000; **47**: 71–9.

65. Elgen I, Sommerfelt K, Markestad T. Population based, controlled study of behavioural problems and psychiatric disorders in low birthweight children at 11 years of age. *Arch Dis Child Fetal Neonatal Ed* 2002; **87**: F128–32.

66. Botting N, Powls A, Cooke RW, Marlow N. Attention deficit hyperactivity disorders and other psychiatric outcomes in very low birthweight children at 12 years. *J Child Psychol Psychiatry* 1997; **38**: 931–41.

67. Limperopoulos C, Bassan H, Sullivan NR, *et al.* Positive screening for autism in ex-preterm infants: prevalence and risk factors. *Pediatrics* 2008; **121**: 758–65.

68. Indredavik MS, Vik T, Heyerdahl S, *et al.* Psychiatric symptoms and disorders in adolescents with low birth weight. *Arch Dis Child Fetal Neonatal Ed* 2004; **89**: F445–50.

69. Gale CR, Martyn CN. Birth weight and later risk of depression in a national birth cohort. *Br J Psychiatry* 2004; **184**: 28–33.

70. Patton GC, Coffey C, Carlin JB, Olsson CA, Morley R. Prematurity at birth and adolescent depressive disorder. *Br J Psychiatry* 2004; **184**: 446–7.

71. Wiles NJ, Peters TJ, Leon DA, Lewis G. Birth weight and psychological distress at age 45–51 years: results from the Aberdeen Children of the 1950s cohort study. *Br J Psychiatry* 2005; **187**: 21–8.

72. Walshe M, Rifkin L, Rooney M, *et al.* Psychiatric disorder in young adults born very preterm: role of family history. *Eur Psychiatry* 2008; **23**: 527–31.

73. Hack M, Youngstrom EA, Cartar L, *et al.* Behavioral outcomes and evidence of psychopathology among very low birth weight infants at age 20 years. *Pediatrics* 2004; **114**: 932–40.

74. Raikkonen K, Pesonen AK, Heinonen K, *et al.* Depression in young adults with very low birth weight: the Helsinki study of very-low-birth-weight adults. *Arch Gen Psychiatry* 2008; **65**: 290–6.

75. Monfils Gustafsson W, Josefsson A, Ekholm Selling K, Sydsjo G. Preterm birth or foetal growth impairment and psychiatric hospitalization in adolescence and early adulthood in a Swedish population-based birth cohort. *Acta Psychiatr Scand* 2009; **119**: 54–61.

76. Cannon M, Jones PB, Murray RM. Obstetric complications and schizophrenia: historical and meta-analytic review. *Am J Psychiatry* 2002; **159**: 1080–92.

77. Hultman CM, Sparen P, Takei N, Murray RM, Cnattingius S. Prenatal and perinatal risk factors for schizophrenia, affective psychosis, and reactive psychosis of early onset: case-control study. *BMJ* 1999; **318**: 421–6.

78. Cnattingius S, Hultman CM, Dahl M, Sparen P. Very preterm birth, birth trauma, and the risk of anorexia nervosa among girls. *Arch Gen Psychiatry* 1999; **56**: 634–8.

79. Allin M, Walshe M, Fern A, *et al.* Cognitive maturation in preterm and term born adolescents. *J Neurol Neurosurg Psychiatry* 2008; **79**: 381–6.

80. Hack M, Flannery D J, Schluchter M, Cartar L, *et al.* Outcomes in young adulthood for very-low-birth-weight infants. *N Engl J Med* 2002; **346**: 149–57.

81. Taylor HG, Klein N, Minich NM, Hack M. Middle-school-age outcomes in children with very low birthweight. *Child Dev* 2000; **71**: 1495–511.

82. Nosarti C, Giouroukou E, Micali N, *et al.* Impaired executive functioning in young adults born very preterm. *J Int Neuropsychol Soc* 2007; **13**: 571–81.

83. Tideman E. Longitudinal follow-up of children born preterm: cognitive development at age 19. *Early Hum Dev* 2000; **58**: 81–90.

84. Peng Y, Huang B, Biro F, *et al.* Outcome of low birthweight in China: a 16-year longitudinal study. *Acta Paediatr* 2005; **94**: 843–9.

85. Taylor HG, Minich N, Bangert B, Filipek PA, Hack M. Long-term neuropsychological outcomes of very low birth weight: associations with early risks for periventricular brain insults. *J Int Neuropsychol Soc* 2004; **10**: 987–1004.

86. Anderson P, Doyle LW. Neurobehavioral outcomes of school-age children born extremely low birth weight or very preterm in the 1990s. *JAMA* 2003; **289**: 3264–72.

87. Waber DP, McCormick MC. Late neuropsychological outcomes in preterm infants of normal IQ: selective vulnerability of the visual system. *J Pediatr Psychol* 1995; **20**: 721–35.

88. Woodward LJ, Edgin JO, Thompson D, Inder TE. Object working memory deficits predicted by early brain injury and development in the preterm infant. *Brain* 2005; **128**: 2578–87.

89. Harvey J M, O'Callaghan MJ, Mohay H. Executive function of children with extremely low birthweight: a case control study. *Dev Med Child Neurol* 1999; **41**: 292–7.

90. Luciana M, Lindeke L, Georgieff M, Mills M, Nelson CA. Neurobehavioral evidence for working-memory deficits in school-aged children with histories of prematurity. *Dev Med Child Neurol* 1999; **41**: 521–33.

91. Taylor HG, Minich NM, Klein N, Hack M. Longitudinal outcomes of very low birth weight: Neuropsychological findings. *J Int Neuropsychol Soc* 2004; **10**: 149–63.

92. Faust ME, Balota DA, Spieler DH, Ferraro FR. Individual differences in information-processing rate and amount: implications for group differences in response latency. *Psychol Bull* 1999; **125**: 777–99.

93. Largo RH, Molinari L, Comenale PL, Weber M, Duc G. Language development of term and preterm children during the first five years of life. *Dev Med Child Neurol* 1986; **28**: 333–50.

94. Largo RH, Molinari L, Kundu S, Lipp A, Duc G. Intellectual outcome, speech and school performance in high risk preterm children with birth weight appropriate for gestational age. *Eur J Pediatr* 1990; **149**: 845–50.

95. Le Normand MT, Cohen H. The delayed emergence of lexical morphology in preterm children: the case of verbs. *J Neurolinguistics* 1999; **12**: 235–46.

96. Sansavini A, Guarini A, Alessandroni R, *et al.* Early relations between lexical and grammatical development in very immature Italian preterms. *J Child Lang* 2006; **33**: 199–216.

97. Magill-Evans J, Harrison MJ, Van deralm ZJ, Holdgrafer G. Cognitive and language development of healthy preterm infants at 10 years of age. *Phys Occup Ther Pediatr* 2002; **22**: 41–56.

98. Hall A, McLeod A, Counsell C, Thomson L, Mutch L. School attainment, cognitive ability and motor function in a total Scottish very-low-birthweight population at eight years: a controlled study. *Dev Med Child Neurol* 1995; **37**: 1037–50.

99. Saavalainen P, Luoma L, Bowler D, *et al.* Naming skills of children born preterm in comparison with their term peers at the ages of 9 and 16 years. *Dev Med Child Neurol* 2006; **48**: 28–32.

100. Jennische M, Sedin G. Gender differences in outcome after neonatal intensive care: speech and language skills are less influenced in boys than in girls at 6.5 years. *Acta Paediatr* 2003; **92**: 364–78.

101. Wolke D, Samara M, Bracewell M, Marlow N. Specific language difficulties and school achievement in children born at 25 weeks of gestation or less. *J Pediatr* 2008; **152**: 256–62.

102. Saavalainen P, Luoma L, Bowler D, *et al.* Spatial span in very prematurely born adolescents. *Dev Neuropsychol* 2007; **32**: 769–85.

103. Gathercole SE, Pickering SJ. Working memory deficits in children with low achievements in the national curriculum at 7 years of age. *Br J Educ Psychol* 2000; **70** (Pt 2): 177–94.

104. Taylor HG, Klein N, Drotar D, Schluchter M, Hack M. Consequences and risks of < 1000-g birth weight for neuropsychological skills, achievement, and adaptive functioning. *J Dev Behav Pediatr* 2006; **27**: 459–69.

105. Chaikind S, Corman H. The impact of low birthweight on special education costs. *J Health Econ* 1991; **10**: 292–311.

106. Aylward GP. Neurodevelopmental outcomes of infants born prematurely. *J Dev Behav Pediatr* 2005; **26**: 427–40.

107. Hack M, Klein NK, Taylor HG. Long-term developmental outcomes of low birth weight infants. *Future Child* 1995; **5**: 176–96.

108. Taylor HG, Burant CJ, Holding PA, Klein N, Hack M. Sources of variability in sequelae of very low birth weight. *Child Neuropsychol* 2002; **8**: 163–78.

109. Gross SJ, Mettelman BB, Dye TD, Slagle TA. Impact of family structure and stability on academic outcome in preterm children at 10 years of age. *J Pediatr* 2001; **138**: 169–75.

110. Msall ME, Buck GM, Rogers BT, *et al.* Risk factors for major neurodevelopmental impairments and need for special education resources in extremely premature infants. *J Pediatr* 1991; **119**: 606–14.

111. Msall ME, Phelps DL, Hardy RJ, *et al.* Educational and social competencies at 8 years in children with threshold retinopathy of prematurity in the CRYO-ROP multicenter study. *Pediatrics* 2004; **113**: 790–9.

112. Vohr BR, Allan WC, Westerveld M, *et al.* School-age outcomes of very low birth weight infants in the indomethacin intraventricular hemorrhage prevention trial. *Pediatrics* 2003; **111**: e340–6.

113. Drillien CM. A longitudinal study of the growth and development of prematurely and maturely born children. II. Physical development. *Arch Dis Child* 1958; **33**: 423–31.

114. Masten AS, Coatsworth JD. The development of competence in favorable and unfavorable environments. Lessons from research on successful children. *Am Psychol* 1998; **53**: 205–20.

115. Allin M, Rooney M, Cuddy M, *et al.* Personality in young adults who are born preterm. *Pediatrics* 2006; **117**: 309–16.

116. Als H, Gilkerson L, Duffy FH, *et al.* A three-center, randomized, controlled trial of individualized developmental care for very low birth weight preterm infants: medical, neurodevelopmental, parenting, and caregiving effects. *J Dev Behav Pediatr* 2003; **24**: 399–408.

117. Campbell F, Ramey C. Effects of early intervention on intellectual development and academic achievement: a follow-up study of children from low-income families. *Child Dev* 1994; **65**: 884–98.

118. Enhancing the outcomes of low-birth-weight, premature infants. A multisite, randomized trial. The Infant Health, and Development Program. *JAMA* 1990; **263**: 3035–42.

119. McCarton CM, Brooks-Gunn J, Wallace IF, *et al.* Results at age 8 years of early intervention for low-birth-weight premature infants. The Infant Health and Development Program. *JAMA* 1997; **277**: 126–32.

120. McCormick MC, Brooks-Gunn J, Buka SL, *et al.* Early intervention in low birth weight premature infants: results at 18 years of age for the Infant Health and Development Program. *Pediatrics* 2006; **117**: 771–80.

121. Spittle AJ, Orton J, Doyle LW, Boyd R. Early developmental intervention programs post hospital discharge to prevent motor and cognitive impairments in preterm infants. *Cochrane Database Syst Rev* 2007; (2): CD005495.

122. Ment LR, Kesler S, Vohr B, *et al.* Longitudinal brain volume changes in preterm and term control subjects during late childhood and adolescence. *Pediatrics* 2009; **123**: 503–11.

123. Parker J, Mitchell A, Kalpakidou A, *et al.* Cerebellar growth and behavioural & neuropsychological outcome in preterm adolescents. *Brain* 2008; **131**: 1344–51.

124. Allin M, Nosarti C, Narberhaus A, *et al.* Growth of the corpus callosum in adolescents born preterm. *Arch Pediatr Adolesc Med* 2007; **161**: 1183–9.

125. Walden RV, Taylor SC, Hansen NI, *et al.* Major congenital anomalies place extremely low birth weight infants at higher risk for poor growth and developmental outcomes. *Pediatrics* 2007; **120**: e1512–19.

126. Schmidt B, Asztalos EV, Roberts RS, *et al*. Impact of bronchopulmonary dysplasia, brain injury, and severe retinopathy on the outcome of extremely low-birth-weight infants at 18 months: results from the trial of indomethacin prophylaxis in preterms. *JAMA* 2003; **289:** 1124–9.

127. Allin M, Rooney M, Griffiths T, *et al*. Neurological abnormalities in young adults born preterm. *J Neurol Neurosurg Psychiatry* 2006; **77:** 495–9.

128. Olsén P, Vainionpää L, Pääkkö E, *et al*. Psychological findings in preterm children related to neurologic status and magnetic resonance imaging. *Pediatrics* 1998; **102:** 329–36.

129. Sullivan MC, Margaret MM. Perinatal morbidity, mild motor delay, and later school outcomes. *Dev Med Child Neurology* 2003; **45:** 104–12.

130. Downie AL, Jakobson LS, Frisk V, Ushycky I. Auditory temporal processing deficits in children with periventricular brain injury. *Brain Lang* 2002; **80:** 208–25.

131. Taylor HG, Klein N, Schatschneider C, Hack M. Predictors of early school age outcomes in very low birth weight children. *J Dev Behav Pediatr* 1998; **19:** 235–43.

132. Aylward GP, Pfeiffer SI, Wright A, Verhulst SJ. Outcome studies of low birth weight infants published in the last decade: a metaanalysis. *J Pediatr* 1989; **115:** 515–20.

133. Aylward GP. Methodological issues in outcome studies of at-risk infants. *J Pediatr Psychol* 2002; **27:** 37–45.

134. Aylward GP. Cognitive and neuropsychological outcomes: more than IQ scores. *Ment Retard Dev Disabil Res Rev* 2002; **8:** 234–40.

135. Curtis WJ, Zhuang J, Townsend EL, Hu X, Nelson CA. Memory in early adolescents born prematurely: a functional magnetic resonance imaging investigation. *Dev Neuropsychol* 2006; **29:** 341–77.

136. Nosarti C, Rubia K, Smith A, *et al*. Altered functional neuroanatomy of response inhibition in adolescent males who were born very preterm. *Dev Med Child Neurol* 2006; **48:** 265–71.

137. Santhouse AM, Ffytche DH, Howard RJ, *et al*. The functional significance of perinatal corpus callosum damage: an fMRI study in young adults. *Brain* 2007; **125:** 1782–92.

138. Rushe TM, Temple CM, Rifkin L, *et al*. Lateralisation of language function in young adults born very preterm. *Arch Dis Child Fetal Neonatal Ed* 2004; **89:** F112–18.

139. Lawrence EJ, Rubia K, Murray RM, *et al*. The neural basis of response inhibition and attention allocation as mediated by gestational age. *Hum Brain Mapp* 2009; **30:** 1038–50.

140. Gimoenez M, Junqué C, Vendrell P, *et al*. Hippocampal Functional magnetic resonance imaging during a face-name learning task in adolescents with antecedants of prematurity. *Neuroimage* 2005; **25:** 561–9.

141. Fitzgerald M. The development of nociceptive circuits. *Nat Rev Neurosci* 2005; **6:** 507–20.

142. Als H, Duffy FH, McAnulty GB, *et al*. Early experience alters brain function and structure. *Pediatrics* 2004; **113:** 846–57.

143. Svensson AC, Pawitan Y, Cnattingius S, Reilly M, Lichtenstein P. Familial aggregation of small-for-gestational-age births: the importance of fetal genetic effects. *Am J Obstet Gynecol* 2006; **194:** 475–9.

144. Cannon TD, Yolken R, Buka S, Torrey EF. Decreased neurotrophic response to birth hypoxia in the etiology of schizophrenia. *Biol Psychiatry* 2008; **64:** 797–802.

145. Allin MP, Walshe M, Shaikh M, *et al*. COMT genotype influences corpus callosum development in adolescents born preterm. *Schizophr Res* 2008; **102:** 47.

146. Cicchetti D, Cannon TD. Neurodevelopmental processes in the ontogenesis and epigenesis of psychopathology. *Dev Psychopathol* 1999; **11:** 375–93.

147. Xu S, Yashchuk VV, Donaldson MH, *et al*. Magnetic resonance imaging with an optical atomic magnetometer. *Proc Natl Acad Sci U S A* 2006; **103:** 12668–71.

Index

VLBW, *See* very low birth weight
(VLBW)
volumetric brain studies, 204
volumetric measurements, 45
voxel-based morphometry (VBM)
adult MRI data, 68, 69
brain developmental changes, 120
DTI analysis, 101, 107
on FA template, 102
VLBW and SGA compared, 107
VPT, *See* very preterm (VPT) infants

water
brain tissue change over time, 102
brain tissue in the infant, 50
diffusion in DTI, 97–8
diffusion in DWI, 44
signal from H atoms in MRI, 43, 44
Weschler Objective Numeric
Dimensions test, 62
white matter
age-related changes in children, 181
anisotropic diffusion, 97
cell damage, 103
development, 71
cognitive function and, 108
DTI and, 102–7
microstructural abnormalities, 107

diffusion changes, 48–9, 98
environment enrichment and, 72–3
fractional anisotropy, 97–8
gender and volume, 55
heterogeneity, 98, 102–3, 104
myelinated, 44–5
plasticity, 107–8
regional cerebral blood flow, 79
resilience and, 108–9
spatial mapping of, 59
studies needed, 182
tract anatomy, 98–101
volume changes, 49, 54–5, 71–2, 257
vulnerability, 73
white matter lesions, 65, 253
cognitive delay, 36, 253
congenital heart disease, 64–5
CP and, 40, 59–60
CUS findings, 40
DEHSI, 48
executive functioning, 198–9, 203
in adolescence, 104–7
long-term findings, 58
mechanisms, 22–3
MRI
in childhood, 59–60
neonatal morbidities, 145–6
parenchymal lesions, 48

pathology detection, 103
pathology missed, 97, 103
periventricular damage, 21
prognostic, 48
qualitative, 58
Williams syndrome, 46–7
Woodcock–Johnson Tests of
Achievement, 212
working memory, 185
changes over time, 202
deficits, 186, 190, 255
executive functioning, 195,
198–9
fMRI studies, 89–90
neural development, 185–7
neuroanatomical factor, 203–4
of adolescents, 179, 202

X-ray beam, in CT, 42

young adults
educational outcomes, 214
executive function, 201–3
functional neuroimaging, 85–90
learning difficulties, 219
young children,
cognitive development, 141–2
neonatal care effects, 6